# Complication

## Research and Practice

# Complication

## Research and Practice

Published by iConcept Press

Complication: Research and Practice

Publisher: iConcept Press Ltd.

ISBN: 978-1-922227-46-1

Printed in the United States of America

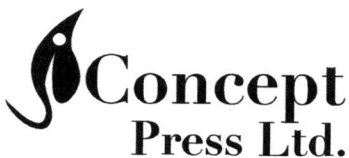

𝒻Concept
Press Ltd.

www.iconceptpress.com

# Contents

Preface . . . . . . . . . . . . . . . . . . . . . . . . . . . . . . . . . . . . . viii

1    A Comprehensive Review of Placental Chorioangioma . . . . . . . . . . . . . .    1
Nabil Abdalla (*Medical University of Warsaw, Warsaw, Poland*), Michal Bachanek
(*Medical University of Warsaw, Warsaw, Poland*), Agnieszka Timorek (*Medical University of Warsaw, Warsaw, Poland*), Krzysztof Cendrowski (*Medical University of Warsaw, Warsaw, Poland*) and Wlodzimierz Sawicki (*Medical University of Warsaw, Warsaw, Poland*)

2    Age-related Oxidative Stress in the Cardiovascular Diseases and Lipoic
Acid as Antioxidant . . . . . . . . . . . . . . . . . . . . . . . . . . . . . .    24
Beata Skibska (*Medical University of Lodz, Łódź, Poland, Poland*) and Anna Goraca
(*Medical University of Lodz, Łódź, Poland, Poland*)

3    Pericytes: Role in Human Atherogenesis and Complicated Plaque . . . . . . .    53
Alexander N Orekhov (*Russian Academy of Sciences, Moscow, Russia / Skolkovo Innovative Center, Moscow, Russia / Lomonosov Moscow State University, Moscow, Russia*)
and Ekaterina A Ivanova (*Katholieke Universiteit Leuven, Leuven, Belgium*)

4    Comparative Cost-Effectiveness of Coflex® Interlaminar Stabilization
vs. Instrumented Fusion . . . . . . . . . . . . . . . . . . . . . . . . . . . .    74
Jordana Kate Schmier (*Exponent Inc., Alexandria, Virgia, United States*), Greg Maislin
(*Biomedical Statistical Consulting, Wynnewood, Pennsylvania, United States*) and Kevin
Ong (*Exponent Inc., Philadelphia, Pennsylvania, United States*)

5    Posterior Reversible Encephalopathy Syndrome . . . . . . . . . . . . . . . .    89
Yashpal Singh (*Banaras Hindu University, Varanasi, India*), Bikram K Gupta (*Banaras Hindu University, Varanasi, India*) and Ram Badan Singh (*Banaras Hindu University, Varanasi, India*)

6    Fluoride: It's Biphasic Behavior . . . . . . . . . . . . . . . . . . . . . .    105

Patricia Vázquez-Alvarado (*Universidad Autónoma del Estado de Hidalgo, Mexico*), Alejandra Hernández-Ceruelos (*Universidad Autónoma del Estado de Hidalgo, Mexico*), Sergio Muñoz-Juárez (*Universidad Autónoma del Estado de Hidalgo, Mexico*), Jesús Ruvalvaba-Ledezma (*Universidad Autónoma del Estado de Hidalgo, Mexico*), Julieta Macías-Ortega (*Universidad Autónoma del Estado de Hidalgo, Mexico*), Juan Carlos Paz-Bautista (*Universidad Autónoma del Estado de Hidalgo, Mexico*), Josefina Reynoso-Vázquez (*Universidad Autónoma del Estado de Hidalgo, Mexico*) and Alejandro Chehue-Romero (*Universidad Autónoma del Estado de Hidalgo, Mexico*)

7     **Bacteria and Fungi Involved in the Diarrheic and Respiratory Diseases in Workers Tanning Process** . . . . . . . . . . . . . . . . . . . . . . . 132

Diana Carolina Castellanos Arévalo (*University of Buenos Aires, Argentina*), Andrea Paola Castellanos Arévalo (*Centro de Investigacion y Estudios Avanzados – IPN, Mexico*), David Alfonso Camarena Pozos (*Centro de Investigacion y Estudios Avanzados – IPN, Mexico*), Juan Colli (*Instituto Tecnologico de Irapuata, Mexico*), Bertha Isabel Arévalo Rivas (*University of Guanajuato, Mexico*), Juan José Peña-Cabriales (*Unidad Irapuato, Mexico*) and Maria Vega Maldonado (*Hospital Regional de Alta Especialidad del Bajio, Mexico*)

8     **Can Glucocorticoids Against Severe Sepsis Act As Causal Drugs?** . . . . . . . 168

Thomas Scior (*Benemérita Universidad Autónoma de Puebla, Mexico*), Itzel Gutierrez-Aztatzi (*Benemérita Universidad Autónoma de Puebla, Mexico*) and Jorge Lozano-Aponte (*Benemérita Universidad Autónoma de Puebla, Mexico*)

9     **Diabetes Mellitus And Hearing Loss** . . . . . . . . . . . . . . . . . . . . . . . 186

Prasanna Venkatesan Eswaradass (*University of Calgary, Calgary, AB, Canada*), Swapna Anandhan (*Griffin Hospital, Derby, CT, United States*), Hari Krishnan Nair (*Tufts University School of Medicine, Boston, MA, United States*) and Mohammed Ismail (*Manipal University, Karnataka, India*)

10     **Unscarred Gravid Uterine Rupture: A Rare Obstetrical Emergency** . . . . . . . 197

Nabil Abdalla (*Medical University of Warsaw, Poland*), Monika Pazura (*Medical University of Warsaw, Poland*), Robert Piorkowski (*Medical University of Warsaw, Poland*), Krzysztof Cendrowski (*Medical University of Warsaw, Poland*) and Wlodzimierz Sawicki (*Medical University of Warsaw, Poland*)

11     **Serum Magnesium Levels and Cardiovascular Outcome in Patients with Advanced Chronic Kidney Disease** . . . . . . . . . . . . . . . . . . . . . . . 215

Olimpia Ortega (*Hospital Severo Ochoa, Leganés, Madrid, Spain*)

12     **Fluid Therapy: Analysis of the Components for a Rational Fluid Management** . . . . . . . . . . . . . . . . . . . . . . . . . . . . . . . . . . . . . . 227

Juan C Grignola (*Universidad de la República, Uruguay*) and Juan P Bouchacourt (*Universidad de la República, Uruguay*)

**13   Sweet Potato: Production Trends And Health Benefits** . . . . . . . . . . . . . . 250
Lowell Dilworth (*The University of the West Indies, Mona, Jamaica*), Dewayne Stennett (*The University of the West Indies, Mona, Jamaica*) and Felix Omoruyi (*Texas A&M University – Corpus Christi, Corpus Christi, Texas, United States*)

# Preface

Complication is usually a consequence of a disease. The disease can become worse in its severity or show a higher number of symptoms or new pathological changes, and widespread throughout the body to affect other organ systems. Depending on the degree of vulnerability, susceptibility, age, health status, immune system condition, etc. complications may arise more easily. This book describes some of the emerging topics in the context of complication. There are totally 13 chapters in this book.

There are totally 13 chapters in this book. Chapter 1 presents a comprehensive review of placental chorioangioma, the most common type of non-trophoblastic placental tumor with no risk of metastasis. They are usually small, single and asymptomatic. Chapter 2 discusses the role of Lipoic acid (LA) as antioxidants in lowering the incidence of some pathologies of cardiovascular diseases as well as for anti-aging. LA is a natural antioxidant which is believed to have a beneficial effect on oxidative stress parameters in relation to diseases of the cardiovascular system. Chapter 3 studies the role of pericytes in human atherogensis. Pericytes are capable of proliferation, active accumulation of lipids, production of various signaling molecules and differentiation into other cell types. Chapter 4 describes a health care economic model to estimate the direct health care costs and quality-adjusted life years of coflex®-treated patients compared to patients treated with instrumented posterolateral fusion over a five-year period using updated clinical inputs and costs.

Chapter 5 discusses posterior reversible encephalopathy syndrome (PRES), a neurotoxic state with a unique imaging appearance on CT or MRI. Worldwide incidence of PRES is unknown and majority of case reported in young to middle-aged adult with marked female predominance. Chapter 6 reviews the effectiveness of using fluoride (F-) for decreasing the prevalence and incidence of tooth decay: on the one hand, small amounts helps prevent dental caries; on the other hand, high concentrations can be potentially toxic and harmful to dental and systemic health. Chapter 7 evaluates and identifies the microbial load in oropharyngeal mucosa of tannery employees. The health risk was estimated based on identification of microorganisms found in the oropharyngeal mucosa samples. Chapter 8 discusses the molecular events to shed new light on the possible causal relationship and mechanism of action for hydrocortisone hormone therapy and the cell surface receptors which are thought of being the first step in triggering endotoxic molecular signaling into the body cells of the patients.

Chapter 9 discusses about sensorineural hearing loss (SNHL) which is a common but under recognised complication of diabetes mellitus. Diabetes is associated with a gradually progressive, bilateral SNHL affecting predominantly higher frequencies. With increasing incidence of diabetes worldwide, diabetes-associated SNHL may become a significant contributor to hearing impairment in future. Chapter 10 reviews a rare disease which is known as unscarred uterine rupture. Many risk factors have been reported to be associated with uterine rupture without history of caesarean section. Chapter 11 analyses the results of some reports which support or not support the possible implication of magnesium in cardiovascular damage and cardiovascular outcome among patients with advanced chronic kidney disease. Chapter 12 provides an overview of the components of a rational fluid management in acute illness, as decisions regarding fluid therapy, whether this is in the operating room (patients undergoing high-risk surgery), intensive care unit, or emergency department, remain a highly challenged tasks. Chapter 13 provides an overview of the production trends and health benefits that may accrue from the consumption of sweet potato.

Editing and publishing a book is never an easy task. Each chapter in this book has gone through a peer review, a selection and an editing process so as to guarantee its quality. Without the supports and contributions of the authors and reviewers, this book can never be able to complete. We would like to thank all of the authors in this book and all of the reviewers who participated in the reviewing process: Nihat Akbulut, Helena Barroso, Marco Matteo Ciccone, Qi Dai, Mohammad FarzUddin, Hailan Feng, Ravindra Kumar Garg, Gary M Ginsberg, Jing-Fei Huang, Anastasios J. Karayiannakis, Panagiotis Korovessis, Irena Levitan, Wesley Luzetti Fotoran, Ioana Mozos, Yuji Naito, Kei Nakajima, Martina PerÅ¡e, Luigi Alberto Pini, Mahmoud Rouabhia, Barbara Ruszkowska, Mohamed A Shawarby, Hsiu-Nien Shen, Akinobu Takaki, Takuji Tanaka, Andrea Tinelli, Gaurav Tomar, Gülcan Turker, Barbara Wegiel, Josef Yayan, B. Linju Yen and Xiaobo Zhang. We hope that you, the reader, will find this book interesting and useful. Any advices please feel free and are always welcome to tell us.

iConcept Press Editorial Office
December 2017

# Chapter 1

# A Comprehensive Review of Placental Chorioangioma

Nabil Abdalla[1], Michal Bachanek[1], Agnieszka Timorek[1],
Krzysztof Cendrowski[1], Wlodzimierz Sawicki[1]

## 1  Introduction

Placental neoplasms can be classified as primary or secondary (Gruca-Stryjak et al., 2011). Primary neoplastic diseases of the placenta include a wide range of conditions that can generally be classified as trophoblastic and non-trophoblastic diseases. Gestational trophoblastic diseases can be further subdivided into complete hydatidiform moles, partial hydatidiform moles, invasive moles, gestational choriocarcinomas and placental site trophoblastic tumors. These diseases arise from the proliferation of abnormal placental trophoblastic tissues, may become malignant, and have the potential to metastasize elsewhere in the body (Alifrangis & Seckl., 2010; Monchek & Wiedaseck, 2012). Non-trophoblastic diseases occur more frequently and are always benign. Chorioangioma, teratoma, hepatocellular adenoma and leiomyoma belong to this group of disorders (Fiutowski & Pawelski, 1996). Chorioangioma is the most common type of non-trophoblastic placental tumor. The pathogenesis of these neoplasms is controversial; however, they can originate from any part of the placenta, excluding trophoblastic tissues (Elsayes et al., 2009; Prashanth et al., 2012; Miliaras et al., 2011; Fiutowski & Pawelski, 1996). Chorioangiomas are benign, and there is no risk of metastasis to either the maternal or fetal tissues (Miliaras et al., 2011). In the literature, the term "giant chorioangioma" has been used to describe large chorioangiomas. An arbitrary size of more than 4 or 5 cm has been used to define these tumors (Jhun et al., 2015). The incidence of maternal cancer during pregnancy is very low. Secondary metastases to the placenta occur very rarely; but when they do, they may originate from different parts of the

[1] Department of Obstetrics, Gynecology and Oncology, Medical University of Warsaw, Warsaw, Poland

body (Miller et al., 2012, Thelmo et al., 2010). Malignant melanoma is the most common malignant maternal neoplasm to metastasize to the products of conception (Eltorky et al., 1995). Melanoma is associated with an increased risk that malignant cells will transfer to the fetus, and deliveries of infants with metastases from mother have been reported (Valenzano Menada et al., 2010).

The term "chorangiocarcinoma" was first used by Jauniaux et al. in 1988. The term was given to a chorioangioma atypical of trophoblastic proliferation (Jauniaux et al., 1988). Khong proposed that chorangiocarcinomas are actually more common than implied in the literature and suggested that the phrase "chorioangioma with trophoblastic proliferation" more appropriately identifies these tumors (Khong, 2000).

Chorioangioma should be differentiated from chorangiomatosis and chorangiosis. Chorangiomatosis is a lesion of abnormally vascularized mature stem villi in which multiple vascular channels are seen. These lesions are located between normal terminal villi, rather than in a single mass (Amer et al., 2010). Chorangiosis is best described as a lesion of terminal villi (Amer et al., 2010) and was first defined by Altshuler as 10 or more vascular channels per 10 terminal villi per 10 non-ischemic/non-infarcted zones in at least three areas, as seen through a 10x microscope (Altshuler, 1984).

# 2   Epidemiology

Placental chorioangioma is the most common type of placental non-trophoblastic tumor and occurs in 1% of births (Fox & Sebire, 2007; Amer et al., 2010). A retrospective study of 22,000 placental examinations showed that chorioangiomas occurred in 0.6% of placentas (Kuhnel, 1933). In another retrospective study of 22,439 placentas, the incidence of chorioangiomas was 0.61% (Guschmann et al., 2003). Giant chorioangiomas (more than 5 cm) have incidence rate between 1:3500 and 1:16,000 births (Kirkpatrick et al., 2007). Chorangiocarcinoma is rare and has only been reported a few times in the literature (Arici et al., 2005; Faes et al.,2012).

# 3   Etiology and Risk Factors

The exact mechanism of the pathogenesis of placental chorioangioma is still undefined. Hypoxia may play a role in the formation of chorioangiomas, and the development of marginal chorioangiomas may be induced by hypoperfusion and hypoxia at the placental margins (Faes et al., 2012; Ogino et al., 2000). Hypobaric hypoxia may be the possible etiologic agent of the higher incidence of placental chorioangiomas at high altitudes. Overexpression of angiogenic cytokines, which are upregulated by this factor, may mediate this effect (Reshetnikova et al., 1996).

In Guschmann et al.'s retrospective study of 22,439 placentas, the rate of chorioangioma occurrence increased linearly with maternal age. Most often, chorioangiomas were found in pregnant women over 30 years old. Chorioangiomas occurred more often in pregnancies associated with hypertension and diabetes than they did in normal pregnancies and were more frequently associated with female fetuses (72%). Arrested and delayed matura-tion of villi was observed in 33% of cases, and premature labor occurred three times more often in pregnancies complicated by chorioangioma than in normal pregnancies. The study also indicated that chorioangiomas are often diagnosed in primipara and multiple gestation (Guschmann et al., 2003).

The pathogenesis of chorangiocarcinoma is still unclear, though some theories have been suggested. These include the occurrence of a chorion carcinoma variant or the appear-ance of a new tumor. These tumors may be collision tumors, in which two separate lesions, chorioangioma and incidental chorion carcinoma, present together. A composition tumor, or a reactive lesion of trophoblasts and a villous vascular tree, has also been suggested (Guschmann et al. 2003). Faes et al. proposed that chorangiocarcinoma is associated with amniocentesis. In that reported case of chorangiocarcinoma, an initial ultrasound diagnosis of a placental tumor was made at 20 weeks of gestation, a considerable time after amniocen-tesis. It was suggested that the process might cause hypoperfusion and hypoxia in the mar-gin of the placenta, which could trigger the release of vascular endothelial growth factors (VEGF) and in turn give rise to the tumor (Faes et al., 2012).

# 4    Pathology

Chorioangioma, originally described by Clarke in 1798, is the most common histological type of placental tumor (Benirschke & Kufmann, 1990). Chorioangioma can also be classified as a hamartoma rather than a neoplastic process (Kodandapani et al., 2012). Chorioangiomas are thought to originate on about the 16th day after fertilization (Bracero et al., 1993). They appear primarily in the fetal part of the placenta, and the feeding vessels arise from fetal circulation (Elsayes et al., 2009).

## 4.1    Macroscopic features

The majority of chorioangiomas are single, small, encapsulated and intraplacental (Zanar-dini et al., 2010). They are found on the fetal surface of the placenta or within the placental parenchyma (Cvjetko et al., 2010). Only 10% of chorioangiomas are macroscopically visible (Duro et al., 2011). Giant chorioangiomas are those measuring more than 5 cm and are asso-ciated with additional obstetrical complications (Cvjetko et al., 2010). The size of the chori-oangioma may increase during pregnancy, or it may remain the same (Mara et al., 2002; Abdalla et al., 2014). Chorioangiomas have no fibrous capsule. On gross examination, these tumors are well demarcated, fleshy and congested. They are usually located near the inser-tion of the umbilical cord and at the margin of the placenta (Ogino et al., 2000; Abdalla et al., 2014) (Figure 1). Most chorioangiomas are red or grayish red. A pale yellow or grey-white color may indicate a low blood supply (He et al., 2004). All reported cases of choran-giocarcinoma have had a single lesion. These tumors are well demarcated and may have a lobulated appearance with numerous small, whitish nodules (Faes et al., 2012). The gross appearance of infarcts on the placenta has been reported (Trask et al. 1994).

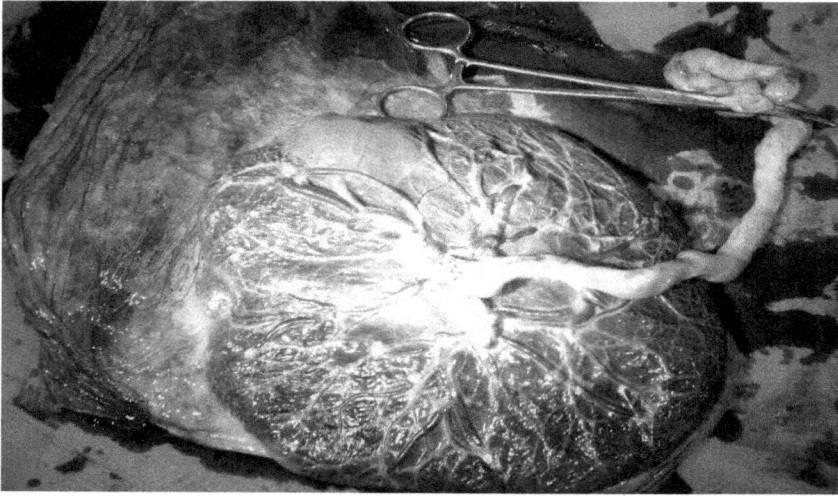

**Figure 1.** The macroscopic appearance of placental chorioangioma at the margin of the placenta.

## 4.2   Microscopic Features

Microscopically, these tumors are composed of numerous blood vessels in various stages of proliferation (Amer et al., 2010). The chorioangioma contains all developmental phases of angioblastema—endotheliomatous, capillary and cavernous. (Cvjetko et al., 2010). Tumor cells show focal staining for cytokeratin 18, which may suggest that chorioangiomas originate from chorionic plate and anchoring villi blood vessels (Lifschitz-Mercer et al., 1989). From a histological perspective, chorioangiomas can be classified as angiomatous (capillary), cellular or degenerative (Marchetti, 1939). Capillary chorioangiomas are the most common histologic type and are analogous to chorioangiomas elsewhere in the body. These masses are composed of multiple capillary channels supported by connective tissue stroma and lined by a layer of trophoblasts. In cellular chorioangiomas, the capillary lumens have collapsed and the surrounding stroma has undergone varying degrees of collagenization and cellularity and consists of fibroblasts, macrophages and collagen. In degenerative chorioangiomas, degradation such as calcification, hemosiderin and the formation of infarcts can be seen (Amer et al., 2010). Placental tumors with combined chorioangioma and leiomyoma features have been reported (Miliaras et al., 2011).

Microscopic evidence of chorangiocarcinoma includes abnormal trophoblast proliferation in combination with abnormal hypervascular chorangiosis of the villous stroma (Guschmann et al. 2003). There may be trophoblastic proliferation in the form of multiple nodules with focal multinucleation, as well as pleomorphic cell nuclei, extensive central necrosis and high mitotic activity. The neoplastic nodules can show dystrophic calcification. In contrast to classic choriocarcinoma, no stromal invasion occurs (Ariel et al., 2009; Faes et al., 2012). Strong immunoreactivity to human chorionic gonadotropin (hCG) has been demonstrated in immuno-histochemical studies of abnormal trophoblasts (Guschmann et al. 2003).

# 5   Clinical Features

Chorioangiomas are usually symptomless and usually overlooked during routine ultra-sound examination. Approximately 80% of chorioangiomas are small and of no clinical importance (Lampe et al., 1995). Abnormalities found elsewhere may arouse suspicion of placental structural abnormalities. Chorioangiomas can be discovered accidently by ultrasound (Quarello et al., 2005). They can also be discovered postnatally. In a clinical study of 136 chorioangiomas, more than half of the cases were only discovered using histologic techniques (Guschmann et al., 2003). Larger masses, especially those more than 5 cm, are more easily diagnosed by ultrasound, and they are more likely to cause complications. Maternal complications include polyhydramnios, preterm labor and placental abruption (Duro & Moussou, 2011; Kodandapani et al., 2012). Fetal congestive heart failure, thrombocytopenia, non-immunologic fetal hydrops, hemolytic anemia, intrauterine growth restriction, congenital anomalies, brain infarction, umbilical vein thrombosis, fatal cerebral embolism and intrauterine fetal and neonatal death associated with chorioangioma have been reported (Kodandapani et al., 2012; Ghidini & Locatelli, 2006; Sivasli et al., 2009). Giant chorioangioma may be associated with uneventful pregnancies if the remaining placental tissues re-compensate for fetal needs (Cvjetko et al., 2010). Spontaneous thrombosis and degeneration may be a cause of large chorioangiomas that are not associated with maternal or fetal complications (Esen et al., 1997).

Congenital malformations were not confirmed in the few reported cases of chorangiocarcinoma (Faes et al., 2012). The reported chorangiocarcinoma cases were associated with preeclampsia, premature labor, vaginal bleeding and intrauterine growth restrictions (Arici et al., 2005; Jauniaux et al,. 1988; Guschmen et al., 2003). One of the cases was associated with a dichorionic diamniotic twin that had a complicated prenatal course (Trask et. al., 1994). One case was discovered during an ultrasound checkup in the second trimester after amniocentesis, which was performed because increased risk of Down syndrome was identified in a first-trimester screening (Faes et al., 2012).

# 6   Diagnostic Techniques

Doppler ultrasound examination is the gold standard in primary prenatal diagnosis of hemangioma. It is also the main method used to differentiate chorioangioma from other types of placental tumors (Gruca-Stryjak et al., 2011). Diagnostic techniques such as magnetic resonance imaging (MRI) and tumor markers may help to detect complications or may be used when there is doubt about a diagnosis. A definitive diagnosis of chorioangioma can be established via a histological examination of the tumor (Abdalla et al., 2014).

## 6.1   Ultrasound

Antenatal ultrasound detection of chorioangioma was first reported in 1978 (Asokan et al, 1978). Chorioangiomas appear in gray-scale ultrasound images as well-demarcated, round, echogenic masses of different sizes protruding into the fetal surface of the placenta, usually near the insertion of the umbilical cord (Abdalla et al., 2014) (Figure 2; figure 3). Cystic lesions inside the tumor are formed by enlarged blood vessels creating a dense vascular network (Gruca-Stryjak et al., 2011). Doppler ultrasound can show the substantial vascularization of these tumors (Elsayes et al., 2009; Chou et al., 1994) (Figure 4). A single feeding blood vessel may be seen on Doppler ultrasound (Zalel et al., 2002). This can be beneficial for certain ultrasound-guided procedures, such as laser photocoagulation (Gajewska et al., 2010). Less common cellular and degenerative chorioangiomas are poorly vascularized and appear as solid or cystic tumors with little vascularity and a gray-scale appearance that ranges from echogenic to hypoechogenic (Shih et al., 2004). The echo pattern of a chorioangioma is stable in comparison to that of a hematoma, which changes over time as a result of its composition (Elsayes et al., 2009). Placental hematomas appear as well-circumscribed masses with echogenicity that varies over time. In the acute phase, these masses are hypoechoic or anechoic. They become heterogeneously echoic in the subacute phase and then anechoic in the chronic phase. Doppler ultrasound can show the presence of blood flow that is continuous with fetal circulation, and this can differentiate chorioangioma from other placental masses such as degenerating liomyoma, placental teratoma, retroplacental hematoma and mesenchymal dysplasia (Caldas et al., 2015; Elsayes et al., 2009). The absence of blood flow in a placental tumor does not exclude a chorioangioma diagnosis, since lack of blood flow is possible in cases of chorioangioma infarction. Spontaneous infarction of a chorioangioma can complicate an ultrasound diagnosis (D'Souza & Olah, 1999). Placental teratomas are similar in appearance to chorioangiomas, but they can be differentiated by the presence of calcification (Harris et al., 1996). However, calcification has also cause reduced blood flow in chorioangiomas, as shown in Doppler ultrasound images (Zalel et al., 2002). Chorangiocarcinoma has the same ultrasound features of chorioangioma. Not all reported cases of chorangiocarcinoma have been discovered prenatally by ultrasound (Faes et al. 2012).

3D ultrasound has also been used to diagnose and monitor placental chorioangioma. 3D ultrasound technology can reveal angioarchitecture and thereby enable confirmation that a tumor's vasculature is continuous with fetal circulation. This process allows to rule out other lesions like placental hemorrhaging, maternal lakes, degenerated myoma or placenta accreta. The mass volume and vascularity index (VI) can also be measured using this method and may be helpful in the monitoring of chorioangioma. A reduction of the vascularity index may suggest spontaneous infarction of the tumor (Shih et al., 2004).

Ultrasound examination can reveal other placental, fetal and amniotic fluid abnormalities as well. An ultrasound scan can be used to detect placental abnormalities associated with chorioangiomas such as a placental abruption, placenta previa, a circumvallated placenta or the velamentous insertion of the umbilical cord (Bracero et al., 1993). The amniotic fluid should be assessed if chorioangioma is suspected, particularly since polyhydramnios is a recognized complication of chorioangioma. Polyhydramnios can be mild, moderate or severe, depending on the amniotic fluid index (AFI) value or the maximum vertical pocket (MVP) level (Harman, 2008). However, polyhydramnios is not a universal effect of chorioangioma, and the presence of oligohydramnios does not exclude the possibility of chorioangioma (Prapas et al, 2000; Lau et al., 2003). Abnormal fetal ultrasound features such as those associated with non-immune hydrops fetalis (NIHF) can be the result of chorioangioma-related NIHF. Features include generalized skin edema, hepatomegaly, ascites and pleural effusion. Skin edema of 20 mm at the back of neck is a common sign of chorioangi-oma-related complications (Kodandapani et al.,2013). Abnormal fetal Doppler ultrasound findings related to circulatory decompensation include pulsatile flow in the umbilical vein, reversed end-diastolic flow and abnormal blood flow in the ductus venosus (Jones et al., 2012). Increased middle cerebral artery peak systolic velocity (MCA-PCV) corresponding to multiple of medians of the expected value is a useful tool to assess fetal anemia. Caution should be used when interpreting MCA-PCV in associated with NIHF. Severe bilateral fetal hydrothorax may cause cardiac compression, leading to impaired ventricular filling and low cardiac output, and resulting in relatively normal MCA-PSV in spite of severe anemia. Drainage of the fetal hydrothorax in this situation will lead to decreased intrathoracic pres-sure and cardiac compression, leading to increased ventricular filling, stroke volume, car-diac output and MCA-PCV. Increased MCA-PCV indicates the actual level of fetal anemia, which had been overlooked previously in the assessment of fetal hemodynamic disturb-ances caused by NIHF (Hellmund et al., 2012). Anatomic fetal abnormalities can be related to congenital fetal abnormalities associated with chorioangiomas (Akercan et al., 2012). A single umbilical artery can be ultrasound-associated evidence of this issue. The incidence of single umbilical artery in pregnancies complicated by chorioangioma was 2.7% compared to 0.7% in the control group (Bracero et al., 1993).

Ultrasound-guided cordocentesis can serve as a diagnostic method to confirm anemia and to diagnose genetic disorders; at the same time, a blood transfusion to the fetus can be performed to correct fetal anemia (Gruca-stryjak et al., 2011). Intervention procedures like embolization or an alcohol injection can be done under ultrasound guidance to localize the tumor in relation to the placenta and the positions of feeding vessels (Babic et al., 2012). A Doppler ultrasound can determine the feeding vessels and their locations. Fetoscopic laser coagulation can be applied in cases in which perfusion of the tumor is derived via superficial feeding vessels that are small in diameter (Quarello et al., 2005). In the case of embolization, it is theoretically better to embolize the distal vessels as close to the tumor as possible to reduce the risk of the formation of collaterals (Lau et al., 2003).

Ultrasound examinations can be used to monitor the effects of certain procedures (e.g., laser photocoagulation and alcohol injections to treat chorioangioma). After these pro-cedures, the absence of blood flow can be noted using a color Doppler evaluation. The tu-mors will be smaller in size, and cystic changes may appear (Jones et al., 2012).

Fetal echocardiography is needed in cases of heart failure. In such cases, a severely dilated and hypertrophied right ventricle, mid-tricuspid regurgitation, decreased systolic right ventricle function, abnormal diastolic function and ductal constriction can be noted (Jones et al., 2012). Use of abdominal ultrasound to identify metastases is not indicated be-cause chorioangiomas are always benign (Harris et al, 1996).

Gray-scale ultrasound and color Doppler imaging are helpful during follow-ups re-lated to chorioangiomas (Durin et al., 2002). The frequency of ultrasound assessment de-pends on many factors, including the tumor's size, gestational age, and fetal and maternal complications. No strict protocol exists to monitor these tumors; however, small tumors may need to be checked every 3-4 weeks, while larger tumors should be monitored every 1-2 weeks (Caldas et al., 2015).

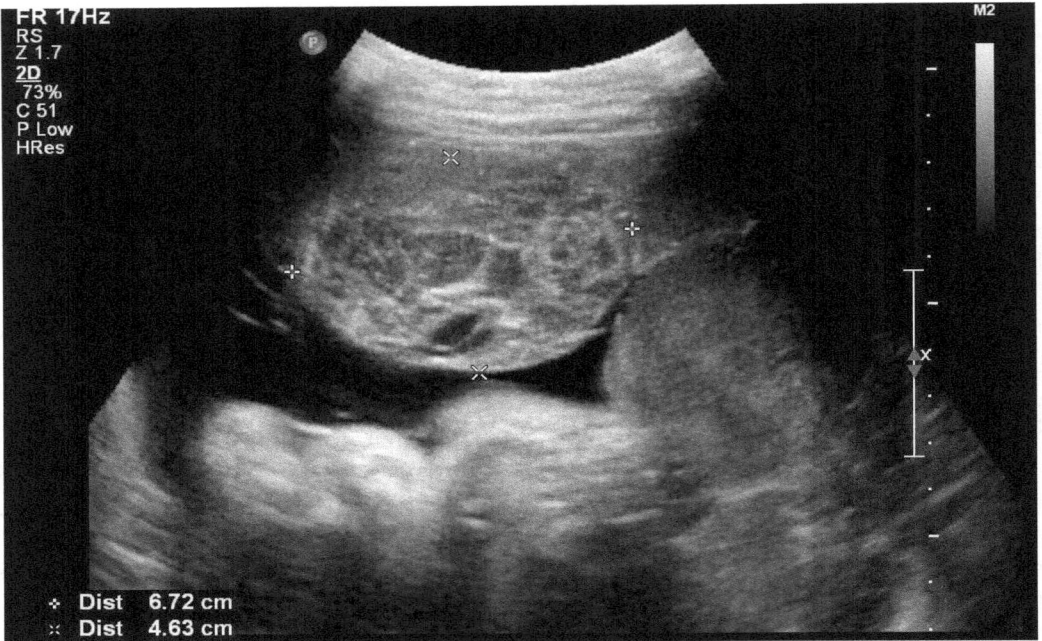

**Figure 2.** Gray-scale ultrasound image of a chorioangioma. The dimensions of the mass are 67x46 mm.

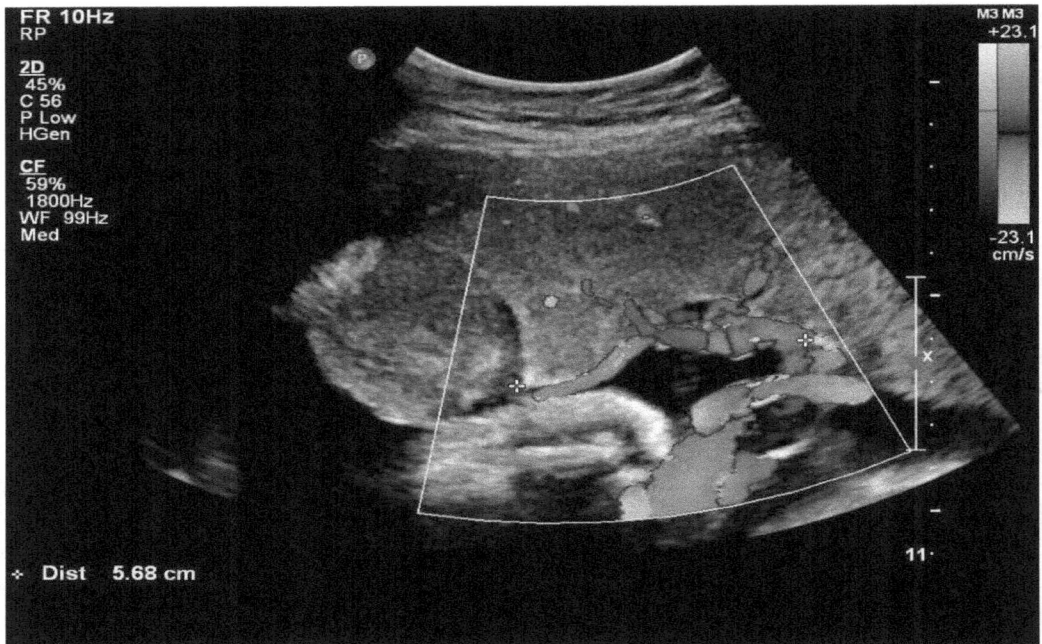

**Figure 3.** The distance of the placental tumor from the umbilical cord insertion is 56 mm.

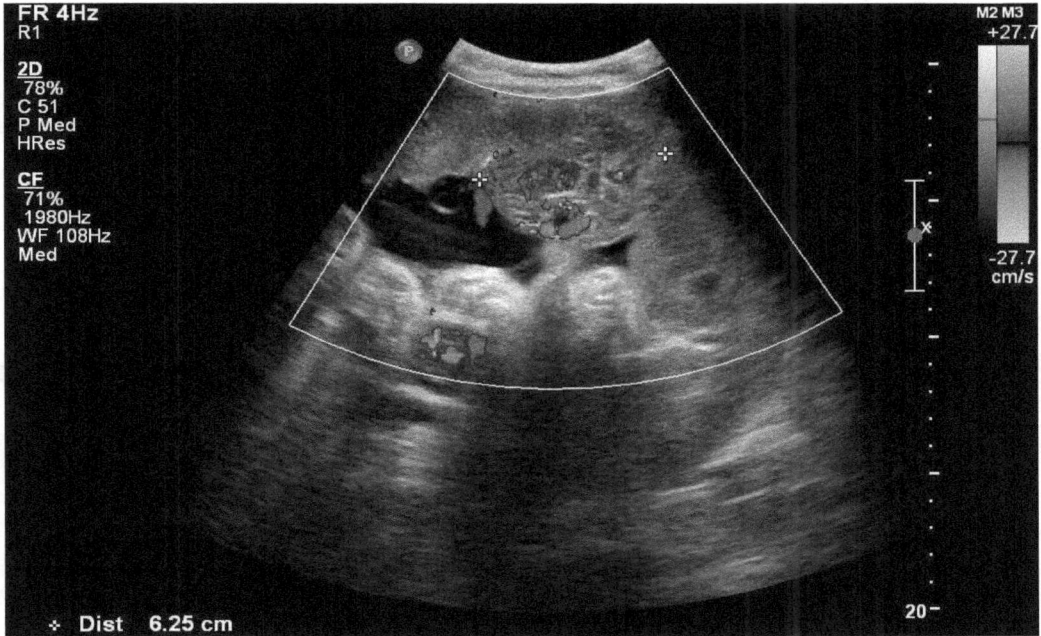

**Figure 4.** Color Doppler ultrasound showing vascularization of the placental tumor.

## 6.2   Other Radiological Techniques

Magnetic resonance imaging is used only in equivocal cases; the placental hemangioma will appear as an isointense mass on T1-weighted images, with increased signal intensity on T2-weighted images. Intralesion hemorrhaging appears as focal areas of increased signal intensity in both T1- and T2-weighted images (Elsayes et al., 2009). MR imaging is sensitive to the presence of bleeding inside the tumor (Caldas et al., 2015).

Computed tomography (CT) may play a limited role in the diagnosis of placental angioma, primarily because of the high radiation risk to the fetus. Use of CT to detect metastases is also not indicated because hemangiomas are always benign (Harris et al., 1996).

## 6.3   Tumor Markers

Increased serum and amniotic fluid alpha feto-protein (AFP) level have been noticed in chorioangioma cases; however, increased AFP is not pathognomonic for chorioangioma since it may be related to other pathologies (Androutsopoulos et al., 2013; Højberg et al., 1994). Feto-maternal hemorrhaging through tumor capillaries may be the causative agent for AFP elevation (Amer et al., 2010). Elevation of AFP in a triple test was one of the findings described in a case of chorangiocarcinoma (Ariel et al. 2009). However, normal or even low AFP does not eliminate the possibility of chorioangioma (Prapas et al., 2000), and AFP returns to normal after delivery (Abdalla et al, 2014).

Beta human chorionic gonadotropin (beta hCG) has no clinical role in the diagnosis or monitoring of non-trophoblastic placental tumors because these tumors do not develop from trophoblastic tissues (Miliaras et al., 2011). A chorioangioma diagnosis occurred during an investigation of increased hCG levels in maternal serum, as reported in Zalel et al. (2002). In a rare case of chorangiocarcinoma, beta HCG dropped to less than 0.1 mIU/ml one month after delivery (Faes et al., 2012).

## 6.4    Histopathological Examination

The definitive diagnosis of a placental tumor is established by the histopathological examination of the placenta. Most chorioangiomas are asymptomatic and are of no clinical significance. Routine placental histological examination is not recommended; as a result the incidence of placental tumors may be underestimated (Gruca-Stryjak et al., 2011). However, placental histopathological examination is recommended when placental tumors are diagnosed prenatally if they give rise to complications (Abdalla et al., 2014). In instances where adverse, unexplained fetal conditions that could be caused by placental tumors are observed, histopathological assessment of the placenta is also recommended to identify the cause of the disease (Kawano et al., 2013). Finally, histopathological assessment is needed to confirm the chorioangioma diagnosis and to exclude other rare conditions such as chorangiocarcinoma (Abdalla et al., 2014).

# 7    Maternal Complications

Chorioangioma causes complications that increase maternal morbidity. Additional diagnostic and therapeutic interventions are needed to ameliorate and treat the symptoms of this disease. Increased rates of induction of labor, termination of pregnancy and caesarean section have been noted due to complications caused by chorioangiomas (Dorman et al. 1995; Caldas et al., 2015).

## 7.1    Polyhydramnios

Polyhydramnios is the most common complication related to chorioangioma and occurs in 14-28% of cases (Gruca-Stryjak et al., 2011). Polyhydramnios can be defined as an increased volume of amniotic fluid in relation to gestational age. Polyhydramnios can be classified as mild, moderate, or severe, according to the AFI relative to gestational age (Harman, 2008). The pathological mechanism of polyhydramnios in cases of chorioangioma is not completely understood, though several theories have been suggested to explain this phenomenon. Placental insufficiency may arise secondarily as a result of a reduction in the placenta's absorption function caused by blood flow to the tumor's vessels. Transudation from the large surface area of the tumor's vessels may contribute to polyhydramnios. Increased transudation into the amniotic cavity may be caused by increased intravascular pressure resulting from an obstruction of blood flow by a tumor located near the umbilical cord insertion point (Abdalla et al., 2014). Intraplacental shunting of blood together with fetal anemia may cause fetal hyperdynamic circulation, which may lead to an increased glomerular filtrate

rate and, consequently, increased urine production and polyhydramnios (Ercan et al., 2012). Fetal hypoxia can stimulate the excretion of metabolites, which leads to increased osmotic pressure from the amniotic fluid and thereby increases the production of said fluid (Gruca-Stryjak et al., 2011). Chorioangioma is a rare cause of polyhydramnios, so other causes of polyhydramnios such as maternal diabetes mellitus or fetal esophageal atresia should be considered when making a diagnosis. Polyhydramnios can cause premature uterine contractions, cervical insufficiency, premature labor, placental abruption due to a sudden drop in intrauterine pressure after membrane rupture, malpresentation, increased risk of a caesarean section and postpartum hemorrhages (Harman, 2008). With increasing gestational age, the overall size and surface area of the placenta will increase. When the tumor size remains the same and the relative surface area of the placenta increases, the relative surface area of the tumor will decrease. This may relatively decrease transudation caused by the tumor and simultaneously increase the absorption of the amniotic fluid by the more viable placenta. This mechanism may explain why polyhydramnios is resolved with the aid of amnioreductions in some cases during pregnancy (Abdalla et al., 2014). The spontaneous resolution of chorioangioma-related polyhydramnios without intervention has also been reported (Caldas et al., 2015).

## 7.2   Threatened Preterm and Preterm Delivery

Placental chorioangioma is associated with significantly higher risk for preterm delivery (Bashiri A et al., 2002). Preterm delivery may be caused by tumor-related complications or procedures performed to treat those tumors (Arici et al., 2005).

## 7.3   Antepartum and Postpartum Hemorrhage

Antepartum bleeding is believed to be caused by a premature separation of the placenta as a result of bleeding from the tumor bed or a rupture of the vascular pedicle. The incidence rate of placental abruption in chorioangioma cases is approximately 4%. Placenta previa is also a cause of antepartum hemorrhage. However, this condition is only loosely associated with chorioangioma, and a true correlation has never been established. Postpartum hemorrhage may be caused by uterine subatony and atony due to over-distention caused by polyhydramnios, the most common chorioangioma complication (Bracero et al., 1993).

## 7.4   Preeclampsia

In a study by Froehlich et al., an increased incidence of preeclampsia (16.4%) was shown when a group of 76 women with chorioangioma was compared to a control group of 44,994 women (4.8%) (Froehlich et al., 1971). The Ballantyne syndrome, known also as triple edema syndrome or mirror syndrome, has been reported as a complication of large chorioangiomas. In this syndrome, the mother mirrors fetal symptoms of severe edema, which can lead to eclamptic convulsions. The pathogenesis of this syndrome with relation to chorioangioma is not yet known (Dorman et al. 1995).

# 8    Fetal Complications

## 8.1    Hemodynamic Changes

Feto-maternal hemorrhaging (FMH) has been reported as a possible consequence of chorioangioma. In this condition, identifying fetal hemoglobin (HbF) in maternal blood improves the diagnosis. Fetal anemia can be severe and can cause the deterioration of the fetus, resulting in the need for a caesarean section. FMH can be chronic and requires serial intrauterine blood transfusions (Kawano et al., 2013). Anemia may be caused by feto-maternal hemorrhage, microangiopathic hemolysis or hemodilution. Similar mechanisms are responsible for thrombocytopenia (Haak et al., 1999; Gruca-Stryjak et al., 2011). Thrombocytopenic purpura of newborns associated with chorioangioma was first described by Froehlich et al. (Froehlich & Housler, 1971).

NIHF was first described by Potter in 1943. The author described an edematous fetus with fluid collection that was not related to iso-immunization in some or all serous cavities (Potter, 1943). Placental hydrops in the absence of rhesus iso-immunization was first described by Earn et al. in 1950 (Earn & Penner, 1950), while NIHF associated with chorioangioma was first described by Mandelbaum et al. (1969). High cardiac output associated with chorioangiomas leads to NIHF. Cardiomegaly associated with chorioangioma was first described by Benson et al. in 1961 (Benson & Joseph, 1961). Cardiomegaly can occur secondarily to high cardiac output from arteriovenous shunting resulting in a left-to-right shunt. High cardiac output may be caused by chronic fetal hypoxia, which is secondary to insufficient placental functioning or anemia. Hypoxia may develop from unoxygenated blood that bypasses maternal circulation and instead passes through the vasculature of the tumor (Duro & Moussou, 2011; Akercan et al., 2012). NIHF can also be associated with chorioangioma and thrombosis of the umbilical vein varix (Sivasli et al., 2009). NIHF is associated with tumors, most commonly cardiac tumors. Cases of NIHF caused by placental chorioangiomas have a better outcome than all other associated tumors (Isaacs, 2008).

## 8.2    Placental Insufficiency and IUGR

Giant chorioangiomas may function as physiological and functional dead space. This may lead to placental insufficiency, resulting in subsequent chronic hypoxia, fetal distress, intrauterine growth restriction and death (Zanardini et al., 2010). Intrauterine growth restriction (IUGR) has been reported as a possible effect of chorioangioma (Zalel et al., 2002; Zanardini et al., 2010).

## 8.3    Congenital Anomalies of the Fetus

The coexistence of placental chorioangioma and several congenital disorders has been reported. Study data reveal an increased incidence of various malformations in infants with placental chorioangioma when compared to controls; however, this finding is probably due to a statistical aberration (Bracero et al., 1993).

Neonatal hemangiomatosis characterized by the presence of multiple congenital hemangiomas have been reported in association with placental chorioangioma (Witters et al., 2003). The incidence of skin hemangioma in such cases is 12.2% vs 2.1% in the control group (Froehlich et al., 1971). Infantile hemangiomas are the most common type of infant tumors (Itinteang et al., 2011). Both the benign and more aggressive forms of the disease have been observed. Disseminated neonatal hemangiomatosis, a rare form with internal organ involvement, has also been reported (Capelle et al., 2009). The pathogenesis of combined fetal hemangiomatosis and placental chorioangioma is still not understood (Witters et al., 2003). Overexpression of angiogenic cytokines in response to hypoxia may explain the coexistence of both pathologies (Witters et al., 2003; Chang et al., 2007). Fetal hypoxia may also be caused by utero-placental insufficiency resulting from giant chorioangiomas (Jhun et al., 2015). The endothelium of a hemangioma expresses a glucose transporter (GLUT1) that is restricted to endothelial cells serving a blood-tissue barrier function, such as in the placenta (North et al., 2001). Histochemical markers like the Lewis Y antigen, FcγRII and merosin present in both pathologies (Jhun et al., 2015). This may support the theory of the placental origin of infantile hemangiomas where an immunologically regulated ectopic locus of placental cells could be the origin of said infantile hemangiomas (Witters et al., 2003). The expression of human chorionic gonadotropin (hCG) and human placental lactogen (hPL), but not cytokeratin 7 (CK7) or human leukocyte antigen G (HLA-G), by the endothelium of proliferating infantile hemangiomas supports the placental chorionic villous mesenchymal core cellular origin of infantile hemangioma over a trophoblastic origin (Itinteang et al., 2011). It has been suggested that obstetric intervention in the form of laser ablation of the feeding vessel may cause fetal hemangioma. The mechanism of possible escape of placental cells may be similar to that which explains the higher rates of infantile benign vascular tumors associated with chorionic villous sampling of the placenta. The presence of both placental and fetal vascular tumors may be coincidental, particularly since the prevalence of both pathologies independent of one another is relatively common (Jhun et al. 2015)

Fetal chromosomal abnormalities have also been reported in association with chorioangioma (Wurster et al., 1969; Verloes et al., 1991). However, research suggests that the simultaneous presence of both pathologies is coincidental (Bracero et al., 1993).

## 8.4    Fetal Cerebral Stroke

Fetal cerebral ischemic strokes that cause permanent brain damage have been described as a possible complication of chorioangioma (Ghidini & Locatelli, 2006). Emboli from the thrombosed vessels are the likely cause (Bermudez et al., 2007). One study indicated that the fetal heart beat was reassuring a few days after a cerebral embolism; however, the non-stress test may not be an adequate method of monitoring pregnancies in which placental chorioangiomas occur (Ghidini & Locatelli, 2006).

## 8.5    Perinatal Morbidity and Mortality

Intrauterine fetal death has been reported as a complication of large chorioangiomas. This can be attributed to complications caused by large chorioangiomas, including hydrops fetalis (Imdad et al., 2009; hadi et al., 1993). The perinatal death rate related to complications caused by chorioangioma may reach 30%-40% (Zanardini et al., 2010).

Large chorioangiomas are associated with increased neonatal morbidity and mortality, especially due to prematurity, congestive heart failure or congenital abnormalities (Akercan et al., 2012; Kodandapani et al., 2012).

# 9   Chorioangioma Changes

Infarction of chorioangiomas has been reported as a cause of severe abdominal pain, a hard uterus, fetal tachycardia and an absence of blood flow mimicking placental abruption (D'Souza & Olah, 1999). Bleeding from ruptured sinusoids within the tumor in the absence of other complications has been reported as a cause of intrauterine death in the second trimester (Batukan et al., 2001). Torsion of rare large pedunculated chorioangiomas has been reported as a cause of premature labor (Enriquez et al., 1994).

# 10   Treatment Modalities

## 10.1   Expectant Management

The majority of chorioangiomas are small and asymptomatic. Expectant management can be reserved for this group of patients. Serial ultrasound check-ups are indicated to monitor the clinical state of the fetus and to detect abnormalities in the early stages (Kirkpatrick et al., 2007). Expectant management of giant chorioangiomas with strict monitoring is adequate in the absence of complications. The spontaneous infarction of chorioangiomas with spontaneous partial resolution of fetal hydrops has been reported (Chazotte et al., 1990).

## 10.2   Treatment of Associated Complications

### 10.2.1   Amnioreduction

Amnioreduction aims to reduce the excess amniotic fluid to prevent preterm labor and relieve maternal discomfort. In some cases, amnioreduction alone is enough to achieve a normal amount of amniotic fluid. This procedure can be repeated during pregnancy if the amount of amniotic fluid increases between procedures (Abdalla et al., 2014). Amnioreduction should be undertaken with caution. Amnioreduction can worsen fetal hemodynamic circulation. Reducing intra-amniotic pressure may increase shift of fetal blood to the chorioangioma and cause high-output cardiac failure, thereby worsening the fetus's condition (Jones et al., 2012). If amnioreduction is planned along with endoscopic laser coagulation, it may be reasonable to perform the laser photocoagulation first. This will minimalize the risk of increasing the size of the chorioangioma due to increased blood flow in the placenta or an open hemorrhage to the tumor caused by the sudden decrease of intrauterine pressure (Mendez-Figueroa et al., 2009).

## 10.2.2    Intrauterine Blood Transfusion

Intrauterine blood transfusion can be used to treat fetal anemia and circulatory failure. Intrauterine blood transfusions can address hematological and hemodynamic disorders caused by hemangioma (Gruca-Stryjak et al., 2011) and can give temporary relief from anemia since red blood cells will be destroyed within the tumor. For this reason, repeated blood transfusions may be necessary to treat fetal anemia throughout pregnancy (Bermudez et al., 2007).

## 10.2.3    Pharmacologic Treatment

Digoxin may be needed to treat fetal cardiac failure (Zalel et al., 2002). In cases of threatened premature labor, steroid administration between weeks 24+0 and 34+6 of gestation is indicated to accelerate fetal lung maturation (RCOG Recommendations 2010; Haak et al., 1999). Indomethacin has been described as a successful treatment for acute polyhydramnios associated with chorioangioma (Kriplani et al., 2001).

## 10.2.4    Planned Delivery

Complications associated with giant chorioangiomas are numerous and serious and can lead to intrauterine death. A planned delivery can be considered for cases complicated by chorioangioma in the third trimester, when the fetus is mature (Shalev et al., 1984). However, most complications manifest themselves in the second trimester, when prematurity is of great concern. Other treatment modalities are more appropriate for these patients (Gruca-Stryjak et al., 2011). Induction of labor even in the second trimester may be appropriate for patients with a poor prognosis for the fetus or the deterioration of the mother (Dorman et al., 1995). Chorioangioma by itself is not an indication for a caesarean section unless there are complications (Abdalla et al., 2014; Babic et al., 2012). The placenta should be examined carefully since the incomplete delivery of the placenta has been reported; in such instances, the placental mass remains inside the uterus and a uterine revision may be needed to remove the mass (Lowenstein et al., 2006). A spontaneous delivery of a chorioangioma mass 6 hours after vaginal delivery has been reported (Dorman et al., 1995).

## 10.3    Chorioangioma-specific Treatments

### 10.3.1    Laser Photocoagulation.

Ultrasound-guided interstitial laser photocoagulation and fetoscopic laser photocoagulation of the feeding vessel to the chorioangioma can be used to treat large chorioangiomas that may cause fetal heart failure. Interstitial laser therapy can be performed under local anesthesia and does not require precise insertion of the needle into the feeding vessel. This technique can be done even if the placenta is located on the anterior uterine wall, a position that makes endoscopic laser coagulation difficult (Bhide et al., 2003; Zanardini et al., 2010). Photocoagulation can cause an infarction of the tumor and cessation of blood flow through the tumor, thereby improving fetal hemodynamic circulation (Bhide et al., 2003; Jones et al.,

2012). However, this procedure has been correlated with complications like preterm labor and the need for intrauterine blood perfusion resulting from bleeding from the coagulation site (Sepulveda et al., 2009). Intrauterine fetal death has also been reported as a complication of this procedure (Zanardini et al., 2010; Mendez-Figueroa et al., 2009). Successful laser photocoagulation depends on the severity of the chorioangioma complication and the anatomy of the blood vessels supplying blood to the placenta and tumor. Endoscopic photocoagulation of the feeding vessel may be more effective in cases were the feeding vessel is a secondary branch from the umbilical artery directly to the tumor. In such a situation, the remaining portion of the placenta will not be affected by the procedure, as the placenta has its own blood supply from branches of the umbilical artery that do not terminate in the tumor; this prevents the risk of placental insufficiency and intrauterine fetal death. Laser photocoagulation before the development of severe hydrops fetalis may also increase the likelihood of a successful procedure (Jones et al., 2012). Laser treatment requires advanced technical equipment and experienced operators (Quarello et al., 2005).

## 10.3.2    Insertion of Microcoils into Feeding Vessels

Lau et al. (2003) tested the potential of inserting microcoils into a feeding vessel to treat placental chorioangioma. The procedure was done under local anesthesia. The microcoils used were made of stainless-steel wire arranged in a helical fashion. The coil contained polyester fibers protruding out perpendicularly from the wire of the coil. The coils obstructed the vessels while the fibers entrapped the platelets that promoted thrombus formation. The procedure is technically simple and has no risk of fetal circulation embolization. Distal embolization as near the tumor as possible was suggested to prevent the formation of collaterals. The failure of this method in the reported case study may be explained by the formation of collateral and the unusually large size of the tumor in question (20 cm) (Lau et al., 2003).

## 10.3.3    Ligation of the Feeding Vessel

Endoscopic suture ligation of the feeding vessel after subchorionic dissection of the vessel has been reported as a method to treat large chorioangiomas. This method may be more appropriate for tumors whose feeding vessel is large and where the risk of the feeding vessel rupturing during the use of Yag laser photocoagulation is high. The remaining blood supply is then coagulated using bipolar electrocautery. Interruption of the blood supply was accomplished in an experimental trial of this method, but the fetus died on the third postoperative day. The cause of fetal death may have been related to increased placental resistance due to the reduced perfusion area, along with an increased afterload, which may have contributed to abrupt hemodynamic changes caused by the procedure (Quintero et al., 1996).

## 10.3.4    Alcohol Injection

Ultrasound-guided absolute alcohol injections can be performed by inserting a needle directly into the chorioangioma away from vascular structures. The procedure can be combined with other procedures such as amnioreduction, cordocentesis and amniotransfusion. This procedure has a theoretical risk of the transfer of alcohol through the umbilical vein to the fetus circulation, which could lead to fetal toxicity and intrauterine death. The fetal blood can be sampled to measure the alcohol level. In the case presented by Ercan et al., no alcohol was transferred to the fetal blood (Eracn et al., 2012). Alcohol injection into the tumor may be the method of choice in conditions where advanced technical laser equipment is not available (Ercan et al., 2012).

### 10.3.5    Embolization

Embolization of the chorioangioma feeding artery using Glubran 2 surgical glue has been reported as a way to manage large chorioangiomas. Glubran 2 is a cyanoacrylate tissue glue widely used in interventional radiology. Embolization of the feeding vessel can be done under percutaneous ultrasound guidance and local anesthesia. Embolization can cause complete and durable devascularization of the tumor (Gajewska et al., 2010). Embolization can also be performed using Histoacryl. The procedure is safe and has no risk of fetal toxicity (Perrotin et al., 2004; Haddad et al., 2010; Babic I et al., 2012).

## 10.4    Psychological Support

Psychological support may be needed for patients with chorioangioma, especially for those with complications that result in increased stress related to serial ultrasound investigations, performance of other procedures and increased hospitalization (Abdalla et al. 2014). The coexistence of lethal diseases in the fetus may be indicate pregnancy termination. If the diagnosis of a lethal disease is not certain, psychologic support should be given to the patients (Akercan et al., 2012).

# 11    Prognosis

The vascularity of a chorioangioma appears to be more important than size in predicting its outcome. This can be explained by the fact that blood flow through the vasculature of a chorioangioma is derived from fetal circulation (Akercan et al., 2012). An increase in the size of a placental chorioangioma does not necessarily correlate with the deterioration of the fetus's clinical state, since simultaneous infarction is possible (Shich et al., 2004). Non-trophoblastic placental tumors are benign diseases. They do not have malignant potential and do not metastasize. Therefore, follow-up with mothers and infants to assess metastasis is unnecessary (Abdalla et al., 2014).

In the few reported cases of chorangiocarcinoma, follow-up of the patients revealed no metastasis at the time of delivery or during follow-up (Faes et al., 2012). This may suggest the benign clinical nature of the disease; however, this disease is very rare and the possibility of metastases cannot be excluded on the basis of a few case reports. Intraplacental choriocarcinoma metastasis to the mother and newborn has been reported (Liu et al., 2006). This fact suggests that follow-up of mothers and infants is sensible when chorangiocarcinoma is present (Faes et al. 2012).

## 12   Summary

Placental chorioangioma is the most common type of non-trophoblastic placental tumor. It is a benign tumor with no risk of metastasis. They are usually small, single and asymptomatic. Large chorioangiomas can cause maternal and fetal complications. Maternal complications include polyhydramnios, premature labor, antepartum hemorrhage, preeclampsia and increased incidence of caesarean sections. Fetal complications include cardiomegaly, non-immunologic hydrops fetalis, anemia, thrombocytopenia, placental insufficiency, intrauterine growth restriction, congenital abnormalities, fetal cerebral stroke and increased perinatal morbidity and mortality. The initial diagnosis of chorioangioma can be performed using a Doppler ultrasound. Expectant management is sufficient for small chorioangiomas without complications. Treatment modalities for larger chorioangiomas may be performed to relieve the effects of the chorioangiomas or may be specific to the tumor. The prognosis depends on the vascularity of the tumors, their sizes and the complications associated with them.

## References

Abdalla, N., Bachanek, M., Trojanowski, S., Cendrowski, K., Sawicki, W. (2014). Placental tumor (chorioangioma) as a cause of polyhydramnios: a case report. Int J Womens Health. 6:955–9.

Akercan, F, Oncul Seyfettinoglu, S., Zeybek, B., Cirpan, T. (2012). High-output cardiac failure in a fetus with thanatophoric dysplasia associated with large placental chorioangioma: case report. J Clin Ultrasound. 40(4):231–3.

Alifrangis, C., Seckl, M.J. (2010). Genetics of gestational trophoblastic neoplasia: an update for the clinician. Future Oncol. 6(12):1915–23.

Altshuler, G. (1984). Chorangiosis. An important placental sign of neonatal morbidity and mortality. Arch Pathol Lab Med. 108(1):71–4.

Amer, H.Z., Heller, D.S. (2010). Chorangioma and related vascular lesions of the placenta —a review. Fetal Pediatr Pathol. 29(4):199–206.

Androutsopoulos, G., Gkogkos, P., Decavalas, G. (2013). Mid-trimester maternal serum HCG and alpha fetal protein levels: clinical significance and prediction of adverse pregnancy outcome. Int J Endocrinol Metab. 11(2):102–6.

Arici, S., Cetin, M., Oztoprak, I., Erden, O/, Kizilgedik. S. (2005). Chorangioma with atypical trophoblastic proliferation. Aust N Z J Obstet Gynaecol. 45(1):86–7.

Ariel, I., Boldes, R., Weintraub, A., Reinus, C., Beller, U., Arbel, R. (2009). Chorangiocarcinoma: a case report and review of the literature. Int J Gynecol Pathol. 28(3):267–71.

Asokan, S., Chad Alavada, K., Gard, R. (1978). Prenatal diagnosis of placental tumor by ultrasound. JCU. 6:180 -181.

Babic, I., Tulbah, M., Kurdi, W. (2012). Antenatal embolization of a large placental chorioangioma: a case report. J Med Case Rep. 6:183.

Bashiri, A., Furman, B., Erez, O., Wiznitzer, A., Holcberg, G., Mazor, M. (2002). Twelve cases of placental chorioangioma. Pregnancy outcome and clinical significance. Arch Gynecol Obstet. 266(1):53–5.

Batukan, C., Holzgreve, W., Danzer, E., Bruder, E., Hösli, I., Tercanli, S. (2001). Large placental chorioangioma as a cause of sudden intrauterine fetal death. A case report. Fetal Diagn Ther. 16(6):394–7.

Benirschke, K., Kufmann, P. (1990). Pathology of the human placenta: benign tumors, pp. 841–51. (New York: Springer-Verlag).

Benson, P.F., Joseph, M.C. (1961). Cardiomegaly in a Newborn Due to Placental Chorioangioma. Br Med J. 1(5219):102–5.

Bermúdez, C., Luengas, O., Pérez-Wulff, J., Genatios, U., García, V., Guevara-Zuloaga, F., Quintero, R.A. (2007). Management of a placental chorioangioma with endoscopic devascularization and intrauterine transfusions. Ultrasound Obstet Gynecol. 29(1):97–8.

Bhide. A., Prefumo, F., Sairam. S., Carvalho. J., Thilaganathan, B. (2003). Ultrasound-guided interstitial laser therapy for the treatment of placental chorioangioma. Obstet Gynecol. 102(5 Pt 2):1189–91.

Bracero, L., Davidian, M., Casiisdy, S. (1993). Chorioangioma: diffuse angiomatous form www.thefetus.net

Caldas, R.T., Peixoto, A.B., Paschoini, M.C., Adad, S.J., Souza, M.L., Araujo Júnior, E. (2015). Giant placental chorioangioma with favorable outcome: a case report and literature review of literature. Ceska Gynekol. 80(2):140–3.

Capelle, X., Syrios, P., Chantraine, F., Rigo, V., Schaaps, J.P., Kridelka, F., Foidart, J.M.. (2009). A rare case of placental chorioangioma associated with neonatal disseminated hemangiomatosis. J Gynecol Obstet Biol Reprod (Paris). 38(3):246–9.

Chang, E.I., Chang, E.I., Thangarajah, H., Hamou, C., Gurtner, G.C. (2007). Hypoxia, hormones, and endothelial progenitor cells in hemangioma. Lymphat Res Biol. 5(4):237–43.

Chazotte, C., Girz, B., Koenigsberg, M., Cohen, W.R. (1990). Spontaneous infarction of placental chorioangioma and associated regression of hydrops fetalis. Am J Obstet Gynecol. 163(4 Pt 1):1180–1.

Chou, M.M., Ho, E.S., Hwang, S.F., Lee, Y.H., Chan, LP., Wen, M.C. (1994). Prenatal diagnosis of placental chorioangioma: contribution of color Doppler ultrasound. Ultrasound Obstet Gynecol. 4(4):332–4.

Cvjetko, L., Rajko, F., Zlatko, H., Stanko, B., Josip, F., Karsten, M. (2010). Chorangioma placentae. Rare Tumors. 2(4):e67.

Dorman, S.L., Cardwell, M.S. (1995). Ballantyne syndrome caused by a large placental chorioangioma. Am J Obstet Gynecol. 173(5):1632–3.

D'Souza, D., Olah, K.S. (1999). Infarction of a placental chorioangioma mimicking placental abruption. J Obstet Gynaecol. 19(4):421–2.

Durin, L., Barjot, P., Herlicoviez, M. (2002). Placental chorioangioma, value of ultrasonography: report of two cases. J Radiol. 83(6 Pt 1):739–41.

Duro, E.A., Moussou, I. (2011). Placental chorioangioma as the cause of non-immunologic hydrops fetalis; a case report. Iran J Pediatr. 21(1):113–5.

Earn, A.A., Penner, D.W. (1950). Five cases of chorioangioma. J Obstet Gynaecol Br Emp. 57(3):442–4.

Elsayes, K.M., Trout, A.T., Friedkin, A.M., Liu, P.S., Bude, R.O., Platt, J.F., Menias, C.O. (2009). Imaging of the placenta: a multimodality pictorial review: Radiographics. 29(5):1371–91.

Eltorky, M., Khare, V.K., Osborne, P., Shanklin, D.R. (1995). *Placental metastasis from maternal carcinoma. A report of three cases. J Reprod Med. 40(5):399–403.*

Enríquez, R., Escalona, J., Oyarzún, E., Chuaqui, R., Soza, A., Contreras, G. (1994). *Complicated placental chorioangioma: infrequent cause of premature labor. Rev Chil Obstet Ginecol. 59(5):390–2.*

Ercan, C.M., Coksuer, H., Karasahin, K.E., Alanbay, I., Baser, I. (2012). *Combined Approach in a Large Placental Chorioangioma Case with Intratumoral Alcohol Injection, Cordocentesis, IU Transfusion, and Amnioreduction. Fetal Pediatr Pathol. 31(6):374–8.*

Esen, U.I., Orife, S.U., Pollard, K. (1997). *Placental chorioangioma: a case report and literature review. Br J Clin Pract. 51(3):181–2.*

Faes, T., Pecceu, A., Van Calenbergh, S., Moerman, P. (2012). *Chorangiocarcinoma of the placenta: a case report and clinical review. Placenta. 33(8):658–61.*

Fiutowski, M. ., Pawelski, A. (1996). *Primary nontrophoblastic tumors of the placenta. Ginekol Pol. 67(10):515–9.*

Fox, H., Sebire, N.J. (2007). *Non trophoblastic tumors of the placenta. In Pathology of the Placenta (3rd edn). Saunders Elsevier: London; 401–430.*

Froehlich, L.A., Fujikura, T., Fisher, P. (1971). *Chorioangiomas and their clinical implications. Obstet Gynecol 37:51(9).*

Froehlich, L.A., Housler, M. (1971). *Neonatal thrombocytopenia and chorangioma. J Pediatr. 78(3):516–9.*

Gajewska, K., Herinckx, A., Holoye, A., D'Haene, N., Massez, A., Cassart, M., Van Rysselberge, M., Donner, C. (2010). *Antenatal embolization of a large chorioangioma by percutaneous Glubran 2 injection. Ultrasound Obstet Gynecol. 36(6):773–5.*

Ghidini, A., Locatelli, A. (2006). *Diffuse placental chorioangiomatosis causing multiple fetal cerebral embolism: a case report. J Reprod Med. 51(4):321–4.*

Gruca-Stryjak, K., Ropacka-Lesiak, M., Breborowicz, G. (2011). *Nontrofoblastic placental tumors. Archieves of perinatal medicine. 17(2):113–117.*

Gruca-Stryjak, K., Ropacka-Lesiak, M., Breborowicz, G. (2011). *Intrauterine blood transfusion in case of placental chorangioma. Ginekol Pol. 82(4):304–8.*

Guschmann, M., Schulz-Bischof, K., Vogel, M. (2003). *Incidental chorangiocarcinoma. Case report, immuno-histochemistry and theories of possible histogenesis. Pathologe. 24(2):124–7.*

Guschmann, M., Henrich, W., Entezami, M., Dudenhausen, J.W. (2003). *Chorioangioma — new insights into a well-known problem. I. Results of a clinical and morphological study of 136 cases. J Perinat Med. 31(2):163–9.*

Haak, M.C., Oosterhof, H., Mouw, R.J., Oepkes, D., Vandenbussche, F.P. (1999). *Pathophysiology and treatment of fetal anemia due to placental chorioangioma. Ultrasound Obstet Gynecol. 14(1):68–70.*

Haddad, G., Herbreteau, D., Simon, E., Develay-Morice, J., Perrotin, F. (2010). *Arterial embolization in arterial venous shunt: about our experience in the management of placental chorioangiomas with fetal hydrops. Ultrasound in Obstetr & Gynecol. 36 (S1): 276–277.*

Hadi, H.A., Finley, J., Strickland, D. (1993). *Placental chorioangioma: prenatal diagnosis and clinical significance. Am J Perinatol. 10(2):146–9.*

Harman, C.R. (2008). *Amniotic fluid abnormalities. Semin Perinatol. 32(4):288–94.*

Harris, R.D., Cho, C., Wells, W.A. (1996). *Sonography of the placenta with emphasis on pathological correlation. Semin Ultrasound CT MR. 17(1):66–89.*

He, X.H., Zhou, H.J., Zheng, W. (2004). Clinical characteristics and pathologic study of placental chorioangioma. Zhonghua Fu Chan Ke Za Zhi. 39(4):227–9.

Hellmund, A., Berg, C., Rösing, B., Gembruch, U., Geipel, A. (2012). Masked anemia due to cardiac tamponade in a hydropic fetus caused by placental chorioangioma. Ultrasound Obstet Gynecol. 39(4):479–80.

Højberg, K.E., Aagaard, J., Henriques, U., Sunde, L. (1994). Placental vascular malformation with mesenchymal hyperplasia and a localized chorioangioma. A rarity simulating partial mole. Pathol Res Pract. 190(8):808–13; discussion 814.

Imdad, A., Sheikh, L., Malik, A. (2009). A large chorioangioma causing intrauterine foetal demise. J Pak Med Assoc. 59(8):580–1.

Isaacs H. Jr. (2008). Fetal hydrops associated with tumors. Am J Perinatol. 25(1):43–68.

Itinteang, T., Tan, S.T., Guthrie, S., Tan, C.E., McIntyre, B.C., Brasch, H.D., Day, D.J. (2011). A placental chorionic villous mesenchymal core cellular origin for infantile haemangioma. J Clin Pathol. 64(10):870–4.

Jauniaux, E., Zucker, M., Meuris, S., Verhest, A., Wilkin, P., Hustin, J. (1988). Chorangiocarcinoma: an unusual tumour of the placenta. The missing link? Placenta. 9(6):607–13.

Jhun, K.M., Nassar, P., Chen, T.S., Sardesai, S., Chmait, R.H. (2015). Giant chorioangioma treated in utero via laser of feeding vessels with subsequent development of multifocal infantile hemangiomas. Fetal Pediatr Pathol. 34(1):1–8.

Jones, K., Tierney, K., Grubbs, B.H., Pruetz, J.D., Detterich, J., Chmait, R.H. (2012). Fetoscopic laser photo-coagulation of feeding vessels to a large placental chorioangioma following fetal deterioration after amnioreduction. Fetal Diagn Ther. 31(3):191–5.

Kawano, R., Takemoto, S., Shimamatsu, K., Hori, D., Kamura, T. (2013). Fetomaternal hemorrhage with intraplacental chorioangioma. J Obstet Gynaecol Res. 39(2):583–7.

Khong, T.Y. (2000). Chorangioma with trophoblastic proliferation. Virchows Arch. 436(2):167–71.

Kirkpatrick, A.D., Podberesky, D.J., Gray, A.E., McDermott, J.H. (2007). Best cases from the AFIP: Placental chorioangioma. Radiographics. 27(4):1187–90.

Kodandapani, S., Roopa, P.S., Muralidhar, V. (2013). Non immune fetal hydrops: an overview. Wyno Journal of Medical Sciences. 2(3): 26–31.

Kodandapani, S., Shreshta, A., Ramkumar, V., Rao, L. (2012). Chorioangioma of placenta: a rare placental cause for adverse fetal outcome. Case Rep Obstet Gynecol. 2012:913878.

Kriplani, A., Abbi, M., Banerjee, N., Roy, K/K., Takkar, D. (2001). Indomethacin therapy in the treatment of polyhydramnios due to placental chorioangioma. J Obstet Gynaecol Res. 27(5):245–8.

Kuhnel, P. (1933). Placental chorioangioma. Acta Obstertricia et Gynecologica Scandinavica 13: 143–145.

Lampe, S., Butterwegge, M., Krech, R.H. (1995). Chorioangiomatosis of the placenta — diagnosis and obstetrical management. Zentralbl Gynakol. 117(2):101–4.

Lau, T.K., Leung, T.Y., Yu, S.C., To, K.F., Leung, T.N. (2003). Prenatal treatment of chorioangioma by microcoil embolisation. BJOG. 110(1):70–3.

Lifschitz-Mercer, B., Fogel, M., Kushnir, I., Czernobilsky, B. (1989). Chorangioma. A cytoskeletal profile. Int J Gynecol Pathol. 8(4):349–56.

Liu, J., Guo, L. (2006). Intraplacental choriocarcinoma in a term placenta with both maternal and infantile metastases: a case report and review of the literature. Gynecol Oncol. 103(3):1147–51.

Lowenstein, L., Solt, I., Drugan, A., Auslander, R., Beloosesky, R., Bronstein, M. (2006). *Prenatal diagnosis of chorioangioma. Harefuah. 145(2):95–7, 167.*

Mandelbaum, B., Ross, M., Riddle, C.B. (1969). *Hemangioma of the placenta associated with fetal anemia and edema. Report of a case. Obstet Gynecol. 34(3):335–8.*

Mara, M., Calda, P., Zizka, Z., Sebron, V., Eretova, V., Dudorkinova, D., Dundr, P., Binder, T., Hajek, Z. (2002). *Fetal anemia, thrombocytopenia, dilated umbilical vein, and cardiomegaly due to a voluminous placental chorioangioma. A case report. Fetal Diagn Ther. 17(5):286–92.*

Marchetti, A.A. (1939). *A consideration of certain types of benign tumors of the placenta. Surg Gynecol Obstet. 68:733 74.*

Mendez-Figueroa, H., Papanna, R., Popek, E.J., Byrd, R.H., Goldaber, K., Moise, K.J. Jr, Johnson, A. (2009). *Endoscopic laser coagulation following amnioreduction for the management of a large placental chorioangioma. Prenat Diagn. 29(13):1277–8.*

Miliaras, D., Anagnostou, E., Papoulidis, I., Miliara, X. (2011). *Non-trophoblastic tumor of the placenta with combined histologic features of chorangioma and leiomyoma. Placenta. 32(1):102–4.*

Miller, K., Zawislak, A., Gannon, C., Millar, D., Loughrey, M.B. (2012). *Maternal gastric adenocarcinoma with placental metastases: what is the fetal risk? Pediatr Dev Pathol. 15(3):237–9.*

Monchek, R., Wiedaseck, S. (2012). *Gestational trophoblastic disease: an overview. J Midwifery Womens Health. 57(3):255–9.*

North, P.E., Waner, M., Mizeracki, A., Mrak, R.E., Nicholas, R., Kincannon, J., Suen, J.Y., Mihm, M.C. Jr. (2001). *A unique microvascular phenotype shared by juvenile hemangiomas and human placenta. Arch Dermatol. 137(5):559–70.*

Ogino, S., Redline, R.W. (2000). *Villous capillary lesions of the placenta: distinctions between chorangioma, chorangiomatosis, and chorangiosis. Hum Pathol. 31(8):945–54.*

Perrotin, F., Herbreteau, D., Waymberger, S., Potin, J., Gallas, S., Arbeille, P. (2004). *Ultrasound-guided embolization for the treatment of symptomatic placental chorioangioma. Ultrasound Obstetr & Gynecol 24(3): 280.*

Potter, E.L. (1943). *Universal oedema of the fetus unassociated with erythroblastosis. Am J Obstet Gynaecol. 46:13904.*

Prapas, N., Liang, R.I., Hunter, D., Copel, J.A., Lu, L.C., Pazkash, V., Mari, G. (2000). *Color Doppler imaging of placental masses: differential diagnosis and fetal outcome. Ultrasound Obstet Gynecol. 16(6):559–63.*

Prashanth, A., Lavanya, R., Girisha, K.M., Mundkur, A. (2012). *Placental Teratoma Presenting as a Lobulated Mass behind the Neck of Fetus: A Case Report. Case Rep Obstet Gynecol. 2012:857230.*

Royal college of Obstetricians and Gynecologists. (2010). *Antenatal Corticosteroids to Reduce Neonatal Morbidity and Mortality. October 2010. Green–top Guideline No. 7.*

Quarello, E., Bernard, J.P., Leroy, B., Ville, Y. (2005). *Prenatal laser treatment of a placental chorioangioma. Ultrasound Obstet Gynecol. 25(3):299–301.*

Quintero, R.A., Reich, H., Romero, R., Johnson, M.P., Gonçalves, L., Evans, M.I. (1996). *In utero endoscopic devascularization of a large chorioangioma. Ultrasound Obstet Gynecol. 8(1):48–52.*

Reshetnikova, O.S, Burton, G.J., Milovanov, A.P., Fokin, E.I. (1996). *Increased incidence of placental chorioangioma in high-altitude pregnancies: hypobaric hypoxia as a possible etiologic factor. Am J Obstet Gynecol. 174(2):557–61.*

Sepulveda, W., Wong, A.E., Herrera, L., Dezerega, V., Devoto, J.C. (2009). *Endoscopic laser coagulation of* feeding vessels in large placental chorioangiomas: report of three cases and review of invasive treatment options. Prenat Diagn. 29(3):201–6.

Shalev, E., Weiner, E., Feldman, E., Zuckerman, H.K. (1984). Prenatal diagnosis of placental hemangioma — clinical implication: a case report. Int J Gynaecol Obstet. 22(4):291–3.

Shih, J.C., Ko, T.L., Lin, M.C., Shyu, M.K., Lee, C.N., Hsieh, F.J. (2004). Quantitative three-dimensional power Doppler ultrasound predicts the outcome of placental chorioangioma. Ultrasound Obstet Gynecol. 24(2):202–6.

Sivasli, E., Tekşam, O., Haliloğlu, M., Güçer, S., Orhan, D., Gürgey, A., Tekinalp, G. (2009). Hydrops fetalis associated with chorioangioma and thrombosis of umbilical vein. Turk J Pediatr. 51(5):515–8.

Trask, C., Lage, J.M., Roberts, D.J. (1994). A second case of "chorangiocarcinoma" presenting in a term asymptomatic twin pregnancy: choriocarcinoma in situ with associated villous vascular proliferation. Int J Gynecol Pathol. 13(1):87–91.

Thelmo, M.C., Shen, E.P., Shertukde, S. (2010). Metastatic pulmonary adenocarcinoma to placenta and pleural fluid: clinicopathologic findings. Fetal Pediatr Pathol. 29(1):45–56.

Valenzano Menada, M., Moioli, M., Garaventa, A., Nozza, P., Foppiano, M., Trimarchi, N., Fulcheri, E. (2010). Spontaneous regression of transplacental metastases from maternal melanoma in a newborn: case report and review of the literature. Melanoma Res. 20(6):443–9.

Verloes, A., Schaaps, J.P., Herens, C., et al. (1991). Prenatal diagnosis of cystic hygroma and chorioangioma in the Wolf-Hirschhorn syndrome. Prenat Diagn 11:129–32.

Witters, I., Van Damme, M.T., Ramaekers, P., Van Assche, F.A., Fryns, J.P. (2003). Benign multiple diffuse neonatal hemangiomatosis after a pregnancy complicated by polyhydramnios and a placental chorioangioma. Eur J Obstet Gynecol Reprod Biol. 106(1):83–5.

Wurster, D.E., Hoetnagel, D., Bernischke, K., et al. (1969). Placental chorangiomata and mental deficiency in a child with 2/15translocations: 46,XX, t(2q -;15 q+). Cytogenetics 8:389–99.

Zalel, Y., Weisz, B., Gamzu, R., Schiff, E., Shalmon, B., Achiron, R. (2002). Chorioangiomas of the placenta: sonographic and Doppler flow characteristics. J Ultrasound Med. 21(8):909–13.

Zanardini, C., Papageorghiou, A., Bhide, A., Thilaganathan, B. (2010). Giant placental chorioangioma: natural history and pregnancy outcome. Ultrasound Obstet Gynecol. 35(3):332–6.

# Chapter 2

# Age-related Oxidative Stress in the Cardiovascular Diseases and Lipoic Acid as Antioxidant

Beata Skibska[1], Anna Goraca[2]

## 1   Introduction

Oxidative stress and chronic inflammation play a key role in the development of many cardiovascular diseases, including atherosclerosis, hypertension, ischemia-reperfusion injury and heart failure (Figure 1). There are many factors associated with oxidative stress, which lead to the development of these diseases. One of the main factors is over-production of ROS and NOS, together with decreased nitric oxide bioavailability and reduced antioxidant capacity in the vasculature (Paravicini & Touyz, 2008).

ROS such as superoxide anions ($O_2\cdot^-$), hydrogen peroxide ($H_2O_2$) and hydroxyl groups ($OH^-$) cause mitochondrial genomic damage. Many studies confirm that mitochondria are a major source of ROS in aging tissues (Lenaz et al., 2002).

It has been estimated that 2-3% of the $O_2\cdot^-$ consumed by mitochondria is incompletely reduced, generating $O_2\cdot^-$, which is a moderately stable free radical anion. $O_2\cdot^-$ may be catalyzed by superoxide dismutase (SOD) to $H_2O_2$ and then to hydroxyl radical by $Fe^{2+}$ depend Fenton reaction. $H_2O_2$ is a relatively stable ROS. $OH^-$ is the most reactive and unstable radical that reacts with a large variety of compounds and membranes. It may be formed upon direct reaction of $H_2O_2$ and $O_2\cdot^-$ (Haber Weiss reaction) or by the cycle of reactions involving oxidation of transition metals, such as $Fe^{2+}$ or $Cu^{2+}$ (Fenton reaction) (Nedelykovic et al., 2003).

---

[1] Department of Applied Pharmacy, Department of Pharmacy, Medical University of Lodz, Łódź, Poland.

[2] Department of Cardiovascular Physiology, Medical University of Lodz, Łódź, Poland.

**Age-related Oxidative Stress**

**ATHEROSCLEROSIS**
Endothelial dysfunction:
– Loss of nitric oxide bioactivity
– Inhibition of endothelial
   activation (i.e. expression
   of adhesion molecules and
   monocyte chemoattractants)

Initiation of faty streak
development

Inury in the arterial wall

**HEART FAILURE**
Qualitative and quantitative
defects in mtDNA

Increased destruction of nitric
oxide

Chronically elevated peripheral
vasoconstriction

**HYPERTENSION**
Vascular dysfunction:
– Increased VSCM proliferation
– Arterial stiffness
– Decreased vasodilation
– Increased vascular tone

**ISCHEMIA/REPERFUSION**
Endothelial dysfunction:
– Impaired tissue perfusion
– Vasoconstriction of conduit
   vessels including coronary
   arteries

Alternations of protective
signaling pathways in cardiac
cells

Impaired oxidative
phosphorylation and
energy transfer

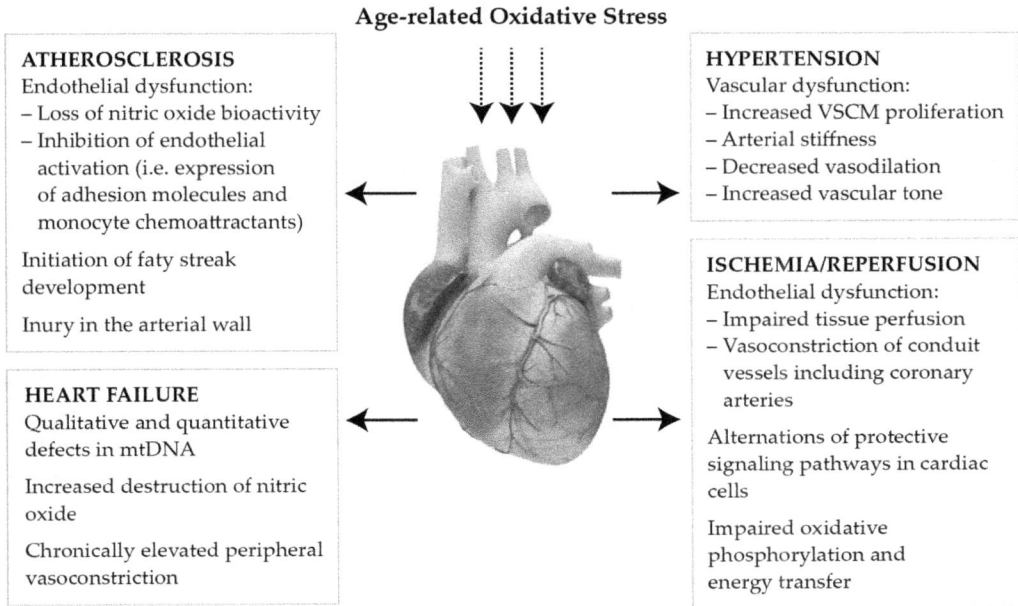

**Figure 1:** The adverse effect of age – related oxidative stress on some cardiovascular diseases: atherosclerosis, hypertension, ischemia/reperfusion and heart failure.

ROS are also generated, e.g. by exposure to air pollutants, industrial chemicals and when a body is exposed to X-rays, to drugs capable of redox cycling, or to xenobiotics that can form free radical metabolites in situ.

High levels of ROS are observed in a variety of cellular components, including proteins, lipids, and DNA, as well as dysfunctional organelles such as mitochondria, ribosomes, peroxisomes, and the endoplasmic reticulum, leading to pathological changes.

Death due to cardiovascular diseases is the cause of mortality in 80% of people aged over 65 years. In addition, the aging process is associated with oxidative stress in the blood vessels and in the heart, which leads to the development of cardiovascular disease (CVD) (Karavidas et al., 2010). Increased oxidative stress produced in the mitochondria and cytosol of the heart is a common denominator to almost all CVDs.

According to the free radical theory of aging developed by Harman, the antioxidant defense mechanisms become less effective in people after the age of 40 (Mei et al., 2015; Harman, 1956). This results in fatty acid oxidation and lipid peroxidation, with consequent changes in the physical properties of cell membranes and phospholipids. As they have long half-lives and increased polarity, phospholipid peroxides are active intermediaries of the oxidation and reduction chain (Bartosz, 2009), which may migrate from point of origin to other places in the organism. Changes in the membrane are sufficient to activate the extracellular phospholipases, leading to cell membrane damage and cell death (apoptosis).

Excessive ROS production and weakened antioxidant mechanisms lead to the occurrence of oxidative stress and induction of apoptosis. ROS reacts with DNA, proteins, and lipids, resulting in the accumulation of products, the onset of degenerative processes, and ultimately, the development of many serious diseases and aging. Although aging is a natural process, it is accelerated by ROS production. Oxidative stress is an imbalance between production of ROS present in cells and the biological ability to detoxify the reactive intermediates or repair the harm caused (Reed, 1957).

To counteract increased levels of ROS, which leads to the development of oxidative stress, cells have antioxidant mechanisms that include superoxide dismutases (SODs) — which are present in mitochondria, such as manganese SOD (MnSOD), cytosol, such as copper zinc SOD (CuZnSOD), and plasma membrane and extracellular spaces (such as extracellular SOD) — catalase, glutathione peroxidases, peroxiredoxins, and thioredoxin (Trx). Trx1 is a protein, which plays an important role in regulating the tissue level of oxidative stress, thereby controlling cardiac myocyte growth responses.

Catalase is also an important enzyme, because it is involved in decomposition/detoxification of $H_2O_2$, thereby increasing cardiac resistance to oxidative stress-induced injury such as ischemia (Yamamoto et al., 2003). Also thiols and thiol-dependent enzymes, such as glutathione peroxidases (GPx) possess significant antioxidant properties. GPx are responsible for the removal of $H_2O_2$ and protect from the development of the oxidative stress. Aging causes genetic depletion of GPx-1 or GPx-4. GPx deficiency leads to increased levels of oxidative stress and senescence of fibroblasts, and vascular dysfunction (Oelze et al., 2014; De Haan et al., 2004).

Many studies show detrimental effects of oxidative stress on functions of physiological organs during the aging process and prove that antioxidant enzymes have a significant effect on the healthspan of human and animals during normal aging. (Mikhed et al., 2015).

Unfortunately, described mechanisms are not sufficient to defend the body from oxidative stress, which plays a key role for the quality of aging. Therefore, we are looking for drugs that would effectively eradicate ROS.

Currently, antioxidants are used in order to reduce the production of ROS in cells and limit their harmful effects on the organism. One effective antioxidant is lipoic acid (LA). LA is a natural antioxidant synthesized in the mitochondria of the liver and other tissues (Dudek, 2013), and it plays a crucial role in metabolism. It is a cofactor in the multienzyme complexes that catalyze the oxidative decarboxylation of $\alpha$-keto acids such as pyruvate, $\alpha$-ketoglutarate dehydrogenase, branched-chain $\alpha$-keto acid dehydrogenase and glycine decarboxylase complex.

Its antioxidant properties were first discovered in the 1950s (Reed, 1957) and later confirmed by subsequent studies (Packer et al., 1995; Navari-Izzo et al., 2002; Ghibu et al., 2009; Rochette et al., 2013). Its strong reduction and low oxidation-reduction potential (-0.29 V) have made it the subject of many studies from various fields of Medicine. It is currently regarded as one of the most potent cellular oxidation regulators (Bilska & Wlodek, 2005). LA is a remarkable compound that appears to slow the process of aging in animal experiments. Considering the strong antioxidant properties of lipoic acid, the purpose of this review is to present the protective role of LA on selected cardiovascular diseases.

# 2  Age-related Oxidative Stress in Cardiovascular Diseases

## 2.1  Endothelial Dysfunction and Atherosclerosis

Endothelium of the blood vessels is involved in many physiological and pathological processes. It plays a very important role in the physiological regulation of vascular tone, vascular smooth muscle cell migration, cellular adhesion resistance to thrombosis, and regulates adhesion and extravasation of leucocytes (Steyers & Miller, 2014).

Pathological processes which occur in blood vessels cause the endothelial balance to become dysregulated. This endothelial dysfunction contributes to the development of atherosclerosis, improper blood circulation, inflammation and even cancer progression (Madamanchi & Runge, 2013). Vascular dysfunction is caused by reduction of nitric oxide levels, production of vasoconstrictor/vasodilator factor imbalances, impaired angiogenesis, endothelial cell senescence and oxidative stress (Rubio-Ruiz et al., 2014) and toxic substances emitted to the environment from solid fuels (Ruiz-Vera et al., 2015). Although there are several conditions that contribute to endothelial dysfunction, increased oxidative stress seems to play an important role.

The overproduction of ROS is a result of the adverse effect of oxidative stress on cellular levels of nitric oxide (NO), an important endothelial factor. Recent studies suggest that NO is an important factor for the proper functioning of endothelial cells, because it controls the function of smooth muscle and exerts an antihypertensive effect at the cardiovascular level (Monti et al., 2014).

NO is synthesized from l-arginine by the enzyme NO synthase - NOS and inhibition of the L-arginine/NO pathway via N-nitro-L-arginine methyl ester (L-NAME) can lead to systemic hypertension (Herman et al., 2006). There are three NOS isoforms: the neuronal isoforms – nNOS, the constitutive endothelial isoform - eNOS, and the inducible isoform - iNOS (Assar et al., 2012). Substrates for all NOS isoforms are L-arginine, NADPH and molecular oxygen, forming ·NO, citruline, and water. Moreover, NOS enzymes need cofactors such as: flavin mononucleotide (FMN), flavin adenine dinucleotide (FAD) tetrahydrobiopterin (BH4), heme and NADPH. After the application of BH4 pool depleted NOS can contribute to $O_2^-$ production (Moncada & Bolanos, 2006; Cobb & Cole, 2015 ). The reduction of NO availability disturbs its vascular homeostasis.

Aging is a physiological process, but it also influences the destabilization of endothelial cells. This process, and its associated increased oxidative stress, is one of the factors which may cause endothelial dysfunction, characterized by impaired endothelium-dependent signaling processes. Aging also leads to arterial stiffness. The consequence of increased oxidative stress in aging is inactivation of NO by high concentrations of $O_2^{·-}$ produced by the reaction of NO with ROS (Oakley & Tharakan, 2014; Csiszar et al., 2002; Kajiya et al., 2007). The reaction between NO and $O_2^{·-}$ forms the peroxynitrite anion (ONOO-). This form is known as a reactive nitrogen species (RNS) and characterized high reactivity with proteins, DNA and lipids. Unlike $O_2^{·-}$, ONOO- can penetrate into the cardiovascular cells and cause oxidative modifications within them (Pacher et al., 2007). Peroxynitrite has also been shown to induce microvascular hyperpermeability by disrupting the adherence junction proteins (Zhang et al., 2005).

One *in vitro* study shows decreased eNOS expression in aged human umbilical vein endothelial cells. This process is associated with dysfunction of cell-cell junctions and microvascular hyperpermeability (Yoon et al., 2010). It leads to severe oxidative injury, which results in cell necrosis or apoptosis. This has been confirmed by many other studies which suggest that the decreased endothelial NO production promotes endothelial cell apoptosis and leads to microvascular rarefaction (Csiszar et al., 2004; Csiszar et al., 2007).

Oxidative stress is known to activate redox-sensitive cellular signaling pathways, which have in turn been implicated in inflammation associated with vasculature subjected to aging (Csiszar et al., 2008). According to *in vitro* studies on endothelial cells, this inflammation induces overproduction of ROS and endothelial dysfunction in older rats (Cai & Harrison, 2000).

In recent years, longevity genes that affect lifespan and the rate at which the body becomes old, have been identified. For example, defects in mouse Klotho gene have been shown to be associated with endothelial dysfunction, leading to the premature development of atherosclerosis and, at the same time, accelerated aging (Saito et al., 2006). Kwon et al. reported that down –regulation of sirtuin 3 (Sirt 3) lead to oxidative damage and mitochondrial dysfunction by ROS and contribute to age-related hearing loss (Kwon et al., 2015). Sirt 3 regulates ROS production at the electron transport chain and detoxification of ROS via activation of antioxidant enzymes (Tao et al., 2010).

Mouse models of mild dyslipidemia have been found to demonstrate endothelial dysfunction, for example, those which are deficient in apolipoprotein E. This endothelial dysfunction is associated with stretch-induced hypercontractility and diminished endothelium-dependent vasorelaxation, accompanied by decreased levels of NO and eNOS, as well as increased plasma levels of IL-6, a pro-inflammatory cytokine that reduces eNOS levels and activity. Endothelial dysfunction was found to precede the appearance of atherosclerosis in a murine model of dyslipidemia (Cavieres et al., 2014).

Atherosclerosis is a pathological state of the vasculature which progresses together with endothelial dysfunction caused by dyslipidemia, leading to the deposition of inflammatory cells and lipids in the vascular wall. The key step in the formation of both atherosclerotic plaques and neointimal thickening is hyperproliferation of smooth muscle cells. Chronic inflammation of the vessel wall, as occurs in atherosclerosis, is initiated by leucocyte recruitment and adhesion to the activated endothelium (Danzaki et al., 2012). Recent studies showed that deficiency of vitamin D play an important role in progression of atherosclerosis. Bozic et al. showed that deletion of vitamin D receptors accelerates atherosclerotic plaque formation, elevates serum lipids (LDL, HDL, triglycerides) levels, leads to augmented expression of proinflammatory mediators (Bozic et al., 2015). In addition, knockdown of VDR increases leucocytes-endothelial cell interactions.

Therefore, the state of the aging blood vessels, which are progressively damaged, primarily impacts the development of atherosclerosis. The oxidative stress theory of atherosclerosis indicates that the production of ROS stimulates oxidized low-density lipoprotein formation (ox-LDL) (Chisolm & Steinberg, 2000). ox-LDL has many important properties which may promote atherosclerosis. It stimulates vascular ROS formation and causes endothelial dysfunction (Mangge et al., 2014). In addition, Meisinger et al. note that it acts as a pro-atherogenic marker (Meisinger et al., 2005), and that elevated levels of oxLDL may predict coronary heart disease events in healthy subjects. Moreover, ox-LDL is known to promote oxygen radical generation in human aortic endothelial cells (HEAC) by phosphorylating the p66Shc adaptor protein at Ser36 (Madamanchi & Runge, 2013). Hence, oxidation of LDL appears to contribute to the pro-oxidant environment in atherosclerotic lesions. Kang et al. confirmed that novel protein in VSMC OLR1 is the endogenous oxidized LDL receptor that mediates the NF-kB activation, and induction of this protein in VSCM may contribute to the inflammation and hyperplasia of VSCM (Kang et al., 2015).

Current research shows that endothelial dysfunction also plays an important role in early and late mechanisms of atherosclerosis development. Atherosclerosis is known to result in vascular events such as hypertension, ischemic heart failure, and heart failure. The recent studies showed that expression of growth differentiation factor -15 (GDF-15) occurs in atherosclerosis, heart failure, ischemia/reperfusion. The above factor responsible for cardioprotection. GDF-15 belongs to the family of protein TGF-β and activates signaling pathways (PI3K/AKT/eNOS/NO) and inhibits epidermal growth factor (EGFR), NF-kB/JNK/caspase-3 pathways (Adela & Banerjee, 2015).

## 2.2  Hypertension

Oxidative stress and aging are involved in hypertension. Both lead to overproduction of reactive oxygen species. The ROS generated in cardiovascular cells cause various forms of pathological vascular damage in blood vessels related to the promotion of cell growth, the accumulation of extracellular matrix protein, inflammation and endothelial dysfunction, all of which are characteristic features of the hypertensive vascular phenotype (Sprague & Khalil, 2005). Pacia et al. reported that hypertension affects two layers of the vascular wall, including the *tunica intima* (endothelium with internal elastic lamina) and *tunica media* (smooth muscle cells with elastin fibers) (Pacia et al., 2015).

As in atherosclerosis, one of the major mechanisms by which oxidative stress may promote hypertension is endothelial dysfunction. Aside from impaired vascular expansion, the most important effects of endothelial dysfunction are those concerned with two substances produced by the endothelium: NO and endothelin-1 (ET-1) (Weseler & Bast, 2010). An imbalance between these substances interferes with vascular homeostasis, leading to vasoconstriction and elevated blood pressure (Watson et al., 2008). Disturbed homeostasis is characterized by an increase in the vasoconstriction factor ET-1, and a reduction of the bioavailability of NO (Herrera et al., 2010).

Experimental evidence indicates that ROS can be also generated in response to ET-1 (Piechota et al., 2010). ET-1 is a vasoconstrictor peptide, which raises blood pressure and induces vascular and myocardial hypertrophy (Versari et al., 2009). ET-1 acts via two G-protein-coupled receptors, ETA and ETB. ETA receptor is located in vascular smooth muscles (VSMCs) and contributes to ET-1-induced contraction and proliferation of VSMCs in hypertension. ETB receptor is predominantly expressed in vascular endothelial cells and their activation with ET-1 induces vasodilation through accelerated production of prostacyclin (PGI2) and nitric oxide (NO). ETB receptor is also located in VSMCs, where it has

vasoconstrictive and proliferative actions (Humbert & Ghofrani, 2015). Application of endothelin receptor antagonists lowered blood pressure and reduced endothelia dysfunction in a number of hypertension animal models such as salt-sensitive hypertension rat
model, the deoxycorticosterone acetate-salt (DOCA) rat model, and angiotensin II-induced hypertensive rat model (Tobe et al., 2015).

ET-1 production is known to be influenced by a number of factors. Oxidative stress
may cause modulation of ET-1 and in ET-1-induced activation of various signaling pathways (Kowalczyk et al., 2015). In addition, aging may increase the release of ET-1 from
endothelial cells in humans and animals (Kumazaki, 1993; Brandes et al., 2005). In turn,
*in vitro* studies have shown that ET-1 itself activates many factors, including NFκB and
TNF-α, which are involved in cell growth, inflammation and proliferation (Canty et al.,
1999; Kleniewska et al., 2013; Bhatt et al., 2014). These processes can also affect the development of hypertension.

Along with NO deficiency and increased ET-1 production, a dysfunctional endothelium also acts as a source of other mediators and factors such as prostaglandin H2,
tromboxane A2, ROS and significantly and angiotensin II (AT II) that damage vascular
cells (Versari et al., 2009). Both angiotensin II and endothelin-1 play important roles in
age - related endothelial dysfunction (Yildiz, 2007). Angiotensin II stimulates ET-1 release
and raises blood pressure by a variety of actions (Kohan et al., 2011), and is a potent activator of nicotinamide adenine dinucleotide phosphate (NAD(P)H) oxidase in vascular
cells (Drummond et al., 2011). NAD(P)H is a major source of ROS in the blood vessels
and is considered to be a critical determinants of the redox state of blood vessels (Seshiah
et al., 2002). Some studies suggest that enhanced NAD(P)H oxidase activity can be observed in hypertension-induced oxidative stress and subsequently, endothelial dysfunction. Another study confirms the role of NAD(P)H-oxidase on the formation of ROS in
blood vessels. The activation of NAD(P)H-oxidase in cerebral blood vessels causes $H_2O_2$-
mediated opening of BKCa channels in cerebral arteries, leading to consequent hyperpo-
larization and vasodilation (Paravicini et al., 2004). In addition, oxidative stress activates
other enzymes, including mitochondrial enzymes, NOS and xanthine oxidase, which are
produced following ROS production and have a damaging influence on blood vessels.

The relationship between oxidative stress and hypertension has been shown in
many experimental models (Touyz, 2004; Dinh et al., 2014; Govender & Nadar, 2014; Ocaranza et al., 2014).

The renin-angiotensin-aldosterone system (RAAS) is a crucial regulator of vascular
homeostasis. RAAS is one of the most important hormonal systems; it controls functions
of cardiovascular, renal, and adrenal glands by regulating blood pressure, fluid volume,
as well as sodium and potassium balance. It is important in the pathogenesis of arterial
ageing (Lee & Park, 2013). Angiotensin II (Ang II) plays a key role in the endothelium
dysfunction and development of atherosclerosis. Ang II induces oxidative stress and creates superoxide anions primarily through the activation of NAD(P)H oxidase in vascular
cells and myocytes. Moreover, Ang II activates intracellular signaling pathways and upregulates many inflammation factors including chemokines, cytokines, and growth factors, which have been implicated in atherosclerotic plaque development (Pacurari et al.,
2014). Anti-inflammatory agents, ANG II receptor blockers and renin inhibitors may slow

down inflammatory processes and the progress of the disease (Husain et al., 2015).

To summarize, hypertension may be triggered by a number of factors. However, oxidative stress and aging both exert a significant influence.

## 2.3   Atherosclerosis-ischemic Heart Disease

Age-related oxidative stress also leads to cardiac ischemic and reperfusion injuries. Aging and oxidative stress play important roles in the senescent heart. The aged myocardium has less tolerance to ischemia and hemodynamic stress than the young myocardium (Dai et al., 2014; Lesnefsky et al., 2001; Pepe, 2000).

Ischemic heart disease is a leading cause of morbidity and mortality among the elderly all over the world (Huang et al., 2015). Many metabolic and biochemical changes in myocardial tissue are the result of oxygen and nutrient deprivation during ischemia. Decreased blood flow causes irreparable damage to cardiomyocytes (Klishadi et al., 2015).

In most cases, the presence of atherosclerotic plaques slowly leads to the narrowing of blood vessels, and impairs the blood supply to the heart. Long-term ischemic heart disease can lead to myocardial infarction due to myocardial hypoxia and accumulation of waste metabolites. This can lead to damage to the cardiovascular and cell death by apoptosis (Khurana et al., 2013).

During reperfusion, the concentration of superoxide anions ($O_2 \cdot^-$) and hydroxyl groups ($OH^-$) from mitochondria is greatly increased. Oxidative stress is then intensified by the increased production of these ROS, which then results in oxidation of mitochondrial proteins and mitochondrial dysfunction (Yamamoto & Sadoshima, 2011).

ROS such as superoxide anions, hydrogen peroxide and hydroxyl groups can cause mitochondrial genomic damage and a gradual decline in mitochondrial function in senescent hearts (Jahangir et al., 2007). Mitochondria from aged hearts have been found to demonstrate reduced membrane potential, which may contribute to lowered adenosine 5'-triphosphate (ATP) synthesis (Di Lisa & Bernardi 2005). This imbalance between the synthesis and consumption of ATP significantly influences the metabolism of the heart muscle, leading to greater oxygen consumption. ATP deficiency is also associated with a rapid loss of myocardial contractility, which can result in dysfunctions of the cardiovascular system and arrhythmias (Avkiran & Marber, 2002).

ROS can also activate some biochemical pathways in blood vessels, resulting in changes in cell function. In response to angiotensin II induction, they can activate protein kinase B in vascular smooth muscle cells (VSMC), leading to VSMC hypertrophy (Gonzaga et al., 2014). The activation of biochemical signaling pathways promotes greater cellular dysfunction and impairs cardiomyocyte functionality (Finkel & Holbrook 2008).

Some research demonstrated that inflammatory process is involved in cardiovascular injury resulting from ischemia and reperfusion (Hohensinner et al., 2011; Linde et al., 2007). Ischemia–reperfusion (I/R) is characterized with increased levels of inflammatory markers, such as CRP IL-6 and TNF-α. TNF-α has a negative inotropic effect, resulting in inhibited myocardial contractility, reduced blood pressure and the above factor may induce cardiomyocyte apoptosis and participate in vascular remodeling (Zhu et al.,

2006).

I/R injury seems to be triggered partly by neutrophil activation and the adhesion of the neutrophils results in decrease blood flow. Neutrophil accumulation and TNF-$\alpha$ production increased following I/R. A removal of neutrophils or administration of drugs inhibiting neutrophil activity appeared to reduce ischemia/reperfusion injury (Sun et al., 2015).

These compounds and other cytokines can increase the production of ROS in atherosclerosis by stimulating vascular myocytes. Conversely, by inducing inflammation, ROS may also further stimulate the production of inflammatory cytokines.

Furthermore, other biomarkers of oxidative stress play important roles in the pathophysiology of ischemia-reperfusion damage in myocardial infarction. Extracellular biomarkers of ischemia-reperfusion damage include lipid peroxidation products, plasma antioxidant vitamin levels, total antioxidant capacity of plasma and protein carbonylation. In addition, such intracellular biomarkers as antioxidant enzyme activity, thiol index (GSH/GSSG ratio), carbonyl levels, and F2-isoprostane level can influence the degree of oxidative stress (Rodrigo et al., 2013).

The lipid peroxidation is one of the significant biomarkers of ischemia-reperfusion damage, because causes inter alia the reduction in the activities of important enzymes: $Na^+$-$K^+$-ATPase and $Ca^{2+}$-ATPase. These enzymes play an essential role in the contraction and relaxation of cardiac muscle by maintaining normal ion levels inside myocytes. Increased levels of $Ca^{2+}$ in myocytes and inhibition of $Na^+$ and $K^+$ transport lead to myocardial oxidative stress and apoptosis (Petrich et al., 1996). Oxidative stress in the heart, damages not only lipids, but also modifies the proteins and DNA. The functions of the proteins and intracellular-signaling mechanisms are modulated by the S-thiolation process (Eaton et al., 2002).

During myocardial reperfusion ischemia, ROS generated by oxidative stress lead to the production of the DNA single-strand breaks, which increases catabolism of NAD, resulting in a reduced level of NAD (Lindahl et al., 1995).

NAD plays a significant role in cellular energy homoeostasis and redox state and can be involved in gene transcription, cell division, calcium signaling and in many other cellular and biological outcomes (Chen et al., 2015).

An imbalance between the demand for oxygen and nutrients and the ability to deliver them to the heart muscle, known as ischemia/reperfusion, is most commonly caused by atherosclerosis, but oxidative stress and related overproduction of ROS also play important roles. They cause lipid, protein, and DNA oxidation, potentially contributing to contractile failure (Ferdinandy et al., 2007).

Ischemia can lead to various diseases of the heart such as heart failure and, ultimately, myocardial infarction, depending on the duration and extent of ischemia.

## 2.4 Heart Failure

The effects of oxidative stress on aging on the vasculature and on the heart muscle are varied, but can lead to the development of heart failure (HF). In myocardial ischemia, hypoxia and reoxygenation elevates ROS production in cardiac tissues, which leads to direct oxidative damage to cellular components.

ROS influence the function of the extracellular matrix, which is demonstrated by greater interstitial and perivascular fibrosis (Maulik & Kumar, 2012). On the cellular level, mitochondria are one of the major sites for the generation of ROS, which is an undesirable side product of the energy production. Therefore, mitochondrial dysfunction increases the risk of heart failure.

It is known that mitochondrial function is critically altered in failing hearts both in animals and humans (Yang et al., 2015).

Overproduction of ROS in mitochondria can lead to a disastrous cycle of mitochondrial DNA (mtDNA) damage and, increase electron leakage from the electron transports chain, which can further lead to radical generation (Tsutsui, 2001). This process causes cellular injury and may contribute to the development of myocardial remodeling and HF.

In experimental models, it has been proven that mtDNA deletions contribute to the phenotype of systolic heart failure through increased mitochondrial ROS (mtROS) (Lesnefsky et al., 2001).

The role of mtROS in the development of HF was also demonstrated by overexpressing mitochondrial-targeted catalase in the heart. These studies showed that the increase in mtDNA damage contributes directly to cardiac hypertrophy and HF (Dai et al., 2011). Other studies also confirm that mtDNA damage contributes to the phenotype of systolic heart failure, through increased mtROS (Dai et al., 2014).

Oxidative stress changes gene expression and influences cell death in heart cells which are now known to exert an influence on heart failure and myocardial remodeling. Heart failure itself, is known to involve a decrease in contractility, myocardial fibrosis, myocyte apoptosis and metabolic remodeling (Zhou et al., 2014). Metabolic remodeling in heart failure is characterized by decreased cardiac energy production, which is the result of a decrease in the level of ATP in cardiomyocytes. This may lead to progressive impairments in substrate utilization and mitochondrial biogenesis and function. In addition to ATP deficiency, metabolic remodeling involves changes in metabolic pathways that regulate essential, non-ATP-generating cellular processes such as growth, redox homeostasis and autophagy (Doenst et al., 2013). A reduced supply of ATP necessary for the contractile function of cardiomyocytes can account for chronic heart failure.

In addition, reduced capacity for energy transduction leads to secondary dysregulation of cellular processes critical for cardiac pump function, including Ca2+ handling and contractile function, which results in increased energy demand and diminished function. It was observed that energy deficiency can be a cause and an effect of heart failure (Huss & Kelly, 2005).

In heart failure, overproduction of ROS may adversely alter cardiac mechanics, leading to further worsening of the systolic and diastolic function. This is connected with vascular endothelial dysfunction.

The vascular endothelial dysfunction due to uncoupling of the nitric oxide synthase, activation of vascular and phagocytic membrane oxidases or mitochondrial oxidative stress may lead to increased vascular stiffness, further compromising cardiac performance (Münzel et al., 2015). It has recently been shown that lipid accumulation is a significant feature of clinical heart failure (Sharma et al., 2004).

Similarly, cardiac hypertrophy is strongly associated with an increased risk of heart failure and sudden cardiac death. ROS influence the function of the extracellular matrix, which is demonstrated by greater interstitial and perivascular fibrosis (Maulik & Kumar, 2012). Hypertrophy can lead to the obstruction of outflow from the left ventricle (LV), resulting in an increased afterload in the ventricular wall.

The abnormal production of ROS in aging plays an important role in the pathogenesis of these cardiovascular diseases, leads to increased oxidative stress on cellular structures and causes changes in molecular pathways. In the failing heart, overproduction of ROS leads to the accumulation of superoxide anions, which may be generated by both metabolic and enzymatic sources, including nitric oxide synthase, NADPH oxidases, mitochondrial respiration, and xanthine oxidase (Douglas & Sawyer 2011). The overproduction of the above factors, affects initiation of the inflammatory response. Xanthine oxidase (XO) in particular exerts an important influence on heart failure. XO can also combine with other compounds and enzymes and create reactive oxidants, as well as oxide substrates. It was observed that the concentration of the XO grew with the degree of heart failure. This upregulation can contribute to the energy disorder in myocardial cells (Elahi et al., 2009).

Similarly, increased NAD(P)H activity has been observed in myocardial cells from humans with heart failure (Venkataraman et al., 2013; Peng et al., 2015). This increase is due partly to the presence of increased concentrations of angiotensin II, which leads to an imbalance in the oxidative/nitrosative system. In addition, ROS generated by NADPH oxidase proteins are also important in redox signaling (Hafstad et al., 2013).

All of these processes are caused by oxidative stress, which leads to a disruption of structures of proteins, lipids, and nucleic acids. Disruption of structures of proteins causes aging due to accumulation of oxidized proteins in cells and leads to damage and dysfunction of molecules in the cells (Shringarpure & Davies, 2002; Tosato et al., 2007), whereas mitochondrial DNA damage leads to disruption of electron transport chain and increased ROS production. As a consequence, it leads to energy depletion in the cell and apoptosis (Mandavilli et al., 2002). Many studies have demonstrated an association between these structural disorders and heart failure (Cameron et al., 2006; Wojciechowska et al., 2006).

In summary, multiple factors are involved in the etiology of heart failure, and oxidative stress is one of them. To reduce or prevent the adverse effects of oxidative stress on the organism, substances with antioxidant properties can be applied. Research indicates that dietary supplementation by exogenous antioxidants can play a key role in ameliorating many of the effects of oxidative stress in cardiovascular diseases.

# 3    Protective Effect of Lipoic Acid (LA) on Cardiovascular Diseases

Lipoic acid (LA) is a specific antioxidant: it can easily quench radicals, has an amphiphilic character and does not exhibit any serious side effects (Goraca et al., 2011). LA is a compound that contains sulfur in the form of two thiol groups (Figure 2) acts as a cofactor for

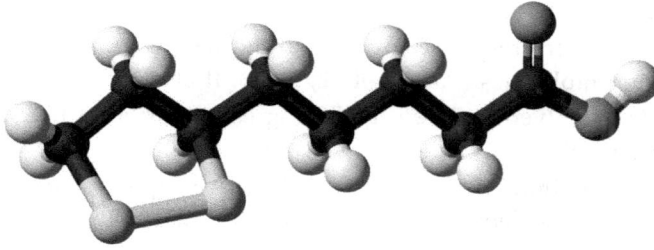

**Figure 2:** The molecular structure of lipoic acid.

several mitochondrial enzymes by catalyzing the $\alpha$-keto acid. The ability of thiol compounds to reduce ROS is associated with the formation of thiol radicals, and the rate and efficiency of thiol radical removal have a critical effect on the antioxidant or pro-oxidant actions of thiols in cells (Glantzounis et al., 2006).

The antioxidant properties of LA are based on its ability to directly scavenge ROS, its metal chelating activity and its potential to react with, and regenerate, other antioxidants such as glutathione, vitamins E and C (Singh & Jialal, 2008). LA also demonstrates anti-inflammatory properties.

An additional advantage of LA is its solubility in both water and in fat, which allows it to travel to all parts of the body (Segall et al., 2004). Because of its special properties, it is able to enter certain parts of the cell that most other antioxidants are not able to reach.

This compound acts by many mechanisms, and can therefore be a very effective antioxidant. Hence, LA is used in various diseases concerning age-depended oxidative stress. It can be particularly effective in cardiovascular diseases including ischemic heart disease, hypertension, heart failure, and atherosclerosis, where it may slow aging and prolong lifespan.

## 3.1   Effect of Lipoic Acid in Atherosclerosis

Many studies have confirmed that LA can improve vascular function and decrease the atherosclerotic plaque burden (Wollin & Jones, 2003; Catapano et al., 2000). By chelating redox-active transition metal ions, LA is thought to inhibit the Fenton-like-reaction mechanism and inhibit the formation of OH $\cdot$. As a consequence, lipid peroxidation is inhibited in mitochondria (Sadowska-Bartosz & Bartosz, 2014).

LA reacts with ROS, such as superoxide anions, normalizes NADPH oxidase activity and can prevent Ang II – induced macrophage, monocyte, and T-cell infiltrations. It is also thought that LA can block AT1 receptors, which improves endothelial function, and reduces plaque area in atherosclerosis (Sola et al., 2005). It has been found that LA increases endogenous antioxidant enzymes, including superoxide dismutase-2, heme oxygenase (HO-1) in rat L skeletal muscle counteracting oxidative stress and aging (Favero et al., 2015).

Many clinical studies have shown that the beneficial effects of LA against Ang II are linked not only to scavenged ROS, but also to NF-kappaB inhibition. LA reduces NF-κB-mediated inflammatory responses by regulating the expression of pro-inflammatory genes, and adhesion molecules (Packer et al., 2001). It also reduces the chemokine and adhesion molecules involved in T cell trafficking to inhibition of monocyte-endothelial interactions by atherosclerotic plaque.

Many animal and human studies report that LA supplementation can result in reduced cholesterol levels (Rideout et al., 2015; Kim et al., 2013). LA may also prevent LDL oxidation by reducing the concentrations of LDL-C, Ox-LDL, serum TC, and lipoprotein (a) [Lp(a)], as well as other oxidative biomarkers (Catapano et al., 2000).

Clinical studies confirm that LA may also reduce the aortic expression of adhesion molecules and the accumulation of aortic macrophages and pro-inflammatory cytokines. resulting in reduced LDL level and triglyceride concentration, and elevated HDL (Carrier et al., 2014; Zhang et al., 2008). In animal models, 12-week administration of LA reduced oxidative stress and improved vascular reactivity in animals fed with a high cholesterol diet (Ying et al., 2010). LA may also be capable of initiating LDL receptor synthesis in the liver, resulting in increased return of cholesterol to the hepatic system and elevated synthesis of apoprotein A component (a HDL particle moiety) for reversed cholesterol transport (Harding et al., 2012; Zhang et al., 2008; Amom et al., 2008).

Moreover, cellular senescence and body aging are associated with shortening of telomere and DNA damage which occur in atherosclerosis. Xiong S. et al. noted that peroxisome proliferator activated receptor $\gamma$ coactivator -1 $\alpha$ (PGC-1$\alpha$) plays an important role in ameliorating senescence and aging. LA increased expression of PGC-1$\alpha$, Nrf2, HO-1 and catalase as well as it inhibited telomerase activity (Xiong et al., 2015).

Finally, it can be concluded that LA has a direct lipid modulating action, and an indirect effect on blood lipid levels, leading to reduced risk of atherosclerosis. Its use as a dietary supplement, either alone or with others oxidants, for example vitamins C and E, may represent a helpful strategy in reducing the adverse effects of oxidative stress. Lipoic acid in combination with other antioxidants or with anti-inflammatory substances may enhance the antioxidant effect. Due to inflammatory nature of atherosclerosis, many studies have recently been conducted in order to search for anti-inflammatory substances which would affect arterial walls. For example, some studies demonstrated the role of carotenoids: β-carotene, α-carotene, β-cryptoxanthin, lycopene, lutein, zeaxanthin, and astaxanthin on cardiovascular risk profile. Unfortunately, literature data are conflicting. There are many data supporting the anti-inflammatory activity of carotenoids and their protective effect on cardiovascular diseases, but there are also unfavorable findings. These results may arise from the use of synthetic molecules, slightly different from natural ones. Thus, further studies are needed to discuss the topic (Ciccone et al., 2013).

## 3.2    Effect of Lipoic Acid in Hypertension

Hypertension increases the production of various inflammatory biomarkers. These include chemokines, such as monocyte chemoattractant protein 1 (MCP-1), adhesion molecules, such as P-selectin, and cytokines, such as tumor necrosis factor-$\alpha$ (TNF-$\alpha$) and interleukin (IL)-6. This elevated production of biomarkers results in reduced NO bioavailability, via NO degradation in vessel cells, and excessive production of endothelin I, which in turn impairs endothelium-dependent vasodilation (Vasdev et al., 2011). ROS, particularly $O_2^{--}$, bind NO and form highly reactive and dangerous ONOO–. This ONOO– produces a cascade of changes, which in turn lead to increased tension within the blood vessels.

Lipoic acid may have a beneficial effect in preventing the development of hypertension by lowering the level of inflammatory cytokines in the blood plasma, thus preventing these pathological changes to vessel cells, and normalizing changes in blood pressure (Leong et al., 2007; Lee et al., 2006).

LA treatment prevents adhesion molecules expression (intercellular adhesion molecule-1 (ICAM-1), vascular cell adhesion molecule-1 (VCAM-1), platelet-endothelial cell adhesion molecule-1 (PECAM-1), which are important markers of inflammation in cardiac and renal vascular endothelium of spontaneously hypertensive rats (Tayebati et al., 2015).

Several clinical trials have shown that LA inhibits the vascular overproduction of endothelin I, the main vasoconstrictor (Takaoka et al., 2001). Furthermore, LA significantly increases the synthesis of NO, the main vasodilator, it may also improve the redox state of the plasma, and improve endothelium-dependent NO-mediated vasodilation. In addition, LA ameliorates the loss of eNOS phosphorylation, which contributes to improved endothelial function (Heitzer et al., 2001; Sena et al., 2008). It is also known to inhibit TNF-alpha activation (Zhang & Frei, 2001). As LA is a good metal chelator, it may also inhibit the production of adhesion molecules by monocytes, thus improving endothelial function. In one study, LA supplementation was found to reduce the aortic expression of adhesion molecules and pro-inflammatory factors, such as lower the accumulation of aortic macrophages (Amom et al., 2008).

Furthermore, LA could potentially regulate intracellular $Ca^{2+}$ levels by preventing the modification of sulfhydryl groups in the $Ca^{2+}$ channels (Gomes & Negrato, 2014). Another study shows that LA increases tissue GSH levels, which otherwise decline with age, by restoring glutathione peroxidase activity (Vasdev et al., 2000; Shay et al., 2009).

The antioxidant properties of LA cause it to exert a "rejuvenative" impact on mitochondria by protecting them against the higher levels of ROS they produce during the aging process. LA increases oxygen consumption and mitochondrial membrane potential, while decreasing the mitochondrial production of oxidants by amplifying the activity of antioxidant mechanisms (Kizhakekuttu & Widlansky, 2010). However, despite LA supplementation not being particularly effective in this regard, it can nevertheless significantly reduce blood pressure when used in combination with other antioxidants such as L-carnitine (McMackin et al., 2007).

## 3.3   Effect of Lipoic Acid in Atherosclerosis — Ischemic Heart Disease

Ischemia injury can follow oxidative stress, and can lead to significant morbidity and mortality. During ischemia, specific changes in the antioxidant system can occur, resulting in injury to organs such as the kidney, liver or heart. In ischemia, oxidative stress causes many complication reactions involving adhesion molecules and cytokines, leading to massive release of ROS. This process increases the production of tumor necrosis factor alpha (TNF-$\alpha$) and interleukin-1 (IL-1) through activation of NF-$\kappa$B. Furthermore, increases in intracellular $Ca^{2+}$ concentration and MDA levels result in decreases in GPx and SOD reactivity (Ozbal et al., 2012), thus inducing contractile dysfunction, hypertrophy, fibrosis and cell death (Frank et al., 2012). Contractile function and arrhythmias may also be depressed (Aiello et al., 1995). Clinical studies indicate that up to 50% of the final infarct may be attributable to ischemia injury in both animals and humans (Rodrigo et al., 2013).

LA counteracts the damage associated with the ischemia experimental model. It can provide protection against ischemia by inhibiting ROS production, blocking inflammation and reducing myocardium apoptosis, as noted above.

Endothelial cells represent an important vascular site of signaling and development of damage during ischemia and inflammation. Overproduction of ROS causes pathological activation of endothelium, including exposure of cell to adhesion molecules. Vascular cell adhesion molecule-1 (VCAM-1), intercellular adhesion molecule-1 (ICAM-1), and platelet-endothelial cell adhesion molecule-1 (PECAM-1) are present on the surface of endothelial cells and represent important markers of endothelial inflammation (Tayebati et al., 2015).

LA prevented adhesion molecules expression in cardiac vascular endothelium and thus may serve as a potential agent on the vascular endothelium (Zygmunt et al., 2013). Recent studies indicate that LA prevents post-reperfusion arrhythmias and protects cardiomyocytes from hypoxia-induced death (Dudek et al., 2014). It induces cardioprotection through a number of routes: inhibition of NOX4 activity leading to NOS recoupling, improved NO bioavailability, reduced oxidative stress, leading ultimately to the preservation of mitochondrial function. In addition, LA limits further damage caused by ischemia by increasing Akt phosphorylation via the activation of the PI3K/Akt pathway and the induction of cytoprotective genes (Deng et al., 2014). It also prevents decreases in ATP content and the activation of pro-inflammatory factor NF-$\kappa$B. In animal models of ischemia, LA was found to ameliorate cardiac dysfunction with reduced infarct size, and lower levels of myeloperoxidase, TNF-$\alpha$, creatinine kinase and lactate dehydrogenase, while upregulating the expression of several antioxidant enzyme genes (Tian et al., 2013). Other studies report that LA administration bestows significant protective effects by raising MDA levels and lowering the activity of glutathione peroxidase (GPx) and superoxide dismutase (SOD) - the enzymatic scavengers of ROS (Ozbal et al., 2012).

Another way to protect the cardiovascular system from oxidative stress is based on its capacity to regenerate endogenous antioxidants such as vitamins C and E. It also regenerates glutathione, which plays a very important role in maintaining the balance between antioxidants and prooxidants. LA may increase the levels of glutathione and other natural antioxidants, thus preventing the progression of ischemia (Gomes & Negrato, 2014).

## 3.4    Effect of Lipoic Acid in Heart Failure

Heart failure (HF) is not simply a single organ disease but it is a complex multi-system clinical syndrome, which influences morbidity and mortality (Warriner et al., 2015). HF may cause severe damage to the heart muscle via myocardial fibrosis, ventricular remodeling, decreased contractility and increased myocyte apoptosis (Madamanchi & Runge, 2013). Mitochondrial damage is central to the pathophysiology of HF. The mechanism of mitochondrial dysfunction is connected with cellular and mitochondrial damage which impairs the mechanical properties of the heart. In age-related oxidative stress, a reduced supply of energy from the mitochondria necessary for the contractile function of cardiomyocytes is often noted (Bayeva et al., 2013). Therefore, one strategy in treating HF is the stimulation of cardiac systolic function by targeting mitochondrial dysfunction.

Cardiomyocyte function is disturbed in HF, but not irreversibly (Ardehali et al., 2012). The cardiomyocytes respond to oxidative stress by increasing antioxidant system activity: increased thioredoxin system (Trx) activity has been observed, together with greater mRNA expression of several antioxidant enzymes (Sawyer, 2011). Myocardial energy efficiency can be improved by up to 30% by using strategies based on increasing glucose oxidation and decreasing fatty acid metabolism (Ardehali et al., 2012).

Many studies on animal models have confirmed that LA can prevent progressive remodeling and even improve cardiac function (Li et al., 2012). By acting as a cofactor for enzymatic reactions within the mitochondria, it can improve mitochondrial function by conserving cellular energy (Packer & Cadenas, 2011). Thus, LA can influence mitochondrial antioxidant status, neutralize ROS and effectively attenuate mitochondrial damage caused by oxidative stress and the aging process (Padmalayam, 2012). Antioxidants such as LA are widely regarded as attractive novel agents which can be employed to prevent oxidative stress when targeted at the mitochondria (Subramanian et al., 2010). Several studies have demonstrated that LA administration effectively attenuates cardiac apoptosis (Li et al., 2009; Cao et al., 2003). It has been found to attenuate oxidative damage to the mitochondria, with increased GSH levels and enhanced SOD activity being observed (Li et al., 2009). It also been seen to mediate the elevation of cellular defense, which may be associated with greater resistance to ROS-elicited cardiac cell injury. Finally, it has also been demonstrated that LA reinforces cellular defenses by inducing endogenous antioxidants and phase 2 enzymes in cultured cardiac cells. These have been associated with markedly increased resistance to ROS-elicited cardiomyocyte injury (Cao et al., 2003).

All the above examples indicate that LA may be helpful in treating HF caused by oxidative stress. It offers a number of benefits concerned with preventing oxidative damage to the mitochondria, both on the molecular and genetic levels, even when applied at low concentrations. The fact that current used therapies of HF are able to relieve symptoms but unable to reverse molecular changes that occur in cardiomyocytes, calls for conducting further studies on the application of LA.

Even if antioxidant supplementation is commonly used in many cardiovascular diseases, some clinical studies showed that the current evidence is insufficient to conclude that antioxidants materially reduce oxidative damage in humans. Some studies simplied that antioxidants administered in high dosages can even lead to human death (Bjelakovic et al., 2012).

Other studies confirmed that antioxidants either have no effect or have a negative effect. For example, results of the GISSI-Prevenzione and HOPE trials showed the absence of relevant clinical effects of vitamin E on the risk of cardiovascular events (Marchioli et al., 2001).

Another study, using vitamin E, showed no effect of this antioxidant on the lifespan (Morley & Trainor, 2001). Table 1 shows the data on the studies involving lipoic acid.

# 4   Summary

In the last years, investigations in humans, and animal models have provided abundant evidence that age-dependent oxidative stress plays an important role in cardiovascular diseases. Studies indicate that antioxidants prevent development many cardiovascular diseases and may even improve course of diseases, such as atherosclerosis, hypertension, ischemia/reperfusion or heart failure. It is therefore disappointing that very few applications have been found for antioxidants in these diseases.

Lipoic acid can provide protection against ROS-induced damage under conditions of elevated oxidative stress brought on by the organism aging. It meets all the criteria for an ideal antioxidant, because may reduce adverse effects of oxidative stress, has an amphiphilic properties and does not exhibit any serious side effects (Huk-Kolega et al., 2011).

However, the results of clinical trials intake of exogenous antioxidant are contradictory. No beneficial effects were reported in several studies in which used only one synthetic antioxidants. Therefore, a better antioxidant effect can be achieved using more than one antioxidant.

# Acknowledgement

The study was supported by a grant 503/0-079-03/503-01 and 503/3-021-01/503-31-003 from the Medical University of Lodz.

# References

Adela, R. & Banerjee, S.K. (2015). GDF-15 as a target and biomarker for diabetes and cardiovascular diseases: A translational prospective. J Diabetes Res, 490842, doi: 10.1155/2015/490842.

Aiello, E.A., Jabr, R.I. & Cole, W.C. (1995). Arrhythmia and delayed recovery of cardiac action potential during reperfusion after ischemia: role of oxygen radical-induced no-reflow phenomenon. Circulation Research, 77(1): 153–162.

Ajith, T.A. (2014). Mitochondria-targeted agents: future perspectives of mitochondrial pharmaceutics in cardiovascular diseases. World Journal of Cardiology, 6(10): 1091–1099.

Amom, Z., Zakaria, Z., Mohamed, J., et al. (2008). Lipid lowering effect of antioxidant alpha-lipoic acid in experimental atherosclerosis. Journal of Clinical Biochemistry and Nutrition, 43(2): 88–94.

Ardehali, H., Sabbah, H.N., Burke, M.A., et al. (2012). Targeting myocardial substrate metabolism in heart failure: potential for new therapies. European Journal of Heart Failure, 14(2): 120–129.

| Studied parameter | Reported effect | Source |
|---|---|---|
| Effect of alpha-lipoic acid (LA) on endothelial function and inflammation in patients with the metabolic syndrome | Improvement of endothelial function and reduction of pro-inflammatory markers, i.e. factors that are implicated in the pathogenesis of atherosclerosis | Sola et al., 2005 |
| Effect of LA on level of cholesterol in rats | Reduction of LDL particle number | Rideout et al., 2015 |
| Effect of LA on atherosclerosis in apolipoprotein E-deficient (apoE-/-) and apoE/low-density lipoprotein receptor-deficient mice | Significant reduction of atherosclerotic lesion formation in the aortic sinus | Zhang et al., 2008 |
| Effect of LA on atherosclerosis in rabbits | Improvement of vascular reactivity (decreased constriction to angiotensin II), decrease in oxidative stress and expression of key adhesion molecules in the vasculature | Ying et al., 2010 |
| Effect of LA on level of cholesterol in rabbits | Reduction of athero-lesion formation in hypercholesterolemic-induced rabbits | Amom et al., 2008 |
| Effect of LA on endothelial function in hypertensive patients | Improvement of endothelial function in hypertensive patients | Lee et al., 2006 |
| Effect of LA on endothelial function in spontaneously hypertensive rats (SHR) | Significant decrease in TBARS levels, the nucleic acid oxidation and prevention from adhesion molecules expression in cardiac and renal vascular endothelium | Tayebati et al., 2015 |
| Preventative effect of LA in hypertension and hypertensive tissue injury induced by deoxycorticosterone acetate (DOCA) in rats | Lower blood pressure and protection against renal and vascular injuries | Takaoka et al., 2001 |
| Effect of LA on NO-mediated vasodilation in diabetic patients | Improvement of NO-mediated vaso dilation | Heitzer et al., 2001 |
| Effect of LA on endothelial function in diabetic and high-fat fed GK diabetic rats | Restoration of endothelial function and significant improvement of systemic and local oxidative stress | Sena et al., 2008 |
| Effect of LA on TNF-alpha -induced adhesion molecule expression and NF-kappaB signaling in human aortic endothelial cells (HAEC) | Inhibition of adhesion molecule expression in HAEC and monocyte adhesion | Zhang & Frei, 2001 |

*Continued on next page...*

...continued from next page

| Effect of LA in spontaneously hypertensive rats (SHR) | Lower blood pressure and normalization of associated biochemical and histopathological changes in SHRs | Vasdev et al., 2000 |
|---|---|---|
| Effect of LA on vasodilator function and blood pressure in subjects with coronary artery disease (CAD) | Decrease in systolic blood pressure | McMackin et al., 2007 |
| Protective effect of LA on testicular damage in rats subjected to testicular ischemia-reperfusion injury | Decrease in the GPx and SOD activity and increase in MDA levels | Ozbal et al., 2012 |
| Effect of LA on sulfane sulfur (S*) level, infiltration of neutrophils and vascular permeability in a model of zymosan-induced peritonitis. | Increase in the sulfane sulfur level, which is probably responsible for anti-inflammatory activity. | Zygmunt et al., 2013 |
| LA as a preventative agent in the occurrence of post-reperfusion arrhythmias in vitro using a Langendorff model of ischemia-reperfusion in rats affecting the K(ATP) channels. | Prevention from post-reperfusion arrhythmias and protection of cardiomyocytes from hypoxia-induced death. | Dudek et al., 2014 |
| Effect and mechanism of LA on myocardial infarct size, cardiac function and cardiomyocyte apoptosis in rat hearts subjected to in vivo myocardial ischemia/reperfusion (MI/R) injury | Reduction of cardiomyoctyes necrosis, apoptosis and inflammation after MI/R | Deng et al., 2014 |
| Effect of LA on cardiac dysfunction, mitochondrial oxidative stress, extracellular matrix remodeling and interrelated signaling pathways in a diabetic rat model | Attenuation of MOS, ECM remodeling and JNK, p38 MAPK activation | Li et al., 2012 |
| Effect of LA on mitochondrion-dependent myocardial apoptosis | Effective attenuation of mitochondria-dependent cardiac apoptosis and protective role against the development of diabetic cardiomyopathy | Li et al., 2009 |
| Effect of LA on endogenous antioxidants and phase 2 enzymes in cultured cardiomyocytes | Increase in endogenous antioxidants. Protection against oxidative cardiac cell injury. | Cao et al., 2003 |

**Table 1:** Effect of lipoic acid on some cardiovascular diseases.

Avkiran, M. & Marber, M.S. (2002). Na+/H+ exchange inhibitors for cardioprotective therapy: progress, problems and prospects. Journal of the American College of Cardiology, 39(5): 747–753.

Bartosz, G. (2009). Reactive oxygen species: destroyers or messengers? Biochemical Pharmacology, 77(8): 1303–1315.

Bayeva, M., Gheorghiade, M. & Ardehali, H. (2013). Mitochondria as a therapeutic target in heart failure. Journal of the American College of Cardiology, 61(6): 599–610.

Bhatt, S.R., Lokhandwala, M.F. & Banday, A.A. (2014). Vascular oxidative stress upregulates angiotensin II type I receptors via mechanisms involving nuclear factor kappa B. Clinical and Experimental Hypertension, 36(6): 367–373.

Bilska, A. & Wlodek, L. (2005). Lipoic acid – the drug of the future? Pharmacological Reports, 57(5): 570–577.

Bjelakovic, G., Nikolova, D., Gluud, L. L., Simonetti, R. G., Gluud, C. (2012). Antioxidant supplements for prevention of mortality in healthy participants and patients with various diseases. Cochrane Database Syst Rev. 310: 1002/14651858. CD007176.

Bozic, M., Alvarez, A., Pablo, C., Maria-Dolores Sanchez-Nino, M.D., Ortiz, A., Dolcet, X., Encinas, M., Fernandez, E. & Valdivielso, J.M. (2015). Impaired vitamin D signaling in endothelial cell leads to an enhanced leukocyte-endothelium interplay: Implications for atherosclerosis development. PLoS One, 10(8), e0136863.

Brandes, R.P., Fleming, I. & Busse, R. (2005). Endothelial aging. Cardiovascular Research, 66(2): 286–294.

Cai, H. & Harrison, D.G. (2000). Endothelial dysfunction in cardiovascular diseases: the role of oxidant stress. Circulation Research, 87(10): 840–844.

Canty, T.G., Jr., Boyle, E.M., Jr., Farr, A., Morgan, E.N., Verrier, E.D. & Pohlman, T. H. (1999). Oxidative stress induces NF-κB nuclear translocation without degradation of IκBα. Circulation, 100(19): 361–364.

Cameron, V.A., Mocatta, T.J., Pilbrow, A.P., et al. (2006). Angiotensin type-1 receptor A1166C gene polymorphism correlates with oxidative stress levels in human heart failure. Hypertension, 47(6): 1155–1161.

Cao, Z., Tsang, M., Zhao, H. & Li, Y. (2003). Induction of endogenous antioxidants and phase 2 enzymes by α-lipoic acid in rat cardiac H9C2 cells: protection against oxidative injury. Biochemical and Biophysical Research Communications, 310(3): 979–985.

Carrier, B., Wen, S., Zigouras, S., et al. (2014). Alpha-lipoic acid reduces LDL-particle number and PCSK9 concentrations in high-fat fed obese zucker rats. PLoS ONE, 9(3), doi: 10.1371/journal.pone.0090863. e90863.

Catapano, A.L., Maggi, F.M. & Tragni, E. (2000). Low density lipoprotein oxidation, antioxidants, and atherosclerosis. Current Opinion in Cardiology, 15(5): 355–363.

Cavieres, V., Valdes, K., Moreno, B., Moore-Carrasco, R. & Gonzalez, D.R. (2014). Vascular hypercontractility and endothelial dysfunction before development of atherosclerosis in moderate dyslipidemia: role for nitric oxide and interleukin-6. American Journal of Cardiovascular Disease, 4(3): 114–122.

Chen, Y., Bang, S., Park, S., Shi, H. & Kim, S.F. (2015). Acyl-CoA-binding domain containing 3 modulates NAD+ metabolism through activating poly(ADP-ribose) polymerase. Biochemical Journal, 469(2): 189-198.

Chisolm, G.M. & Steinberg, D. (2000). *The oxidative modification hypothesis of atherogenesis: an overview.* Free Radical Biology and Medicine, 28(12): 1815–1826.

Ciccone M. M., Cortese, F., Gesualdo, M., Carbonara, S., Zito, A., Ricci, G., De Pascalis, F., Scicchitano, P., Riccioni, G. (2013). *Dietary intake of carotenoids and their antioxidant and anti-inflammatory effects in cardiovascular care.* Mediators Inflamm. 2013:782137.

Cobb, C.A., Cole, M.P. (2015). *Oxidative and nitrative stress in neurodegeneration.* Neurobiology Disease, 1(15), doi: 10.1016/j.nbd.2015.04.020

Csiszar, A., Labinskyy, N., Orosz, Z., Xiangmin, Z., Buffenstein, R. & Ungvari, Z. (2007). *Vascular aging in the longest-living rodent, the naked mole-rat.* American Journal of Physiology, 293(2): 919–927.

Csiszar, A., Ungvari, Z., Edwards, J.G., Kaminski, P., Wolin, M.S., Koller, A. et al. (2002). *Aging-induced phenotypic changes and oxidative stress impair coronary arteriolar function.* Circulation Research, 90(11): 1159–1166.

Csiszar, A., Ungvari, Z., Koller, A., Edwards, J.G. & Kaley, G. (2004). *Proinflammatory phenotype of coronary arteries promotes endothelial apoptosis in aging.* Physiological Genomics, 17(1): 21–30.

Csiszar, A., Wang, M., Lakatta, E.G. & Ungvari, Z.I. (2008). *Inflammation and endothelial dysfunction during aging: role of NF-{kappa}B.* Journal of Applied Physiology, 105(4): 1333–1341.

Dai, D.F., Chiao, Y.A., Marcinek, D.J., Szeto, H.H. & Rabinovitch, P.S. (2014). *Mitochondrial oxidative stress in aging and healthspan.* Longevity & Healthspan, 3, article 6, doi: 10.1186/2046-2395-3-6.

Dai, D.F., Johnson, S.C., Villarin, J.J., Chin, M.T., Nieves-Cintron, M., Chen, T. et al. (2011). *Mitochondrial oxidative stress mediates angiotensin II-induced cardiac hypertrophy and Galphaq overexpression-induced heart failure.* Circulation Research, 108: 837–846.

Danzaki, K., Matsui, Y., Ikesue, M., Ohta, D., Ito, K., Kanayama, M. et al. (2012). *Interleukin-17A deficiency accelerates unstable atherosclerotic plaque formation in apolipoprotein E-deficient mice.* Arteriosclerosis, Thrombosis and Vascular Biology, 32(2): 273–280.

De Haan, J.B. Bladier, C. Lotfi-Miri, M. Taylor, J. Hutchinson, P. Crack, P.J. Hertzog, P. Kola, I.(2004). *Fibroblasts derived from Gpx1 knockout mice display senescent-like features and are susceptible to $H_2O_2$-mediated cell death.* Free Radic. Biol. Med., 36: 53-64.

Deng, C., Sun, Z., Tong, G., et al. (2013). *α-Lipoic acid reduces infarct size and preserves cardiac function in rat myocardial ischemia/reperfusion injury through activation of PI3K/Akt/Nrf2 pathway.* PLoS ONE, 8(3) doi: 10.1371/journal.pone.0058371.e58371

Di Lisa, F. & Bernardi, P. (2005). *Mitochondrial function and myocardial aging. A critical analysis of the role of permeability transition.* Cardiovascular Research, 66(2): 222–232.

Dinh, Q.N., Drummond, G.R., Sobey, C.G. & Chrissobolis, S. (2014). *Roles of inflammation, oxidative stress, and vascular dysfunction in hypertension.* BioMed Research International, 2014:1–11. doi: 10.1155/2014/406960.

Doenst T., Nguyen T.D. & Abel E.D. (2013). *Cardiac metabolism in heart failure: implications beyond ATP production.* Circulation Research, 113(6): 709–724.

Douglas, B. & Sawyer, M.D. (2011). *Oxidative stress in heart failure: what are we missing?* American Journal of the Medical Sciences, 342(2): 120–124.

Drummond, G.R., Selemidis, S., Griendling, K.K., & Sobey, C.G. (2011). *Combating oxidative stress in vascular disease: NADPH oxidases as therapeutic targets.* Nature Reviews Drug Discover, 10(6): 453–471.

Dudek, M., Bilska-Wilkosz, A., Knutelska, J., Mogilski, S., Bednarski, M. & Zygmunt, M. (2013). Are anti-inflammatory properties of lipoic acid associated with the formation of hydrogen sulfide? Pharmacological Reports, 65(4): 1018–1024.

Dudek, M., Knutelska, J., Bednarski, M., et al. (2014). Alpha lipoic acid protects the heart against myocardial post ischemia-reperfusion arrhythmias via KATP channel activation in isolated rat hearts. Pharmacological Reports, 66(3): 499–504.

Eaton, P., Byers, H.L., Leeds, N., Ward, M.A. & Shattock, M.J. (2002). Detection, quantitation, purification, and identification of cardiac proteins S-thiolated during ischemia and reperfusion. Journal of Biological Chemistry, 277: 9806–9811.

Elahi, M.M., Kong, Y.X. & Matata, B.M. (2009). Oxidative stress as a mediator of cardiovascular disease. Oxidative Medicine and Cellular Longevity, 2(5): 259–269.

El Assar, M., Angulo, J., Vallejo, S., Peiró, C., Sánchez-Ferrer, C.F. & Rodríguez-Mañas, L. (2012). Mechanisms involved in the aging-induced vascular dysfunction. Frontiers of Physiology, 3, article 132: 1-13.

Favero, G., Rodella, L.F., Nardo, L., Giugno, L., Cocchi, M.A., Borsani, E., Reiter, R.J., & Rezzani, R. (2015). A comparison of melatonin and α-lipoic acid in the induction of antioxidant defences in L6 rat skeletal muscle cells. Age (Dordr), 37(4): 9824.

Ferdinandy, P., Schulz, R. & Baxter, G.F. (2007). Interaction of cardiovascular risk factors with myocardial ischemia/reperfusion injury, preconditioning, and postconditioning. Pharmacological Reviews, 59(4): 418–458.

Finkel, T. & Holbrook, N.J. (2000). Oxidants, oxidative stress and the biology of ageing. Nature, 408(6809): 239–247. doi: 10.1038/35041687.

Frank, A., Bonney, M., Bonney, S., Weitzel, L., Koeppen, M. & Eckle, T. (2012). Myocardial ischemia reperfusion injury: from basic science to clinical bedside. Seminars in Cardiothoracic and Vascular Anesthesia, 16(3): 123–132.

Ghibu, S., Richard, C., Vergely, C., Zeller, M., Cottin, Y. & Rochette, L. (2009). Antioxidant properties of an endogenous thiol: Alpha-lipoic acid, useful in the prevention of cardiovascular diseases. Journal of Cardiovascular Pharmacology, 54(5): 391–398.

Glantzounis, G.K., Yang, W., Koti, R.S., Mikhailidis, D.P., Seifalian, A.M. & Davidson, B.R. (2006). The role of thiols in liver ischemia-reperfusion injury. Current Pharmaceutical Design, 12(23): 2891–2901.

Gomes, M.B. & Negrato, C.A. (2014). Alpha-lipoic acid as a pleiotropic compound with potential therapeutic use in diabetes and other chronic diseases. Diabetology & Metabolic Syndrome, 6(1): 80, doi: 10.1186/1758-5996-6-80.

Gonzaga, N., Callera, G.E., Yogi, A., et al. (2014). Acute ethanol intake induces mitogen-activated protein kinase activation, platelet-derived growth factor receptor phosphorylation, and oxidative stress in resistance arteries. Journal of Physiology and Biochemistry, 70(2): 509–523.

Goraca, A., Huk-Kolega, H., Piechota, A., Kleniewska, P., Ciejka, E. & Skibska, B. (2011). Lipoic acid— biological activity and therapeutic potential. Pharmacological Reports, 63(4): 849–858.

Govender, M.M., & Nadar, A. (2015). A subpressor dose of angiotensin II elevates blood pressure in a normotensive rat model by oxidative stress. Physiological Research, 64(2):153–159.

Hafstad, A.D., Nabeebaccus, A.A. & Shah, A.M. (2013). Novel aspects of ROS signalling in heart failure. Basic Research in Cardiology, 108(4, article 359) doi: 10.1007/s00395-013-0359-8.

Harding, S.V., Rideout, T.C. & Jones, P.J.H. (2012). *Evidence for using alpha-lipoic acid in reducing lipoprotein and inflammatory related atherosclerotic risk. Journal of Dietary Supplements, 9(2): 116–127.*

Heitzer, T., Finckh, B., Albers, S., Krohn, K., Kohlschütter, A. & Meinertz, T. (2001). *Beneficial effects of α-lipoic acid and ascorbic acid on endothelium-dependent, nitric oxide-mediated vasodilation in diabetic patients: relation to parameters of oxidative stress. Free Radical Biology and Medicine, 31(1): 53–61.*

Herman, M., Flammer, A. & Luscher, T.F. (2006). *Nitric oxide in hypertension. Journal of Clinical Hypertension, 8, 17–29.*

Herrera, M.D., Mingorance, C., Rodríguez-Rodríguez, R. & Alvarez de Sotomayor, M. (2010). *Endothelial dysfunction and aging: an update. Ageing Research Reviews, 9(2): 142–152.*

Hohensinner, P.J., Niessner, A., Huber, K., Weyand, C.M., & Wojta, J. (2011). *Inflammation and cardiac outcome. Current Opinion of Infectious Diseases, 24: 259–264.*

Huang, J., Zhang, X., Qin, F., Li, Y., Duan, X., JianLi Y., Chen, J. & Huang, R. (2015). *Protective effects of Millettia Pulchra flavonoids on myocardial ischemia in vitro and in vivo. Cellular Physiology and Biochemistry, 35: 516–528*

Huk-Kolega, H., Skibska, B., Kleniewska, P., Piechota, A., Michalski, Ł. & Goraca, A. (2011). *Role of lipoic acid in health and disease. Polski Merkuriusz Lekarski, 31(183):183–185.*

Humbert, M. & Ghofrani, H.A. (2015). *The molecular targets of approved treatments for pulmonary arterial hypertension. Thorax, doi: 1136/thoraxjnl-2015-207170.*

Husain, K., Hernandez, W., Ansari, R.A., Ferder, L. (2015). *Inflammation, oxidative stress and renin angiotensin system in atherosclerosis. World Journal of Biological Chemistry, 6(3): 209–217.*

Huss, J.M. & Kelly, D.P. (2005). *Mitochondrial energy metabolism in heart failure: a question of balance. Journal of Clinical Investigation, 115(3): 547–555.*

Jahangir, A., Sagar, S. & Terzic, A. (2007). *Aging and cardioprotection. Journal of Applied Physiology, 103(6): 2120–2128.*

Kajiya, M., Hirota, M., Inai, Y., et al. (2007). *Impaired NO-mediated vasodilation with increased superoxide but robust EDHF function in right ventricular arterial microvessels of pulmonary hypertensive rats. The American Journal of Physiology—Heart and Circulatory Physiology, 292(6): H2737–H2744.*

Kang, D.H., Choi, M., Chang, S., Lee, M.Y., Lee, D.J., Choi, K., Park, J., Han, E.C., Hwang, D., Kwon, K., Jo, H., Choi, C. & Kang, S.W. (2015). *Vascular proteomics reveal novel proteins involved in SMC phenotypic change: OLR1 as a SMC receptor regulating proliferation and inflammatory response. PLoS One, 10(8), e0133845.*

Karavidas, A., Lazaros, G., Tsiachris, D. & Pyrgakis, V. (2010). *Aging and the cardiovascular system. Hell Journal of Cardiology, 51(5): 421–427.*

Khurana, S., Venkataraman, K., Hollingsworth, A., Piche, M. & Tai, T.C. (2013). *Polyphenols: benefits to the cardiovascular system in health and in aging. Nutrients, 5(10): 3779–3827.*

Kim, D.C., Jun, D.W., Jang, E.C., et al. (2013). *Lipoic acid prevents the changes of intracellular lipid partitioning by free fatty acid. Gut and Liver, 7(2): 221–227.*

Kizhakekuttu, T.J. & Widlansky, M.E. (2010). *Natural antioxidants and hypertension: promise and challenges. Cardiovascular Therapeutics, 28(4): e20–e32.*

Kleniewska, P., Piechota-Polanczyk, A., Michalski, L., et al. (2013). *Influence of block of NF-kappa B signaling pathway on oxidative stress in the liver homogenates. Oxidative Medicine and Cellular*

*Longevity, 2013:8. doi: 10.1155/2013/308358.308358.*

Klishadi, M.S., Zarei, F., Hejazian, S.H., Moradi, A., Hemati, M. & Safari, F. (2015). *Losartan protects the heart against ischemia reperfusion injury: sirtuin3 involvement. Journal of Pharmacy and Pharmaceutical Sciences, 18(1): 112–123.*

Kohan, D.E., Inscho, E.W., Wesson, D. & Pollock, D.M. (2011). *Physiology of endothelin and the kidney. Comprehensive Physiology, 1(2): 883–919.*

Kowalczyk, A., Kleniewska, P., Kolodziejczyk, M., Skibska, B. & Goraca, A. (2015). *The role of endothelin-1 and endothelin receptor antagonists in inflammatory response and sepsis. Archivum Immunologiae et Therapiae Experimentalis, 63(1): 41–52.*

Kumazaki, T. (1993). *Modulation of gene expression during aging of human vascular endothelial cells. Hiroshima Journal of Medical Sciences, 42(2): 97–100.*

Kwon, D.N., Park, W.J., Choi, Y.J., Gurunathan, S. & Kim, J.H. (2015). *Oxidative stress and ROS metabolism via down-regulation of sirtuin 3 expression in Cmah-null mice affect hearing loss. Aging (Albany NY), 7(8): 579–594.*

Lee, S.J. & Park, S.H. (2013). *Arterial ageing. Korean Circulation Journal, 43(2): 73–79.*

Lee, S.R., Jeong, M.H., Lim, S.Y., et al. (2006). *The effect of alpha lipoic acid (Thioctacid HR) on endothelial function in diabetic and hypertensive patients. Korean Circulation Journal, 36(8): 559–564.*

Lenaz G., Bovina, C., D'Aurelio, M., Fato, R., Formiggini, G., Genova, M.L., Giuliano, G., Pich, M.M., Paolucci, U.,Castelli G.P., et al. (2002). *Role of mitochondria in oxidative stress and aging. Ann. N. Y. Acad. Sci. 959: 199–213.*

Leong, J., Pepe, S., Van der Merwe, J., et al. (2007). *Preoperative metabolic therapy improves cardiac surgical outcomes: a prospective randomized clinical trial. Heart, Lung and Circulation, 16(supplement 2): S178.*

Lesnefsky, E.J., Moghaddas, S., Tandler, B., Kerner, J. & Hoppel, C.L. *Mitochondrial dysfunction in cardiac disease: ischemia—reperfusion, aging, and heart failure. (2001). Journal of Molecular and Cellular Cardiology, 33(6): 1065–1089.*

Li, C.J., Lv, L., Li, H. & Yu, D.M. (2012). *Cardiac fibrosis and dysfunction in experimental diabetic cardiomyopathy are ameliorated by alpha-lipoic acid. Cardiovascular Diabetology, 11, article 73, doi: 10.1186/1475-2840-11-73.*

Li, C.J., Zhang, Q.M., Li, M.Z., Zhang, J.Y., Yu, P. & Yu, D.M. (2009). *Attenuation of myocardial apoptosis by alpha-lipoic acid through suppression of mitochondrial oxidative stress to reduce diabetic cardiomyopathy. Chinese Medical Journal, 122(21): 2580–2586.*

Lindahl, T., Satoh, M.S., Poirier, G.G. & Klungland, A. (1995). *Posttranslational modification of poly (ADP-ribose) polymerase induced by DNA single strand breaks. Trends Biochemical Sciences, 20: 405–411.*

Linde, A., Mosier, D., Blecha, F. & Melgarejo, T. (2007). *Innate immunity and inflammation: new frontiers in comparative cardiovascular pathology. Cardiovascular Research, 73: 26–36.*

Madamanchi, N.R. Runge, M.S. (2013). *Redox signaling in cardiovascular health and disease. Free Radical Biology and Medicine, 61: 473–501.*

Mandavilli, B. S., Santos, J.H., Van Houten, B. (2002). *Mitochondrial DNA repair and aging. Mutat Res. 509(1–2): 127–151.*

Mangge, H., Becker, K., Fuchs, D. & Gostner, J.M. (2014). *Antioxidants, inflammation and cardiovascular disease. World Journal of Cardiology, 6(6): 462–477.*

Marchioli, R., Schweiger, C., Levantesi, G., Tavazzi, L., Valagussa, F. (2001). *Antioxidant vitamins and prevention of cardiovascular disease: epidemiological and clinical trial data. Lipids. 36 Suppl: S53–63.*

Maulik, S.K. & Kumar, S. (2012). *Oxidative stress and cardiac hypertrophy: a review. Toxicology Mechanisms and Methods, 22(5): 359–366.*

McMackin, C.J., Widlansky, M.E., Hamburg, N.M., et al. (2007). *Effect of combined treatment with α-Lipoic acid and acetyl-L-carnitine on vascular function and blood pressure in patients with coronary artery disease. The Journal of Clinical Hypertension, 9(4): 249–255.*

Mei, Y., Thompson, M.D., Cohen, R.A., & Tong, X. (2015). *Autophagy and oxidative stress in cardiovascular diseases. Biochimica and Biophysica Acta, 2; (1852): 243–351.*

Meisinger, C., Baumert, J., Khuseyinova, N., Loewel, H. & Koenig, W. (2005). *Plasma oxidized low-density lipoprotein, a strong predictor for acute coronary heart disease events in apparently healthy, middle-aged men from the general population. Circulation, 112(5): 651–657.*

Mikhed, Y., Daiber, A., Steven, S. (2015). *Mitochondrial oxidative stress, mitochondrial DNA damage and their role in age-related vascular dysfunction. Int. J. Mol. Sci. 16: 15918–15953.*

Moncada, S. & Bolanos, J.P. (2006). *Nitric oxide, cell bioenergetics and neurodegeneration. Journal of Neurochemistry, 97(6): 1676–1689.*

Monti, M., Solito, R., Puccetti, L., Pasotti, L., Roggeri, R., Monzani, E. et al. (2014). *Protective effects of novel metal-nonoates on the cellular components of the vascular system. Journal of Pharmacology and Experimental Therapeutics, 351(3): 500–509.*

Morley, A. A , Trainor, K. J. (2001). *Lack of an effect of vitamin E on lifespan of mice. Biogerontology. 1; 2(2): 109–112.*

Münzel, T., Gori, T., Keaney, J.F., Jr., Maack, C. & Daiber, A. (2015). *Pathophysiological role of oxidative stress in systolic and diastolic heart failure and its therapeutic implications. European Heart Journal, 4: ehv305.*

Navari-Izzo, F., Quartacci, M.F. & Sgherri, C. (2002). *Lipoic acid: a unique antioxidant in the detoxification of activated oxygen species. Plant Physiology and Biochemistry, 40(6–8): 463–470.*

Nedeykovic, Z.S., Gokce, N., Loscalzo, J. (2003). *Mechanisms of oxidative stress and vascular dysfunction. Postgrad Med J, 79: 195–200.*

Oakley, R. & Tharakan, B. (2014). *Vascular hyperpermeability and aging. Aging Disease, 5(2): 114–125.*

Ocaranza, M.P., Moya, J., Barrientos, V., et al. (2014). *Angiotensin-(1–9) reverses experimental hypertension and cardiovascular damage by inhibition of the angiotensin converting enzyme/Ang II axis. Journal of Hypertension, 32(4): 771–783.*

Oelze, M., Kroller-Schon, S., Steven, S., Lubos, E., Doppler, C., Hausding, M., Tobias, S., Brochhausen, C., Li, H., Torzewski, M. et al. (2014). *Glutathione peroxidase-1deficiency potentiates dysregulatory modifications of endothelial nitric oxide synthase and vascular dysfunction in aging. Hypertension, 63: 390–396.*

Ozbal, S., Ergur, B.U., Erbil, G., Tekmen, I., Bagryank, A. & Cavdar, Z. (2012). *The effects of α-lipoic acid against testicular ischemia-reperfusion injury in rats. The Scientific World Journal, 2012:8. doi: 10.1100/2012/489248.489248*

Pacher, P., Beckman, J.S. & Liaudet, L. (2007). *Nitric oxide and peroxynitrite in health and disease. Physiological Reviews, 87(1): 315–424.*

Pacia, M.Z., Mateuszuk, L., Chlopicki, S., Baranska, M. & Kaczor, A. (2015). *Biochemical changes of the* endothelium in the murine model of NO-deficient hypertension. Analyst, 140(7): 2178–2184.

Packer, L. & Cadenas, E. (2011). Lipoic acid: energy metabolism and redox regulation of transcription and cell signaling. Journal of Clinical Biochemistry and Nutrition, 48(1): 26–32.

Packer, L., Kraemer, K. & Rimbach, G. (2001). Molecular aspects of lipoic acid in the prevention of diabetes complications. Nutrition, 17(10): 888–895.

Packer, L., Witt, E.H. & Tritschler, H.J. (1995). Alpha-lipoic acid as a biological antioxidant. Free Radical Biology and Medicine, 19(2): 227–250.

Pacurari, M., Kafoury, R., Tchounwou, P.B. & Ndebele, K. (2014). The renin-angiotensin-aldosterone system in vascular inflammation and remodeling. International Journal of Inflammation, 2014:13. doi: 10.1155/2014/689360.689360

Padmalayam, I. (2012). Targeting mitochondrial oxidative stress through Lipoic acid synthase: a novel strategy to manage diabetic cardiovascular disease. Cardiovascular and Hematological Agents in Medicinal Chemistry, 10(3): 223–233.

Paravicini, T.M., Chrissobolis, S., Drummond, G.R. & Sobey, C.G. (2004). Increased NADPH-oxidase activity and Nox4 expression during chronic hypertension is associated with enhanced cerebral vasodilatation to NADPH in vivo. Stroke, 35(2): 584–589.

Paravicini, T.M. & Touyz, R.M. (2008). NADPH oxidases, reactive oxygen species, and hypertension: clinical implications and therapeutic possibilities. Diabetes Care, 31(2): 170–180.

Peng, J., Liu, B., Ma, Q.L. & Luo, X.J. (2015). Dysfunctional endothelial progenitor cells in cardiovascular diseases: role of NADPH oxidase. Journal of Cardiovascular Pharmacology, 65(1): 80–87.

Pepe, S. (2000). Mitochondrial function in ischaemia and reperfusion of the ageing heart. Clinical and Experimental Pharmacology and Physiology, 27(9): 745–750.

Petrich, E.R., Schanne, O.F. & Zumino, A.P. (1996). Electrophysiological responses to ischemia and reperfusion. In myocardial ischemia: mechanisms, reperfusion, protection. Birkhäuser Basel: 115–133.

Piechota, A., Polańczyk, A. & Goraca, A. (2010). Role of endothelin-1 receptor blockers on hemodynamic parameters and oxidative stress. Pharmacological Reports, 62(1): 28–34.

Reed, L.J. (1957). The chemistry and function of lipoic acid. Advances in Enzymology and Related Subjects of Biochemistry, 8: 319–347.

Rideout, T.C., Carrier, B., Wen, S., Raslawsky, A., Browne, R.W. & Harding, S.V. (2015). Complementary cholesterol-lowering response of a phytosterol/alpha-Lipoic acid combination in obese zucker rats. Journal of Dietary Supplements, 2015 doi: 10.3109/19390211.2015.1008616.

Rochette, L., Ghibu, S., Richard, C., Zeller, M., Cottin, Y. & Vergely, C. (2013). Direct and indirect antioxidant properties of α-lipoic acid and therapeutic potential. Molecular Nutrition and Food Researcg, 57(1): 114–125.

Rodrigo, R., Libuy, M., Feliú, F. & Hasson, D. (2013). Oxidative stress-related biomarkers in essential hypertension and ischemia-reperfusion myocardial damage. Disease Markers, 35(6): 773–790.

Rubio-Ruiz, M.E., Pérez-Torres, I., Soto, M.E., Pastelín, G. & Lans, V.G. (2014). Aging in blood vessels. Medicinal agents FOR systemic arterial hypertension in the elderly. Ageing Research Reviews, 18: 132–147.

Ruiz-Vera, T., Pruneda-Alvarez, L.G., Ochoa-Martinez, A.C., Ramirez-GarciaLuna, J.L., Pierdant-Perez, M., Gordillo-Moscoso, A.A., Perez-Vazquez, F.J., Perez-Maldonado, I.N. (2015). Assessment of vascular function in Mexican women exposed to polycyclic aromatic hydrocarbons from wood smoke.

*Environmental Toxicology and Pharmacology, 40(2): 423–429.*

Sadowska-Bartosz, I. & Bartosz, G. (2014). *Effect of antioxidants supplementation on aging and longevity. BioMed Research International, 2014:17. doi: 10.1155/2014/404680.404680*

Saito, Y., Kurabayashi, M., Nakamura, T. & Nagai, R. (2006). *Klotho gene and endothelial function. Nihon Ronen Igakkai Zasshi, 43(3): 342–344.*

Sawyer, D.B. (2011). *Oxidative stress in heart failure: what are we missing? The American Journal of the Medical Sciences, 342(2): 120–124.*

Segall, A., Sosa, M., Alami, A., et al. (2004). *Stability study of lipoic acid in the presence of vitamins A and E in o/w emulsions for cosmetic application. Journal of Cosmetic Science, 55(5): 449–461.*

Sena, C.M., Nunes, E., Louro, T., et al. (2008). *Effects of α-lipoic acid on endothelial function in aged diabetic and high-fat fed rats. British Journal of Pharmacology, 153(5): 894–906.*

Seshiah, P.N., Weber, D.S., Rocic, P., Valppu, L., Taniyama, Y. & Griendling, K.K. (2002). *Angiotensin II stimulation of NAD(P)H oxidase activity: upstream mediators. Circulation Research, 91(5): 406–413.*

Sharma, S., Adroque, J.V., Golfman, L., Urav, I., Lemm, J., Youker, K., et al. (2004). *Intramyocardial lipid accumulation in the failing human heart resembles the lipotoxic rat heart. FASEB J, 18(14): 1692–1700.*

Shay, K.P., Moreau, R.F., Smith, E.J., Smith, A.R. & Hagen, T.M. (2009). *Alpha-lipoic acid as a dietary supplement: molecular mechanisms and therapeutic potential. Biochimica et Biophysica Acta, 1790(10): 1149–1160.*

Shringarpure, R., Davies, K. J. (2002). *Protein turnover by the proteasome in aging and disease. Free Radic Biol Med. 1,32(11): 1084–1089.*

Singh, U. & Jialal, I. (2008). *Alpha-lipoic acid supplementation and diabetes. Nutrition Reviews, 66(11): 646–657.*

Sola, S., Mir, M.Q.S., Cheema, F.A., et al. (2005). *Irbesartan and lipoic acid improve endothelial function and reduce markers of inflammation in the metabolic syndrome: results of the Irbesartan and Lipoic Acid in Endothelial Dysfunction (ISLAND) study. Circulation, 111(3): 343–348.*

Sprague, A.H. & Khalil, R.A. (2009). *Inflammatory cytokines in vascular dysfunction and vascular disease. Biochemical Pharmacology, 78(6): 539–552.*

Steyers, C.M. & Miller, F.J. (2014). *Endothelial dysfunction in chronic inflammatory diseases. Int J Mol Sci, 15(7): 11324–11349.*

Subramanian, S., Kalyanaraman, B. & Migrino, R.Q. (2010). *Mitochondrially targeted antioxidants for the treatment of cardiovascular diseases. Recent Patents on Cardiovascular Drug Discovery, 5(1): 54–65.*

Sun, G., Li, Y., Ji, Z. (2015) *Atorvastatin attenuates inflammation and oxidative stress induced by ischemia/reperfusion in rat heart via the Nrf2 transcription factor. Int J Clin Exp Med. 15, 8(9): 14837–14845.*

Takaoka, M., Kobayashi, Y., Yuba, M., Ohkita, M. & Matsumura, Y. (2001). *Effects of α-lipoic acid on deoxycorticosterone acetate-salt-induced hypertension in rats. European Journal of Pharmacology, 424(2): 121–129.*

Tao, R., Coleman, M.C., Pennington, J.D., Ozden, O., Park, S.H., Jiang, H., Kim, H.S., Flynn, C.R., Hill, S., Hayes, McDonald W., Olivier, A.K., Spitz, D.R. & Gius, D. (2010). *Sirt3-mediated deacetylation of evolutionarily conserved lysine 122 regulates MnSOD activity in response to stress. Mol Cell, 40(6): 893–904.*

Tayebati, S.K., Tomassoni, D., Di Cesare Mannelli, L., Amenta, F. (2015). *Effect of treatment with the antioxidant alpha-lipoic (thioctic) acid on heart and kidney microvasculature in spontaneously hypertensive rats. Clin Exp Hypertens, 2015 Aug 19:1–9.*

Tian, Y.F., He, C.T., Chen, Y.T. & Hsieh, P.S. (2013). *Lipoic acid suppresses portal endotoxemia-induced steatohepatitis and pancreatic inflammation in rats. World Journal of Gastroenterology, 19(18): 2761–2771.*

Tobe, S., Kohan, D.E. & Singarayer, R. (2015). *Endothelin receptor antagonists: new hope for renal protection? Curr Hypertens Rep, 17(7): 57.*

Tosato M., Zamboni, V., Ferrini, A., Cesari, M. (2007). *The aging process and potential interventions to extend life expectancy. Clinical interventions in aging. 2(3): 401–412.*

Touyz, R.M. (2004). *Reactive oxygen species, vascular oxidative stress, and redox signaling in hypertension. What is the clinical significance? Hypertension, 44(3): 248–252.*

Tsutsui, H. (2001). *Oxidative stress in heart failure: the role of mitochondria. Intern Med, 40: 1177–1182.*

Vasdev, S., Ford, C.A., Parai, S., Longerich, L. & Gadag, V. (2000). *Dietary α-lipoic acid supplementation lowers blood pressure in spontaneously hypertensive rats. Journal of Hypertension, 18(5): 567–573.*

Vasdev, S., Stuckless, J. & Richardson, V. (2011). *Role of the immune system in hypertension: modulation by dietary antioxidants. International Journal of Angiology, 20(4): 189–212.*

Venkataraman, K., Khurana, S. & Tai, T.C. (2013). *Oxidative stress in aging-matters of the heart and mind. International Journal of Molecular Sciences, 14(9): 17897–17925.*

Versari, D., Daghini, E., Virdis, A., Ghiadoni, L. & Taddei, S. (2009). *Endothelial dysfunction as a target for prevention of cardiovascular disease. Diabetes Care, 32(2): 314–321.*

Versari, D., Daghini, E., Virdis, A., Ghiadoni, L. & Taddei, S. (2009). *Endothelium-dependent contractions and endothelial dysfunction in human hypertension. British Journal of Pharmacology, 157(4): 527–536.*

Warriner, D., Sheridan, P., Lawford, P. (2015). *Heart failure: not a single organ disease but a multisystem syndrome. Br J Hosp Med (Lond), 76(6): 330–336.*

Watson, T., Goon, P.K.Y., & Lip, G.Y.H. (2008). *Endothelial progenitor cells, endothelial dysfunction, inflammation, and oxidative stress in hypertension. Antioxidants and Redox Signaling, 10(6): 1079–1088.*

Weseler, A.R., & Bast, A. (2010). *Oxidative stress and vascular function: implications for pharmacologic treatments. Current Hypertension Reports, 12(3): 154–161.*

Wojciechowska, C., Romuk, E., Tomasik, A., et al. (2014). *Oxidative stress markers and C-reactive protein are related to severity of heart failure in patients with dilated cardiomyopathy. Mediators of Inflammation, 2014;2014:10. doi: 10.1155/2014/147040.147040*

Wollin, S.D. & Jones, P.J.H. (2003). *Alpha-lipoic acid and cardiovascular disease. Journal of Nutrition, 133(11): 3327–3330.*

Xiong, S., Patrushev, N., Forouzandeh, F., Hilenski, L., Alexander, R.W. (2015). *PGC-1α Modulates telomere function and DNA damage in protecting against aging-related chronic diseases. Cell Rep, 12(9): 1391–1399.*

Yamamoto, T. & Sadoshima, J. (2011). *Protection of the heart against ischemia/reperfusion by silent information regulator 1. Trends in Cardiovascular Medicine, 21(1): 27–32.*

Yamamoto, M., Yang, G., Hong, C., Liu, J., Holle, E., Yu, X., Wagner, T., Vatner, S.F. & Sadoshima, J.

(2003). *Inhibition of endogenous thioredoxin in the heart increases oxidative stress and cardiac hypertrophy. J Clin Invest, 112(9): 1395–1406.*

Yang, Y.K., Wang, L.P., Chen, L., Yao, X.P., Yang, K.Q., Gao, L.G. & Zhou, X.L. (2015). *Coenzyme Q10 treatment of cardiovascular disorders of ageing including heart failure, hypertension and endothelial dysfunction. Clin Chim Acta, 450: 83–89.*

Yildiz, O. (2007). *Vascular smooth muscle and endothelial functions in aging. Annals of the New York Academy of Sciences, 1100: 353–360.*

Ying, Z., Kherada, N., Farrar, B., et al. (2010). *Lipoic acid effects on established atherosclerosis. Life Sciences, 86(3–4): 95–102.*

Yoon, H.J., Cho, S.W., Ahn, B.W. & Yang, S.Y. (2010). *Alterations in the activity and expression of endothelial NO synthase in aged human endothelial cells. Mech Ageing Dev, 131(2): 119–123.*

Zhang, W.J., Bird, K.E., McMillen, T.S., LeBoeuf, R.C., Hagen, T.M. & Frei, B. (2008). *Dietary α-lipoic acid supplementation inhibits atherosclerotic lesion development in apolipoprotein E-deficient and apolipoprotein E/low-density lipoprotein receptor-deficient mice. Circulation, 117(3): 421–428.*

Zhang, W.J. & Frei, B. (2001). *α-Lipoic acid inhibits TNF-α-induced NF-κB activation and adhesion molecule expression in human aortic endothelial cells. FASEB J, 15(13): 2423–2432.*

Zhang, Y., Han, P., Wu, N., et al. (2011). *Amelioration of lipid abnormalities by α-lipoic acid through antioxidative and anti-inflammatory effects. Obesity, 19(8): 1647–1653.*

Zhang, Y., Zhao, S., Gu, Y., Lewis, D.F., Alexander, J.S. & Wang, Y. (2005). *Effects of peroxynitrite and superoxide radicals on endothelial monolayer permeability: potential role of peroxynitrite in preeclampsia. J Soc Gynecol Investig, 12(8): 586–592.*

Zhou, S., Sun, W., Zhang, Z. & Zheng, Y. (2014). *The role of Nrf2-mediated pathway in cardiac remodeling and heart failure. Oxidative Medicine and Cellular Longevity, 2014:16. doi: 10.1155/2014/260429. 260429*

Zhu, J., Liu, M., Kennedy, R. H., Liu, S. J. (2006). *TNFalpha-induced impairment of mitochondrial integrity and apoptosis mediated by caspase-8 in adult ventricular myocytes. Cytokine. 34: 96–105.*

Zygmunt, M., Dudek, M., Bilska-Wilkosz, A., Bednarski, M., Mogilski, S., Knutelska, J. & Sapa, J. (2013). *Anti-inflammatory activity of lipoic acid in mice peritonitis model. Acta Pol Pharm, 70(5): 899–904.*

# Chapter 3

# Pericytes: Role in Human Atherogenesis and Complicated Plaque

Alexander N. Orekhov[1,2,3], Ekaterina A. Ivanova[4]

## 1   Introduction

First events that lead to atherosclerosis development take place in the arterial wall (Rafieian-Kopaei et al., 2014; Weber & Noels, 2011). The disease affects large and medium arteries, with some areas more prone to lesion formation than others. Areas with disturbed laminar blood flow, such as branching points, are especially vulnerable (Moore & Tabas, 2011). Despite considerable progress during the recent decades, the pathogenesis of atherosclerosis remains to be studied in full details. One of the established risk factors of the disease is altered lipoprotein profile of the blood plasma, including the increase of the cholesterol and low density lipoprotein (LDL), as well as atherogenic modifications of LDL particles (Martin et al., 2012; Krauss, 2010). Another known pathological mechanism in atherosclerosis is the response of the arterial wall cells resulting in lipid accumulation and local inflammatory process (Hansson & Hermansson, 2011; Yuan et al., 2012). Atherosclerosis is characterized by a slow progress. Early stages of the disease, which can start already at young age, usually remain clinically silent. At the same time, first manifestations if atherosclerosis can be acute or even fatal, when thrombus formation initiated at the atherosclerotic lesion site leads to occlusion of vital arteries (McGill et al., 2002; Tuzcu et al., 2001). Later stages of atherosclerotic lesion development, are characterized

[1] Laboratory of Angiopathology, Institute of General Pathology and Pathophysiology, Russian Academy of Sciences, Moscow, Russia.

[2] Institute for Atherosclerosis Research, Skolkovo Innovative Center, Moscow, Russia.

[3] Department of Biophysics, Faculty of Biology, Lomonosov Moscow State University, Moscow, Russia

[4] Department of Development and Regeneration, Katholieke Universiteit Leuven, Leuven, Belgium

by the formation of complicated plaques associated with calcinosis, vascular remodeling, intraplaque vascularization and in increased risk of thrombus formation. Resident vascular wall cells likely play the key role in these processes.

Atherosclerotic lesion development is associated with dysfunction of the endothelial lining of the arterial wall. However, subendothelial cells also play a crucial role on the process, actively participating in lipid accumulation and the development of local inflammatory process. Histological studies of the arterial wall revealed the presence of pericyte-like cells with stellate morphology that later have been identified as true pericytes (Andreeva et al., 1998; Juchem et al., 2010). Pericyte-containing subendothelial layer was also found in the walls of large veins (Andreeva et al., 1998). The role of macrovascular pericytes in the development of such pathologies as saphenous vein graft disease, thrombosis and atherosclerosis soon became evident. Pericytes are pluripotent cells capable of rapid proliferation. In culture, they can be stimulated to differentiate into various cell types including osteoblasts, chondrocytes and adipocytes. Moreover, pericytes can participate in immune reactions promoting the local inflammation and in thrombus formation, being a local source of thrombogenic tissue factor (Juchem et al., 2010). Taken together, these facts indicate that pericytes, together with other cell types of the arterial wall, actively participate in the progression of atherosclerotic lesions and the development of complicated plaques.

## 2    Structure of human aortic intima

The intima of the adult human arterial wall consists of two distinct layers (Movat et al., 1958; Geer & Haust, 1972; Velican & Velican, 1977). Immediately below the endothelial lining lies a layer containing collagen fibers without a definite orientation and a heterogeneous population of cells including stellate-shaped pericytes. This layer has been defined as connective-tissue (Haust, 1989; Stary, 1989) or proteoglycan-rich layer (Stary, 1989). It is separated by the internal limiting membrane from the muscular-elastic layer, which is built of several layers of elongated bipolar smooth muscle cells and longitudinally-oriented collagen fibers. Internal elastic membrane separates this layer from the media of the arterial wall (Figure 1).

The intimal layers differ from each other by both cellular and fibre content. In the proteoglycan-rich layer, collagen and reticulin fibres prevail, whereas muscular-elastic layer contains more elastic fibres. The layers are also characterized by different composition of glycosaminoglycans (Velican & Velican, 1977). The arterial intima affected by atherosclerosis is thicker than that of grossly normal blood vessels, reaching its maximum in atherosclerotic plaques.

Our group has performed measurement of the intimal thickness in grossly normal areas and in atherosclerotic lesions of human aorta (Orekhov et al., 1987). Different stages of atherosclerotic lesion development include initial lesion, fatty streak, intermediate lesion, atheroma, fibrolipid plaque and fibrotic plaque (Stary, 1994). Thickness of the muscular-elastic layer in fatty streak areas was not altered in comparison with uninvolved tissue, while in atherosclerotic plaques it was 11% greater. In contrast to the muscular-

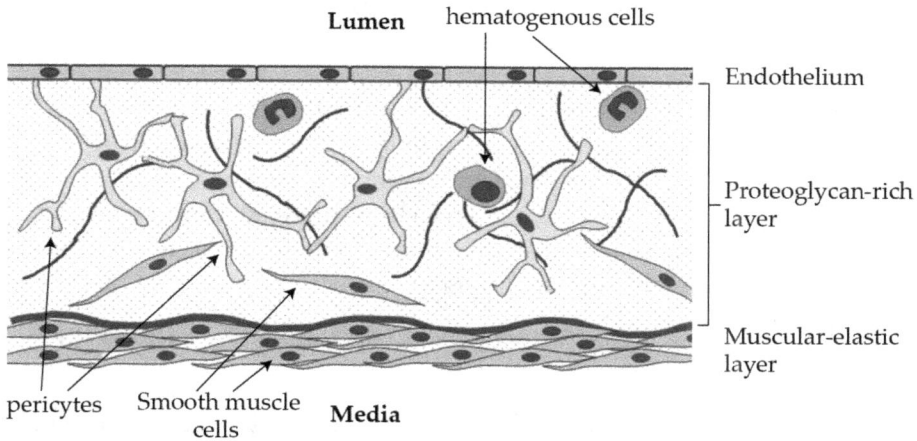

**Figure 1. Schematic presentation of different layers of human arterial intima** (reproduced from Ivanova E.A., Orekhov A.N. Cellular model of atherogenesis based on pluripotent vascular wall pericytes (2015) Stem Cells International, submitted for publication).

elastic layer, proteoglycan-rich layer had a considerably increased thickness in atherosclerotic plaques, forming an intimal protrusion into the lumen, which reduced the blood flow through the vessel. Average thickness of proteoglycan-rich layer in fatty streaks was almost 2 folds higher and in atherosclerotic plaques – almost 4 folds higher than in normal tissue (Orekhov et al., 1987).

The collagen content of the proteoglycan-rich and muscular-elastic intimal layers was similar in uninvolved intima. However, in atherosclerotic lesions, the collagen content was increased predominantly in the proteoglycan-rich layer. Muscular-elastic layer of normal intima contained interstitial collagens type I and III in the form of longitudinally-oriented fibers. On the other hand, proteoglycan-rich layer contains predominantly collagens type IV and V (the basal membrane collagens).

Microscopic analysis of the fatty streak area revealed empty spaces between the interstitial collagen fibres corresponding to lipid droplets that perturbed their normal orientation. Areas of atherosclerotic plaques were characterized by accumulation of all types of collagen, especially in the plaque cap, where the type I and type III collagens were identified. Type IV and V collagens formed a thick layer beneath the endothelial basal membrane. The collagen fibres formed thick capsules around subendothelial cells. At the same time, no visible change in collagen organization could be observed in the muscular-elastic layer of the intima with atherosclerotic lesions.

Lipid accumulation in the arterial wall varied between the two layers. In fatty streaks, Oil Red O staiing revealed both intra- and extracellular lipids located predominantly in the juxtaluminal intimal layer. The lipid content decreased in the deeper layers of the intima. In fibrolipid plaques, lipids were confined to the proteoglycan-rich layer in the plaque core and margins. Total lipid content of the proteoglycan-rich layer was 3.2-

fold higher in fatty streaks and 8-fold higher in atherosclerotic plaques in comparison to healthy tissue. In the muscular-elastic layer the corresponding values were 2.6 and 4.4 (Orekhov et al., 1987).

Taken together, these observations demonstrate that the juxtaluminal proteogly-can-rich layer of human aortic intima is susceptible to atherosclerotic changes to a much greater extent than the muscular-elastic layer. Intimal thickening associated with lesion development occurs mostly due to the outgrowth of proteoglycan-rich layer. Collagen deposition and lipid accumulation also take place predominantly in this area. The observed differences between the intimal layers are likely to be explained by their distinct cellular composition.

# 3   Cellular Composition of Normal and Atherosclerotic Intima of Human Aorta

Cellular content of intimal layers has been analyzed using the method of alcohol-alkaline dissociation (Krushinsky et al., 1983). Grossly normal areas were compared to atherosclerotic lesions at different stages of development. In fatty streaks and atherosclerotic plaques, the proteoglycan-rich mayer contained 1.5- and 2.0-fold increased total amount of cells respectively. At the same time, in the muscular-elastic layer in the atherosclerotic lesion areas, the number of cells remained virtually unchanged in comparison with normal intima (Orekhov et al., 1987). The results of aortic cross-sections study were consostent: cellularity of the muscular-elastic layer of uninvolved and atherosclerotic intima was similar, while the number of cells in the proteoglycan-rich layer of atherosclerotic lesions was increased by 2 folds. Therefore, proteoglycan-rich layer plays the major role in the development of atherosclerotic lesions.

The population of cells inhabiting the proteoglycan-rich layer is heterogeneous and can be divided into two groups: resident cells and round cells morphologically similar to peripheral blood lymphocytes (inflammatory cells). Resident cells of the intima were found to be different from typical smooth muscle cells of the media. These cells have been described by some researchers as modified smooth muscle cells (Campbell & Campbell, 1989). Immunocytochemical analysis allowed performing a more detailed study of cellular composition of normal and atherosclerotic arterial intima. In addition to smooth muscle cells positive for smooth muscle $\alpha$-actin ($\alpha$-SMA) (Nakamura & Sakurai, 1992), the following inflammatory cells were identified in the intima: macrophages and lymphocytes (Munro et al., 1987), mast cells (Kaartinen et al., 1994) and dendritic cells (Bobryshev & Lord, 1995).

# 4   Identification and Characterization of Pericytes in the Arterial wall

Early studies have identified pericytes as mostly microvascular cells. They are important for maintenance of capillary wall and the endothelial barrier function. They also play a prominent role in angiogenesis and vessel branching (van Dijk et al., 2015; Hall, 2006) and contribute to embryonic development of aorta (Nicosia, 2009). Accordingly, it has been proposed that pericytes participate in various conditions associated with microvascular dysfunction, such as diabetes, inflammation, wound healing, hypertension, tumor growth and others (Juchem et al., 2010; Sims, 1991). Pericytes regulate the endothelial function, including endothelial cell proliferation and ion and molecule exchange (Diaz-Flores et al., 1991; Shepro & Morel, 1993). However, pericytes were also found in the walls of large blood vessels (Campagnolo et al., 2010; Orekhov et al., 2014; Rekhter et al., 1992). According to current consensus, the main function of pericytes is to serve as precursors for other cell types of mesenchymal origin: smooth muscle cells (Sims, 1991), osteoblasts (Brighton et al., 1992; Diaz-Flores et al., 1992; Shepro & Morel, 1993), chondrocytes (Sims, 1991) and adipocytes (Iyama et al., 1979). Differentiation into these cell types is a characteristic feature of cultured pericytes *in vitro*.

Accurate identification of pericytes remains quite challenging because of the high phenotypical flexibility of these cells. A number of pericyte marker proteins have been established. However, these proteins are often shared between several cell types and their expression may vary significantly depending on the location of cells and their exposure to certain stimuli (van Dijk et al., 2015). Pericytes can express $\alpha$-smooth muscle actin ($\alpha$-SMA) when stimulated with endothelin-1. The expression of this marker also varies depending on the cell position: pericytes from non-contractile capillaries can be $\alpha$-SMA-negative (Boado & Pardridge, 1994; Dore-Duffy et al., 2011). Other commonly used pericyte markers include platelet-derived growth factor receptor $\beta$ (PDGFR$\beta$), CD146, aminopeptidases A and N (CD13), endoglin, neuron-glial 2 (NG2), non-muscle myosin, desmin, vimentin and nestin (Armulik et al., 2005; van Dijk et al., 2015). Most of these proteins are shared with other cell types, hindering the accurate identification of pericytes. Antigen 3G5 is an *O*-sialoganglioside, which can be used for identification of microvascular pericytes (Nayak et al., 1988). Another antigen, 2A7, also known as chondroitin sulphate proteoglycan or melanoma-associated high molecular weight antigen (HMW-MAA), was found to be typical for pericytes, especially during angiogenesis (Andreeva et al., 1992). The expression of this antigen increases during formation of granulation tissues and healing wounds. 2A7 is expressed on pericytes in "activated" state, with proliferation ability.

A detailed analysis of cellular composition on normal and atherosclerotic intima was performed by our group using a set of specific markers for cell type identification. The majority of cells in normal and atherosclerotic intima were $\alpha$-SMA-positive cells (Table 1). About two-thirds of cells in the muscular-elastic layer expressed $\alpha$-SMA, while in the proteoglycan-rich layer the proportion of positive cells was much lower. Inflammatory cells (lymphocytes and macrophages) were confined to the juxtaluminal part of the proteoglycan-rich layer. Their proportion increased in atherosclerotic lesions, reaching 20% of the total cell content.

Some of the resident subendothelial cells appeared to be $\alpha$-SMA-negative. This could be explained by phenotypic modulation of intimal cells during physiological adaptation and/or pathological changes of the vascular wall. Indeed, a well-developed con-

| Area | % of positive cells | | | | | | |
|---|---|---|---|---|---|---|---|
| | α-SMA | CDLC | CD68 | 3G5 | 2A7 | CDLC+CD14 inflammatory cells | Resident cells |
| Grossly normal 0[a] | 47.6±2.3 (n=4) [b] | 2.2±0.4 (n=3) | 3.9±0.4 (n=5) | 31.3±7.0 (n=4) | 0.0±0.0 (n=3) | 5.5±1.2 (n=8) | 97.3±0.6 (n=8) |
| Initial lesions I | 47.2±3.1 (n=3) | 6.2±1.2 (n=4) | 6.1±1.4 (n=4) | 6.3±1.0* (n=3) | 1.2±0.3 (n=3) | 9.6±1.4* (n=6) | 90.9±1.2 (n=6) |
| Fatty streaks II | 42.2±3.1 (n=4) | 5.0±0.9* (n=3) | 13.2±0.8* (n=5) | 11.7±2.0* (n=8) | 3.0±0.7 (n=3) | 13.4±1.5* (n=10) | 89.4±1.1 (n=10) |
| Fibrolipid plaques Va | 47.0±10.9 (n=5) | 6.2±1.8* (n=9) | 13.1±2.3* (n=4) | 5.0±0.7* (n=5) | 27.0±3.1 (n=3) | 18.7±2.0* (n=8) | 84.7±1.4 (n=8) |
| Fibrotic plaques, Vc | ND | ND | ND | ND | ND | 6.4±1.9 (n=6) | 94.9±1.6 (n=6) |

[a] Lesion type according to AHA Counsil on Atherosclerosis is indicated in the square brackets

[b] The number of cases examined

* Significant difference from the % of positive cells in grossly normal areas, $p < 0.05$.

**Table 1.** Immunocytochemical identification of cells in human aortic intima

tractile apparatus is not highly significant for intimal cells of the aorta and other large arteries, because their tone is maintained by other mechanisms. In large arteries, resident intimal cells may perform other functions, such as trophic function and maintenance of metabolism of the vascular wall cells. It can also be suggested that these cells represent a population, which is functionally and, probably, ontogenetically different from the typical smooth muscle cells. For instance, stellate cells expressing S-100 and CD1a antigens of dendritic cells have been identified in human aortic intima (Bobryshev & Lord, 1995).

We found that some of the resident intimal cells express antigens unusual for medial smooth muscle cells. For instance, 3G5 antigen, typical for quiescent pericytes (Nayak et al., 1988), was present on pericyte-like resident cells in the aortic intima. 3G5-positive cells have been identified in bovine aorta, in healthy human intima and in complicated atherosclerotic plaques with ectopic osteogenesis (Bostrom et al., 1993). According to our results, these cells account for more than 30% of total intimal cell population. Noteworthy, these cells were only present in the uppermost subendothelial layer of the intima, where they formed a network (Andreeva et al., 1997).

In atherosclerotic plaques, the number of 3G5 antigen-positive cells was much lower than in uninvolved intima, while the number of resident α-SMA-positive cells increased. At the same time, the expression of 2A7 antigen typical for "activated" pericytes was increased in atherosclerotic lesions (Table 1). Together these observations indicate that atherosclerotic lesion development is associated with changes of the functional state of intimal cells.

Atherosclerotic lesion development is tightly associated with lipid accumulation in the arterial wall. We tested whether lipid accumulation can influence the expression of pericyte antigens by the subendothelial cells in primary culture. The increase of the intracellular lipid content by 1.5 to 2 folds induced by treatment with atherogenic modified LDL (mLDL) led to a decrease of 3G5 antigen-positive cells, while the total cell number remained unchanged (Figure 2).

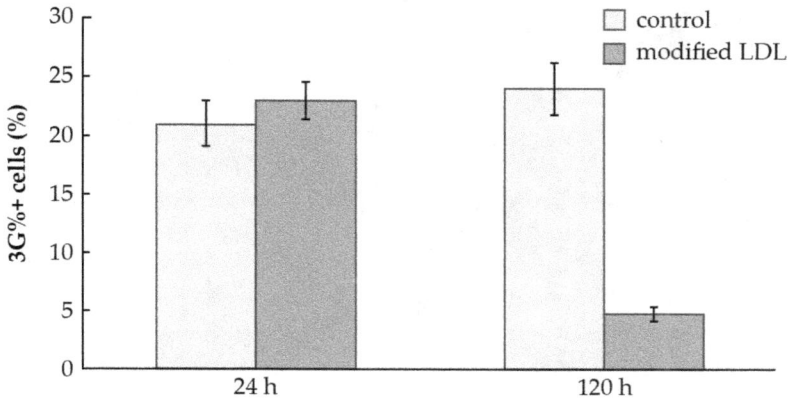

**Figure 2.** The effect of intracellular lipid accumulation on the expression of 3G5 pericyte-associated antigen. On day 4 in primary culture, cells were treated with 100 µg/ml modified (desialylated) LDL. After the incubation, cells were stained with anti-3G5 antibody and total cell number and the number of positive cells were counted. Presented are the results of 3 independent experiments, $p < 0.05$.

Another interesting finding was the presence of macrophage-associated antigen CD68, which is a scavenger receptor, on resident subendothelial cells (Nazarova et al., 1995). In primary culture of intimal cells, the proportion of $\alpha$-SMA-CD68 double positive cells increased after induction of intracellular lipid accumulation with atherogenic mLDL (Andreeva et al., 1997). The expression of CD68 can be therefore regarded as a marker of phagocytic activity rather than of monocytic origin of cells.

# 5   Role of Arterial Cells in Atherosclerosis

As described above, the proteoglycan-rich layer contains a heterogeneous population of resident and inflammatory cells. In atherosclerotic lesions, the proportion of resident cells positive for $\alpha$-SMA was similar to that in uninvolved intima, while the proportion of inflammatory cells increased. The development of atherosclerotic lesion was associated with the increase of the cell number in the area (cellularity), which followed a bell-shape curve along the lesion progression stages (initial lesions – fatty streaks – fibrolipid plaques – fibrous plaques). The increase of cellularity was registered both for resident and inflammatory cells.

Using the method of alcohol-alkaline dissociation of fixed tissue (Orekhov et al., 1986), we studied the cellula composition of normal human arterial intima and atherosclerotic plaques. Cell suspension obtained after dissociation of the extracellular matrix was morphologically heterogeneous (Figure 3).

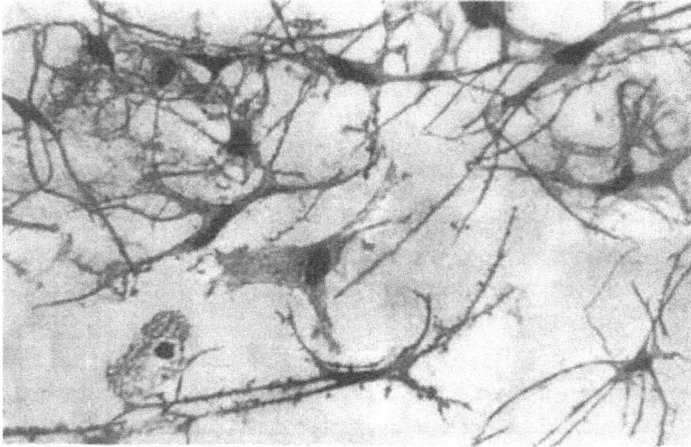

**Figure 3. Cell heterogeneity in the proteoglycan-rich layer of human aortic intima**. Cell suspension prepared by alcohol-alkaline dissociation of fixed tissue. Toluidine blue staining. Magn. X350.

In the cell suspension, different forms of resident subendothelial cells can be seen, including elongated bipolar cells, stellate cells and intermediate forms. Stellate (pericyte-like) cells with round body and three or more long processes are unevenly distributed in the loose connective tissue matrix of the intima. Some of them express pericyte markers 3G5 and 2A7 and CD68. In atherosclerotic plaques, these cells appear to be filled with lipids and can be classified as foam cells (Andreeva et al., 1991). The number of stellate cells increases by 6 folds in atherosclerotic lesions, while the total number of cells and the number of elongated cells increase only by 2 folds. Moreover, the number of stellate cells correlated with total lipids and cholesterol esters contents (correlation coefficients 0.95 and 0.96 respectively, $p < 0.01$), underscoring the important role that these cells play in lipid accumulation. The number of stellate cells also correlated with the amount of collagen content and intimal thickness, although the correlation coefficients were somewhat lower (0.80 and 0.73 respectively) (Andreeva et al., 1992).

Lipid accumulation (lipidosis) is one of the key processes in atherosclerotic lesion development. In grossly normal areas of intima, lipids are mostly present in the extracellular space. However, initial atherosclerotic lesions are characterized by the appearance of cells with lipid inclusions. Our group performed a quantitative study of the proportion of cells with lipid inclusions in uninvolved intima and atherosclerotic lesions at different stages (Andreeva et al., 1991). Fatty streaks had the highest content of lipid-laden cells (up to 25%) located predominantly in the upper part of the proteoglycan-rich layer and comprising approximately two-thirds of it. In atherosclerotic plaques, the majority of cells with lipid inclusions were located in the part of proteoglycan-rich layer adjacent to the internal limiting membrane. Cells with lipid inclusions were found in all cell populations of the aortic intima. However, the proportion of stellate cells accumulating lipids was higher than that of other cell types, reaching 30% (Figure 4).

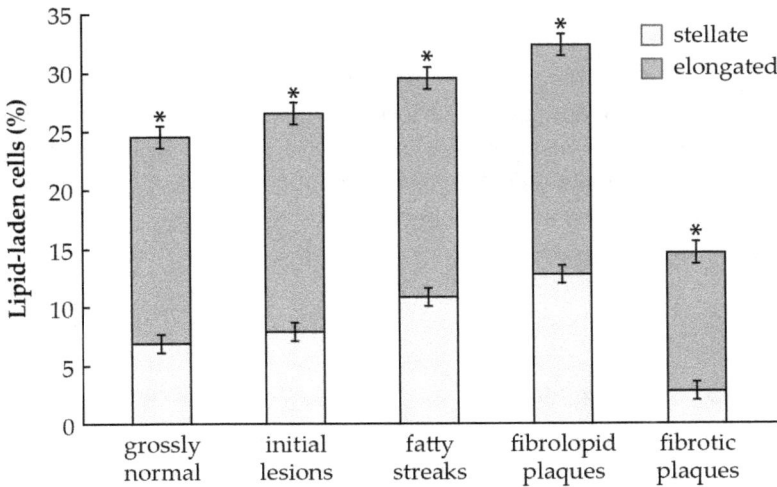

Figure 4. Cells with lipid inclusions among stallate and elongated cells in human aortic intima. The percent of lipid-laden cells in populations of stellate and elongated cells was determined in cell suspension prepared by alcohol-alkaline dissociation of fixed tissue. *, significant difference from elongated cells, $p < 0.05$.

Another process, which plays a prominent role in the pathogenesis of atheroslcerosis is the increase of cellularity in the lesion area leading to the lesion growth. Cell count on cross-sections and in suspension of primary cells obtained after dissociation of tissue samples was 2-fold higher in atheroslcerotic lesions compared to uninvolved intima. The maximum cell count was registered in lipid-rich lesions (fatty streaks and fibrolipid plaques). Both resident and inflammatory cell counts were increased, however, as the proportion of resident cells is higher, they make the major contribution into the increased cellularity of atherosclerotic lesions.

To test whether the increased cell count can be explained by enhanced proliferation, cells were stained with antibody to proliferating cell nuclear antigen (PCNA), which is expressed in the S-phase of cell cycle. The number of proliferating cells in lipid-rich atherosclerotic lesions (fatty streaks and fibrolipid plaques) was 10 to 20 folds higher than in uninvolved intima (Figures 5 and 6) (Orekhov et al., 1998, 2010).

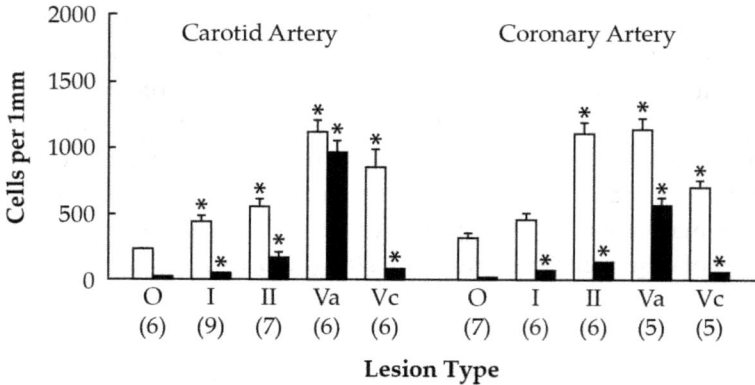

**Figure 5. Number of resident (white bars) and inflammatory (black bars) cells in the intima of coronary and carotid arteries at different stages of atherosclerotic lesion development.** 0, grossly normal unaffected intima; I, initial lesions; II, fatty streaks; Va, lipofibrous plaques; Vc, fibrous plaques. * - statistically significant difference compared to normal unaffected intima with $p < 0.05$. The number of analyzed autopsy cases is indicated in brackets. (Reproduced from: Orekhov et al. 2010)

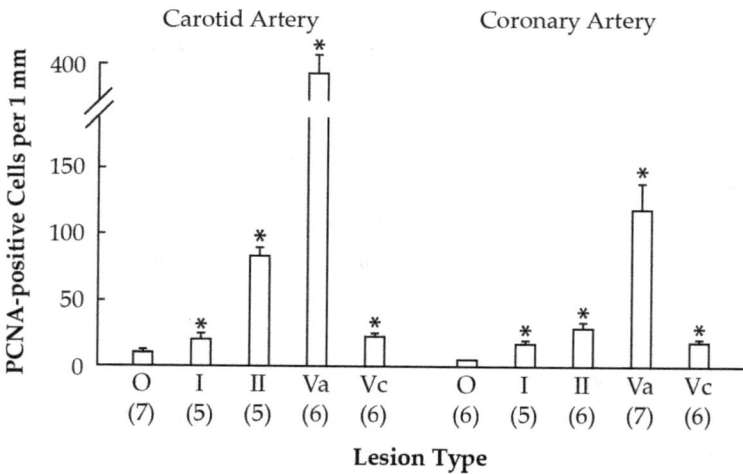

**Figure 6. Number of PCNA-positive cells in the intima of coronary and carotid arteries at different stages of atherosclerotic lesion development.** 0, grossly normal unaffected intima; I, initial lesions; II, fatty streaks; Va, lipofibrous plaques; Vc, fibrous plaques. * - statistically significant difference compared to normal unaffected intima with $p < 0.05$. The number of analyzed autopsy cases is indicated in brackets. (Reproduced from: Orekhov et al. 2010)

The proliferative index (the ratio between proliferating cells and the total cell number) for resident cells was considerably higher in atherosclerotic lesions at all stages than in uninvolved intima, reaching its maximum (8-fold increase) in fibrous plaques. Proliferative index of ininflammatory cells, although being higher than that of the resident cells, was similar to proliferative index of peripheral blood leukocytes and was not significantly different in uninvolved intima and atherosclerotic lesions. It is therefore likely that proliferation of resident cells, along with migration of inflammatory cells, makes an important contribution into the atherosclerotic lesion growth.

Accumulation of extracellular matrix and formation of the connective-tissue can are the most clinically significant manifestations of atherosclerosis. Noteworthy, total collagen content in the atherosclerotic lesion area is increased predominantly in the proteoglycan-rich layer. Collagen type I is the main interstitial collagen accumulated in atherosclerotic plaques. In uninvolved intima, no cells producing this type of collagen can be observed. However in atherosclerotic lesions, as much as 6% (in initial lesions) and 18% (in fatty streaks) of total cell population produce collagen type I (Andreeva et al., 1997). The highest content of collagen-producing cells is in fibrolipid plaques, and there is a splash of synthetic activity in lipid-reach lesions.

It is likely that the described manifestations of atherosclerosis: splash of proliferative activity, increased collagen production and lipid accumulation are tightly linked with each other. In vitro experiments with induced lipid accumulation in primary cultured cells helped revealing some details of this relationship. It was demonstrated that cells deriving from atherosclerotic lesions were characterized by altered lipid metabolism, with the rate of lipid synthesis higher than that in cells obtained from grossly normal intima (Orekhov et al., 1985). In primary cultured cells, prominent lipid accumulation can be induced by incubation with modified LDL, which is prone to self-association and complex formation (Tertov et al., 1992). Elevated level of modified LDL is typical for patients with atherosclerosis. Blood serum and modified LDL isolated from blood of atherosclerosis patients, which induces intracellular lipid accumulation also causes other atherogenic manifestations in cultured cells. Pre-incubation of cells with atherogenic serum or LDL stimulated cell proliferation and synthesis of collagen, glycosaminoglycans and total protein (Orekhov et al., 1990). Another important aspect of the atherosclerotic process is the disturbance of intercellular communication, which is also affected by lipid accumulation induced by atherogenic LDL.

# 6   Cellular Network and Communication in the Intima

Histological studies revealed the presence of three-dimensional cellular network in the proteoglycan-rich payer of human arterial intima formed by stellate pericyte-like cells that can be identified as true pericytes. Cells with long processes connect with processes or bodies of adjacent cells (Rekhter et al., 1991). Such network is not present in the muscular-elastic layer, where densely packed cells formed strata oriented at a small angle to each other. The observed network may have important functions in the vascular wall, since intercellular contacts have been demonstrated to be important for microvascular pericytes that directly communicate with endothelial cells (Juchem et al., 2010). The development of atherosclerotic lesion is associated with considerable changes in the cellular composition of intima. Stellate cells actively accumulate lipids in fatty streaks, which leads to functional and morphological changes (Andreeva et al., 1991). Changes of cellular shape are accompanied by disruption of intercellular contacts and dissociation of the cellular network. Microscopic analysis of atherosclerotic plaque tissue demonstrated that in superficial layers of lesions stellate cells were mostly present as individual cells or small groups that lost contacts with each other. Some of them contained prominent lipid inclusions. In the deeper layers, the number of branched cells with long processes was higher, but the normal network was not observed.

Gap junctions play a key role in the intercellular communication (Trautmann et al., 1988). They are important for tissue homeostasis, as they participate in intercellular transport of metabolites, signalling molecules and other factors. Presence of gap junctions is a specific feature of differentiated cell systems (Beny et al., 1992; Davies, 1986). In particular, this type of cell contact is essential for normal function of pericytes (Larson et al., 1987). Dysfunction of gap junctions has been reported in angiopathologies associated with diabetes (Oku et al., 2001). It is likely that functional disturbance of gap junctions can contribute to the disintegration of the cellular network of the proteoglycan-rich layer observed in atherosclerotic lesions. Connexin 43 (Cx43) is the major protein forming gap junctions. It is localized on the cell surface in structures called connexin plaques. Microscopic study of different stages of atherosclerotic lesion development demonstrated that in fatty streaks the number of Cx43 plaques decreased by 3 folds in comparison to uninvolved intima. Moreover, the number of Cx43 plaques per cell decreased towards the lumen consistent with the hypothesis that the cellular network is less damaged in deep layers of atherosclerotic lesions and is especially affected in the superficial layers (Figures 7 and 8).

Study of perturbed cell communication was performed on primary culture of aortic cells. In addition to Cx43 localization, intercellular communication can be visualized by the transfer of fluorescent dye from the injected cell to adjacent cells. Fluorescent dye is specifically transferred via gap junctions, and the rate of communication can be estimated by the number of contacting fluorescent cells. Studies of cultures obtained from atherosclerotic lesions demonstrated that the rate of communication was decreased by 1.5 folds in cultures obtained from atherosclerotic lesions as compared to cells derived from grossly normal regions of the intima (Andreeva et al., 1995). Moreover, selective injection of the fluorescent dye into lipid-laden (foam) cells demonstrated that these cells were characterized by a 2-fold lower rate of communication than lipid-free cells. The number of Cx43 plaques on such cells was also decreased. It is therefore plausible that lipid accumulation in pericytes impairs cell communication and is the cause of cellular network dissociation in atherosclerotic plaques.

# 7    Resident Vascular Wall Cells and Local Inflammation

The development of atherosclerotic lesions is associated at all stages with inflammatory

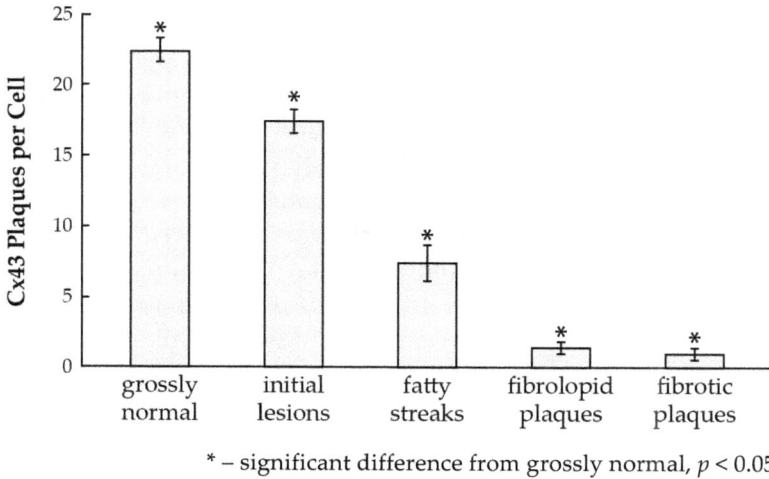

* – significant difference from grossly normal, $p < 0.05$

**Figure 7. The number of Cx43 plaques on the cells in grossly normal and atherosclerotic areas of human aorta.** Cx43 was revealed immunocytochemically on the horizontal sections of the human aorta. The number of Cx43 plaques per cell was calculated on each tissue section and then the mean value of the data obtained on several sections were combined.

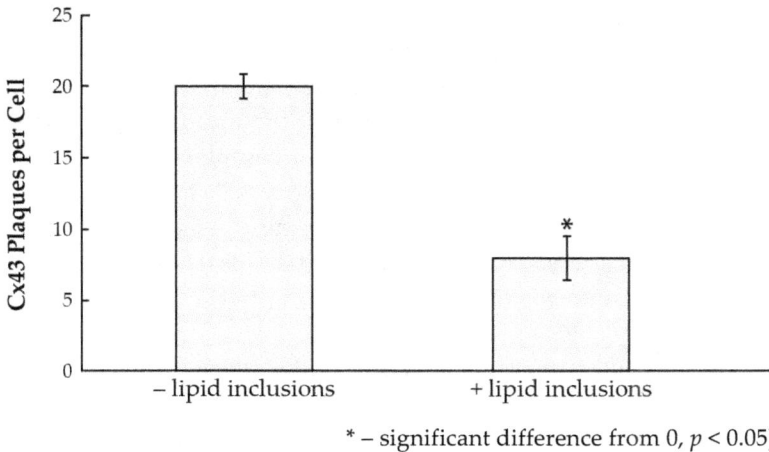

* – significant difference from 0, $p < 0.05$)

**Figure 8. The number of Cx43 plaques on the cells without lipid inclusions and lipid-laden cells in the human aortic intima.** Cx43 was revealed immunocytochemically on the horizontal sections of the human aorta. Lipid-laden cells were revealed with filipin staining. The number of Cx43 plaques per cell without lipid inclusions and lipid-laden cells was calculated on each tissue section and then the mean value of the data obtained on several sections were combined.

Study of perturbed cell communication was performed on primary culture of aortic cells. In addition to Cx43 localization, intercellular communication can be visualized by the transfer of fluorescent dye from the injected cell to adjacent cells. Fluorescent dye is specifically transferred via gap junctions, and the rate of communication can be estimated by the number of contacting fluorescent cells. Studies of cultures obtained from atherosclerotic lesions demonstrated that the rate of communication was decreased by 1.5 folds in cultures obtained from atherosclerotic lesions as compared to cells derived from grossly normal regions of the intima (Andreeva et al., 1995). Moreover, selective injection of the fluorescent dye into lipid-laden (foam) cells demonstrated that these cells were characterized by a 2-fold lower rate of communication than lipid-free cells. The number of Cx43 plaques on such cells was also decreased. It is therefore plausible that lipid accumulation in pericytes impairs cell communication and is the cause of cellular network dissociation in atherosclerotic plaques.

# 7    Resident Vascular Wall Cells and Local Inflammation

The development of atherosclerotic lesions is associated at all stages with inflammatory process (Ross. 1999). The recruitment of circulating leukocytes to the lesion site contributes significantly to the lesion growth and maintains the local pro-inflammatory environment in the arterial wall by secreting cytokines and chemokines. Macrophages participate in lipid uptake and accumulation giving rise to some of the foam cells. Lipid accumulation and local inflammatory process appear to be tightly linked, and modified atherogenic LDL not only causes lipid accumulation in the arterial wall, but also creates pro-inflammatory conditions , stimulating both adaptive and innate immunity (Hansson, 2005). Lipid accumulation in the proteoglycan-rich layer of the arterial intima positively correlated with the expression of major histocompatibility complex class II (MHC II) molecule HLA-DR and the number of the immune-inflammatory cells in the region (Handunnetthi et al., 2010). HLA-DR is a marker of antigen-presenting cells (APCs) of hematogenous origin that include macrophages, B cells and dendritic cells (Geissmann et al., 2010). Dendritic cell are especially important for antigen presentation and are generally regarded as "professional" APCs.

According to recent studies, resident cells of the arterial wall can also contribute to the development of local inflammatory process. Some of the arterial wall cells of non-hematogeneous origin, including endothelial cells and pericytes, are capable of antigen presentation. Endothelial cells can activate T cells and basally express both MHCI and MHCII, although the expression is less prominent in large arteries (von Willebrand et al., 1985). Stellate cells corresponding to pericytes were demonstrated to express HLA-DR. In some areas, up to 15% of total cell population of the intima was HLA-DR-positive (Bobryshev et al., 2012). Moreover, some of the HLA-DR-positive cells contained apoB in the perinuclear space, possibly reflecting the early stage of intracellular lipid accumulation (Figure 9).

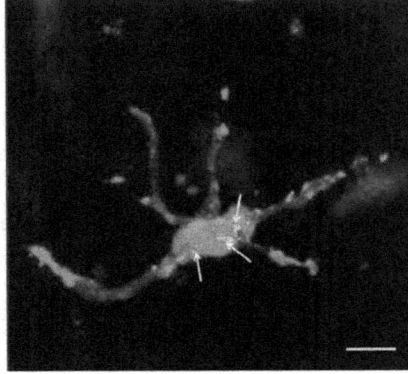

**Figure 9. ApoB (red staining, arrows) in the perinuclear cytoplasm of a HLA-DR+ (green staining) cell.** Scale bar = 10 μm. (Reproduced from Bobryshev et al., 2012).

The accumulating evidence indicates that pericytes may participate in the production of cytokines and therefore contribute to the local inflammatory process in the atherosclerotic lesion. Further investigation of the role of pericytes in the immune reactions is a topic of future studies (Pober & Tellides, 2012). It is likely that the three-dimentional network formed by pericytes in the arterial wall may play important protective functions.

# 8    Role of the Pericytes in Complicated Plaque

At later stages, atherosclerotic lesion can be associated with vascular wall remodelling, calcification, neovascularization of the growing plaque and the increased risk of thrombus development. Because of their high plasticity and pluripotency, macrovascular pericytes are likely to participate in these processes resulting in complicated plaque formation. Pro-inflammatory environment of the growing lesion and lipid accumulation can result in activation of quiescent macrovascular pericytes and their differentiation into other cell types. The exact mechanisms of such induced differentiation remain to be studied; however, some recent results contribute to the improved understanding of these processes. For instance, phenotypic changes and activation of pericytes induced by LDL may be mediated by T-cadherin, an unusual member of the cadherin family, which is up-regulated in atherosclerotic lesion sites (Ivanov et al., 2001). T-cadherin signalling involves the activation of Erk1/2 tyrosine kinase and nuclear translocation of the transcription factor NF-κB (Takeuchi et al., 2001). Pericytes may also play a prominent role in plaque neovascularization. It has been demonstrated that pericytes can be recruited to the vascularization sites through activation of surface c-Met receptors followed by PI3K/Akt signalling (Liu et al., 2007). The ability of pericytes to differentiate into chondrocytes may be important for vascular wall remodelling observed in atherosclerosis. Such differentiation can be mediated by Wnt/β-catenin signalling pathway, since several Wnt receptors could be detected in pericytes, including LDL receptor-like proteins 5 and 6 (Kirton et al., 2007).

Chondrogenic differentiation of pericytes can be enhanced by TGF-$\beta_3$, which is produced by macrophages, foam cells and vascular smooth muscle cells in the atherosclerotic lesion site (Bobik et al., 1999). Pericytes can also participate in vascular calcification, which is also controlled by TGF-$\beta_3$ (Shao et al., 2006). Cultured pericytes were demonstrated to spontaneously form multicellular nodules containing mineralized matrix, osteopontin, osteocalcin, matrix Gla protein and collagen type I typical for calcified vessels (Brighton et al., 1992). On the other hand, cells from the vascular mineralized nodules were shown to express the pericyte antigen 3G5 (Bostrom et al., 1993). It has been demonstrated that 3G5-positive pericytes in atherosclerotic lesion site were able to express vascular calcification-associated factor, which regulates osteogenic differentiation of pericytes (Shao et al., 2006). Together these observations indicate that pericytes may be actively involved in the calcification process in atherosclerotic plaques.

Thrombus formation on the surface of vulnerable plaque accounts for the majority of acute ischemia episodes associated with atherosclerosis. Importantly, pericytes appear to be the major cell type providing thrombogenic tissue factor in the arterial wall (Juchem et al., 2010). A population of pericyte-like subendothelial cells with thrombogenic potential was found in the central region of atherosclerotic lesion. Possible pathogenic pathways of pericyte contribution to atherosclerosis process are presented on Figure 10.

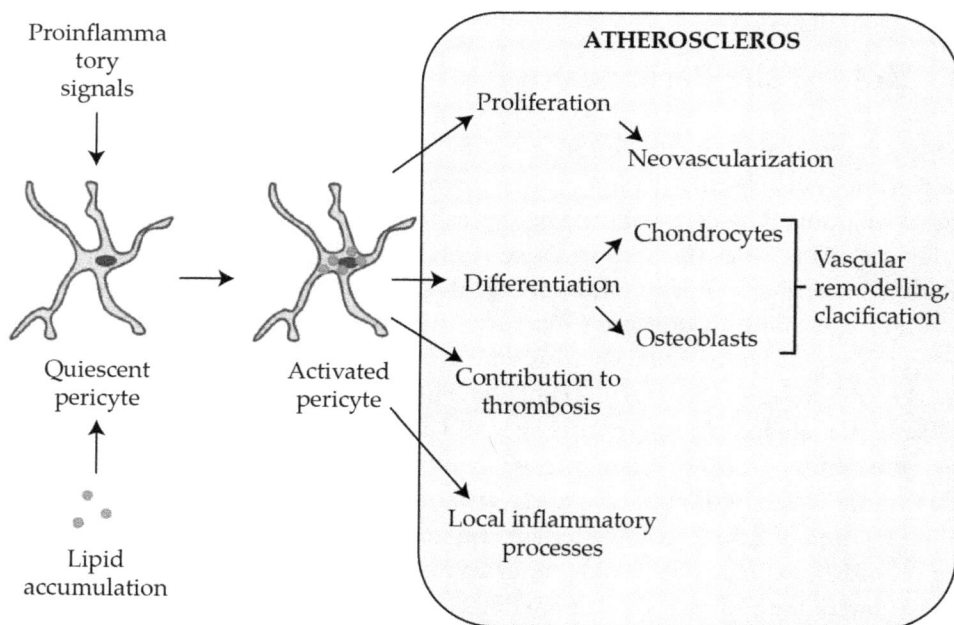

**Figure 10. Schematic presentation of potential roles of pericytes in the pathogenesis of atherosclerosis.** (Adapted from Orekhov at al., 2014).

# 9   Conclusion

The unique location and properties of pericytes make these pluripotent cells especially interesting in the context of atherosclerotic lesion development. Pericytes are capable of proliferation, active accumulation of lipids, production of various signaling molecules and differentiation into other cell types, including chondrocytes and osteoblasts. These cells can therefore participate in the atherosclerotic lesion growth, formation of local pro-inflammatory environment and the development of complicated plaque. Moreover, the cellular network formed by pericytes in the subendothelial layer of arterial intima may have important protective functions that remain to be fully understood. It is likely that pericytes represent a second line of defense (after the endothelial barrier) against the lesion formation. However, macrovascular pericytes remain currently insufficiently studied, partly due to the flexible nature of these cells, which hinders their accurate identification. The development of advanced cell culture and microscopy techniques may help improving our understanding of this cell type, which is an exciting target of future research.

# References

Andreeva ER, Orekhov AN, Smirnov VN. (1991). Quantitative estimation of lipid-laden cells in atherosclerotic lesions of the human aorta. Acta anatomica, 141(4):316–23.

Andreeva ER, Pugach IM, Gordon D, Orekhov AN. (1998). Continuous subendothelial network formed by pericyte-like cells in human vascular bed. Tissue & cell, 30(1):127–35.

Andreeva ER, Pugach IM, Orekhov AN. (1997). Collagen-synthesizing cells in initial and advanced atherosclerotic lesions of human aorta. Atherosclerosis, 130(1–2):133–42.

Andreeva ER, Pugach IM, Orekhov AN. (1997). Subendothelial smooth muscle cells of human aorta express macrophage antigen in situ and in vitro. Atherosclerosis, 135(1):19–27.

Andreeva ER, Rekhter MD, Romanov Yu A, Antonova GM, Antonov AS, Mironov AA, et al. (1992). Stellate cells of aortic intima: II. Arborization of intimal cells in culture. Tissue & cell,  24(5):697–704.

Andreeva ER, Serebryakov VN, Orekhov AN. (1995). Gap junctional communication in primary culture of cells derived from human aortic intima. Tissue & cell, 27(5):591–7.

Armulik A, Abramsson A, Betsholtz C. (2005). Endothelial/pericyte interactions. Circulation research, 97(6):512–23.

Beny JL, Connat JL. (1992). An electron-microscopic study of smooth muscle cell dye coupling in the pig coronary arteries. Role of gap junctions. Circulation research, 70(1):49–55.

Boado RJ, Pardridge WM. (1994). Differential expression of alpha-actin mRNA and immunoreactive protein in brain microvascular pericytes and smooth muscle cells. Journal of neuroscience research, 39(4):430–5.

Bobik A, Agrotis A, Kanellakis P, Dilley R, Krushinsky A, Smirnov V, et al. (1999). Distinct patterns of transforming growth factor-beta isoform and receptor expression in human atherosclerotic lesions. Colocalization implicates TGF-beta in fibrofatty lesion development. Circulation, 99(22):2883–91.

Bobryshev YV, Lord RS. (1995). Ultrastructural recognition of cells with dendritic cell morphology in human aortic intima. Contacting interactions of Vascular Dendritic Cells in athero-resistant and athero-prone areas of the normal aorta. Archives of histology and cytology, 58(3):307–22.

Bobryshev YV, Moisenovich MM, Pustovalova OL, Agapov, II, Orekhov AN. (2012). Widespread distribution of HLA-DR-expressing cells in macroscopically undiseased intima of the human aorta: a possible role in surveillance and maintenance of vascular homeostasis. Immunobiology, 217(5):558–68.

Bostrom K, Watson KE, Horn S, Wortham C, Herman IM, Demer LL. (1993). Bone morphogenetic protein expression in human atherosclerotic lesions. The Journal of clinical investigation, 91(4):1800–9.

Brighton CT, Lorich DG, Kupcha R, Reilly TM, Jones AR, Woodbury RA, 2nd. (1992). The pericyte as a possible osteoblast progenitor cell. Clinical orthopaedics and related research, 275:287–99.

Campagnolo P, Cesselli D, Al Haj Zen A, Beltrami AP, Krankel N, Katare R, et al. (2010). Human adult vena saphena contains perivascular progenitor cells endowed with clonogenic and proangiogenic potential. Circulation, 121(15):1735–45.

Campbell JH, Campbell GR. (1989). Biology of the vessel wall and atherosclerosis. Clinical and experimental hypertension Part A, Theory and practice, 11(5–6):901–13.

Davies PF. (1986). Vascular cell interactions with special reference to the pathogenesis of atherosclerosis. Laboratory investigation; a journal of technical methods and pathology. 55(1):5–24.

Diaz-Flores L, Gutierrez R, Lopez-Alonso A, Gonzalez R, Varela H. (1992). Pericytes as a supplementary source of osteoblasts in periosteal osteogenesis. Clinical orthopaedics and related research, 275:280–6.

Diaz-Flores L, Gutierrez R, Varela H, Rancel N, Valladares F. (1991). Microvascular pericytes: a review of their morphological and functional characteristics. Histology and histopathology, 6(2):269–86.

Dore-Duffy P, Wang S, Mehedi A, Katyshev V, Cleary K, Tapper A, et al. (2011). Pericyte-mediated vasoconstriction underlies TBI-induced hypoperfusion. Neurological research, 33(2):176–86.

Geer JC, Haust MD. (1972). Smooth muscle cells in atherosclerosis. Monographs on atherosclerosis, 2(0):1–140.

Geissmann F, Manz MG, Jung S, Sieweke MH, Merad M, Ley K. (2010). Development of monocytes, macrophages, and dendritic cells. Science, 327(5966):656–61.

Hall AP. (2006). Review of the pericyte during angiogenesis and its role in cancer and diabetic retinopathy. Toxicologic pathology, 34(6):763–75.

Handunnetthi L, Ramagopalan SV, Ebers GC, Knight JC. (2010). Regulation of major histocompatibility complex class II gene expression, genetic variation and disease. Genes and immunity, 11(2):99–112.

Hansson GK, Hermansson A. (2011). The immune system in atherosclerosis. Nature immunology, 12(3):204–12.

Hansson GK. (2005). Inflammation, atherosclerosis, and coronary artery disease. The New England journal of medicine, 352(16):1685–95.

Haust MD. (1989). Recent concepts on the pathogenesis of atherosclerosis. CMAJ : Canadian Medical Association journal = journal de l'Association medicale canadienne, 140(8):929.

Ivanov D, Philippova M, Antropova J, Gubaeva F, Iljinskaya O, Tararak E, et al. (2001). Expression of cell adhesion molecule T-cadherin in the human vasculature. Histochemistry and cell biology, 115(3):231–42.

Iyama K, Ohzono K, Usuku G. (1979). Electron microscopical studies on the genesis of white adipocytes:

*differentiation of immature pericytes into adipocytes in transplanted preadipose tissue. Virchows Archiv B, Cell pathology including molecular pathology, 31(2):143–55.*

Juchem G, Weiss DR, Gansera B, Kemkes BM, Mueller-Hoecker J, Nees S. (2010). *Pericytes in the macrovascular intima: possible physiological and pathogenetic impact. American journal of physiology Heart and circulatory physiology, 298(3):H754–70.*

Kaartinen M, Penttila A, Kovanen PT. (1994). *Mast cells of two types differing in neutral protease composition in the human aortic intima. Demonstration of tryptase- and tryptase/chymase-containing mast cells in normal intimas, fatty streaks, and the shoulder region of atheromas. Arteriosclerosis and thrombosis : a journal of vascular biology / American Heart Association, 14(6):966–72.*

Kirton JP, Crofts NJ, George SJ, Brennan K, Canfield AE. (2007). *Wnt/beta-catenin signaling stimulates chondrogenic and inhibits adipogenic differentiation of pericytes: potential relevance to vascular disease? Circulation research, 101(6):581–9.*

Krauss RM. (2010). *Lipoprotein subfractions and cardiovascular disease risk. Current opinion in lipidology, 21(4):305–11.*

Krushinsky AV, Orekhov AN, Smirnov VN. (1983). *Stellate cells in the intima of human aorta. Application of alkaline dissociation method in the analysis of the vessel wall cellular content. Acta anatomica, 117(3):266–9.*

Larson DM, Carson MP, Haudenschild CC. (1987). *Junctional transfer of small molecules in cultured bovine brain microvascular endothelial cells and pericytes. Microvascular research, 34(2):184–99.*

Liu Y, Wilkinson FL, Kirton JP, Jeziorska M, Iizasa H, Sai Y, et al. (2007). *Hepatocyte growth factor and c-Met expression in pericytes: implications for atherosclerotic plaque development. The Journal of pathology, 212(1):12–9.*

Martin SS, Blumenthal RS, Miller M. (2012). *LDL cholesterol: the lower the better. The Medical clinics of North America, 96(1):13–26.*

McGill HC, Jr., Herderick EE, McMahan CA, Zieske AW, Malcolm GT, Tracy RE, et al. (2002). *Atherosclerosis in youth. Minerva pediatrica, 54(5):437–47.*

Moore KJ, Tabas I. (2011). *Macrophages in the pathogenesis of atherosclerosis. Cell, 145(3):341–55.*

Movat HZ, More RH, Haust MD. (1958). *The diffuse intimal thickening of the human aorta with aging. The American journal of pathology, 34(6):1023–31.*

Munro JM, van der Walt JD, Munro CS, Chalmers JA, Cox EL. (1987). *An immunohistochemical analysis of human aortic fatty streaks. Human pathology, 18(4):375–80.*

Nakamura H, Sakurai I. (1992). *Intimal cell population and location in arteries of Japanese children and youth. Angiology, 43(3 Pt 1):229–43.*

Nayak RC, Berman AB, George KL, Eisenbarth GS, King GL. (1988). *A monoclonal antibody (3G5)-defined ganglioside antigen is expressed on the cell surface of microvascular pericytes. The Journal of experimental medicine, 167(3):1003–15.*

Nazarova VL, Andreeva ER, Tertov VV, Gel'dieva BS, Orekhov AN. (1995). *Immunocytochemical study to localize a scavenger receptor in human aorta smooth muscle cells. Biulleten' eksperimental'noi biologii i meditsiny, 120(8):195–8.*

Nicosia RF. (2009). *The aortic ring model of angiogenesis: a quarter century of search and discovery. Journal of cellular and molecular medicine, 13(10):4113–36.*

Oku H, Kodama T, Sakagami K, Puro DG. (2001). *Diabetes-induced disruption of gap junction pathways within the retinal microvasculature. Investigative ophthalmology & visual science, 42(8):1915–20.*

*Orekhov AN, Andreeva ER, Andrianova IV, Bobryshev YV. (2010). Peculiarities of cell composition and cell proliferation in different type atherosclerotic lesions in carotid and coronary arteries. Atherosclerosis. 212(2):436–43.*

*Orekhov AN, Andreeva ER, Krushinsky AV, Novikov ID, Tertov VV, Nestaiko GV, et al. (1986). Intimal cells and atherosclerosis. Relationship between the number of intimal cells and major manifestations of atherosclerosis in the human aorta. The American journal of pathology, 125(2):402–15.*

*Orekhov AN, Andreeva ER, Mikhailova IA, Gordon D. (1998). Cell proliferation in normal and atherosclerotic human aorta: proliferative splash in lipid-rich lesions. Atherosclerosis, 139(1):41–8.*

*Orekhov AN, Andreeva ER, Tertov VV. (1987). The distribution of cells and chemical components in the intima of human aorta. Soc Med Rev A Cardiol,1:75–100.*

*Orekhov AN, Bobryshev YV, Chistiakov DA. (2014). The complexity of cell composition of the intima of large arteries: focus on pericyte-like cells. Cardiovascular research, 103(4):438–51.*

*Orekhov AN, Tertov VV, Kudryashov SA, Smirnov VN. (1990). Triggerlike stimulation of cholesterol accumulation and DNA and extracellular matrix synthesis induced by atherogenic serum or low density lipoprotein in cultured cells. Circulation research, 66(2):311–20.*

*Orekhov AN, Tertov VV, Smirnov VN. (1985). Lipids in cells of atherosclerotic and uninvolved human aorta. II. Lipid metabolism in primary culture. Experimental and molecular pathology, 43(2):187–95.*

*Pober JS, Tellides G. (2012). Participation of blood vessel cells in human adaptive immune responses. Trends in immunology, 33(1):49–57.*

*Rafieian-Kopaei M, Setorki M, Doudi M, Baradaran A, Nasri H. (2014). Atherosclerosis: process, indicators, risk factors and new hopes. International journal of preventive medicine. 5(8):927–46.*

*Rekhter MD, Andreeva ER, Andrianova IV, Mironov AA, Orekhov AN. (1992). Stellate cells of aortic intima: I. Human and rabbit. Tissue & cell. 24(5):689–96.*

*Rekhter MD, Andreeva ER, Mironov AA, Orekhov AN. (1991). Three-dimensional cytoarchitecture of normal and atherosclerotic intima of human aorta. The American journal of pathology, 138(3):569–80.*

*Ross R. (1999). Atherosclerosis — an inflammatory disease. The New England journal of medicine, 340(2):115–26.*

*Shao JS, Cai J, Towler DA. (2006). Molecular mechanisms of vascular calcification: lessons learned from the aorta. Arteriosclerosis, thrombosis, and vascular biology, 26(7):1423–30.*

*Shepro D, Morel NM. (1993). Pericyte physiology. FASEB journal : official publication of the Federation of American Societies for Experimental Biology, 7(11):1031–8.*

*Sims DE. (1991). Recent advances in pericyte biology — implications for health and disease. The Canadian journal of cardiology, 7(10):431–43.*

*Stary HC. (1994). Changes in components and structure of atherosclerotic lesions developing from childhood to middle age in coronary arteries. Basic research in cardiology, 89 Suppl 1:17–32.*

*Stary HC. (1989). Evolution and progression of atherosclerotic lesions in coronary arteries of children and young adults. Arteriosclerosis, 9(1 Suppl):I19–32.*

*Takeuchi T, Ohtsuki Y. (2001). Recent progress in T-cadherin (CDH13, H-cadherin) research. Histology and histopathology, 16(4):1287–93.*

*Tertov VV, Sobenin IA, Gabbasov ZA, Popov EG, Jaakkola O, Solakivi T, et al. (1992). Multiple-modified* desialylated low density lipoproteins that cause intracellular lipid accumulation. Isolation, fractionation and characterization. Laboratory investigation; a journal of technical methods and pathology, 67(5):665–75.

Trautmann A. (1988). Functions of gap junction channels in the open and closed states. Biochemical Society transactions, 16(4):534–6.

Tuzcu EM, Kapadia SR, Tutar E, Ziada KM, Hobbs RE, McCarthy PM, et al. (2001). High prevalence of coronary atherosclerosis in asymptomatic teenagers and young adults: evidence from intravascular ultrasound. Circulation, 103(22):2705–10.

Van Dijk CG, Nieuweboer FE, Pei JY, Xu YJ, Burgisser P, van Mulligen E, et al. (2015). The complex mural cell: Pericyte function in health and disease. International journal of cardiology, 190:75–89.

Velican D, Velican C. (1977). Histochemical study on the glycosaminoglycans (acid mucopolysaccharides) of the human coronary arteries. Acta histochemica, 59(2):190–200.

Von Willebrand E, Lautenschlager I, Inkinen K, Lehto VP, Virtanen I, Hayry P. (1985). Distribution of the major histocompatibility complex antigens in human and rat kidney. Kidney international, 27(4):616–21.

Weber C, Noels H. (2011). Atherosclerosis: current pathogenesis and therapeutic options. Nature medicine, 17(11):1410–22.

Yuan Y, Li P, Ye J. (2012). Lipid homeostasis and the formation of macrophage-derived foam cells in atherosclerosis. Protein & cell, 3(3):173–81.

# Chapter 4

# Comparative Cost-Effectiveness of Coflex® Interlaminar Stabilization vs. Instrumented Fusion

Jordana Kate Schmier[1], Greg Maislin[2] and Kevin Ong[3]

## 1  Introduction

Lumbar spinal stenosis (LSS), which involves narrowing of the spinal canal and sympto-matic neurogenic compression, affects as much as 38.8% of adults 60 years and older in the United States (Kalichman et al., 2009). This symptomatology, including patients with neuropathic pain, has been shown to have substantial effects on quality of life and func-tioning, with severe low back pain having a particularly extensive impact on patients (Schaefer et al., 2014; Battie et al., 2012; Sigmundsson et al., 2013). As the population ages, the prevalence and overall burden of LSS is likely to increase (Otani et al., 2013). A trend towards increased hospitalization is already evident, although changes in the demo-graphic characteristics of LSS patients suggest the rate of increase may slow in coming years (Skolasky et al., 2013). There is some evidence of the effectiveness of nonsurgical treatments such as pharmacologic therapy, intramuscular calcitonin and epidural steroid injections, yet there is concern that the design and quality of existing studies limits the understanding of these treatments and that they may be minimally beneficial in most patients and are much as three times more expensive than open surgical decompression (Harrop et al., 2014). It is noteworthy that after seeking conservative treatment for LSS, many patients do not progress to surgery immediately; in fact, only one-fifth of Medicare

[1] Health Sciences, Exponent Inc., Alexandria, Virgia, USA.

[2] Biomedical Statistical Consulting, Wynnewood, Pennsylvania, USA.

[3] Biomedical Engineering, Exponent Inc., Philadelphia, Pennsylvania, USA.

beneficiaries diagnosed in 2003 with LSS underwent surgery wthin the three years after diagnosis (Chen et al., 2010). When conservative care fails, surgical decompression, with or without instrumented fusion, is effective for the majority of LSS patients (North American Spine Society, 2007), however, newer surgical options such as interspinous implants have also demonstrated clinical effectiveness in patients for whom conservative treatments have failed (Bono & Vaccaro, 2007).

Several studies have quantified the costs of surgical treatment for LSS. Some of these studies limit their analyses to surgical costs and do not identify any differences in treatment expenditures past the initial hospitalization (Katz et al., 1997; Deyo et al., 2010). Others suggest that there is a short-term increase in post-surgical health care resource, although over time it returns to pre-surgery levels (Andersen et al., 2013). Decompression surgery appeared much more cost-effective than fusion when each was compared to nonsurgical intervention among stenosis patients enrolled in the Spine Patient Outcomes Research Trial (SPORT) (Tosteson et al., 2008), while a Swedish study found fusion to be cost-effective compared to nonsurgical treatment (Fritzell et al., 2004). Overall, though, cost-effectiveness of treatment strategies remains uncertain partly due to the heterogeneity of studies and difficulty in aggregating findings (Harrop et al., 2014). While the overall rates of surgery for LSS have decreased from 2002 to 2007, the rate of multi-level fusion procedures increased by 15-fold (Deyo et al., 2010). Multi-level fusion procedures were shown to be more costly and associated with significantly more life-threatening complications and re-hospitalizations than decompression alone, particularly within 30 days post-surgery (Deyo et al., 2010). Yet, limited data on multi-level fusion procedures makes it challenging to evaluate cost-effectiveness of treatments for LSS (Harrop et al., 2014) in light of the shift to more multi-level procedures.

The coflex® interlaminar stabilization device has been approved as an alternative to spinal fusion in the treatment of spinal stenosis with or without low grade spondylolisthesis. The 2-year clinical and radiographic results (Davis R et al., 2013; Davis RJ et al., 2013) and a comparative cost-effectiveness of these treatments (Schmier et al., 2014) have been reported. The cost study found that coflex "dominated" the alternative of fusion, that is, it had lower costs and better outcomes than fusion. Other studies appear to confirm its clinical value (Kumar et al., 2014; Roder et al., 2014). In this chapter, we describe a health care economic model to estimate the direct health care costs and quality-adjusted life years of coflex®-treated patients compared to patients treated with instrumented posterolateral fusion over a five-year period using updated clinical inputs and costs.

# 2  Methods

Multiple sources of data were utilized as inputs to the economic model. The model incorporates clinical and patient-reported data, treatment patterns and costs into an Excel spreadsheet. The model presents costs (presented in 2014 dollars) both based on the US Medicare fee schedule and from a commercial payer perspective. Five-year costs and outcomes were estimated and discounted annually at 3% in the base case. The structure of the model is illustrated in Figure 1.

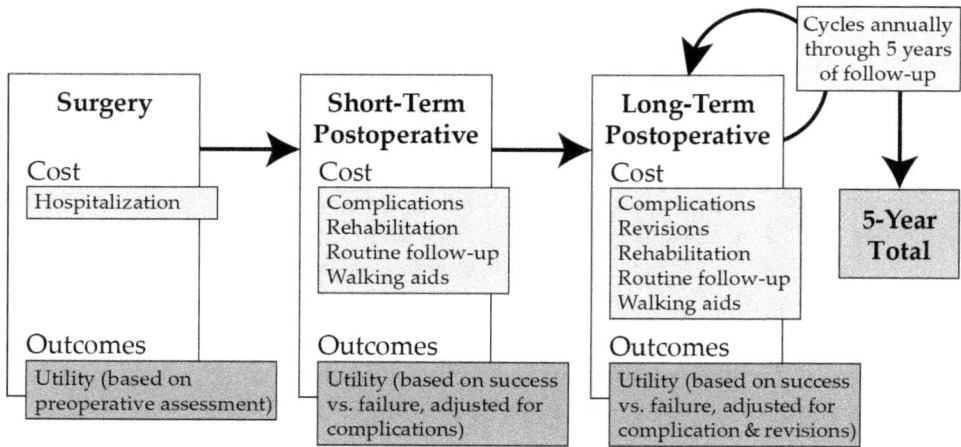

**Figure 1:** Model Structure.

The clinical data inputs were based on 4-year follow-up of patients enrolled in a randomized Investigational Device Exemption (IDE) clinical trial comparing coflex® to instrumented fusion. Two- and three-year results have been previously reported by Davis et al (Davis R *et al.*, 2013; David RJ *et al.*, 2013; Davis RJ *et al.*, 2014). Patients included in the trial had LSS in one or two vertebral levels from L1 to L5 and had undergone at least 6 months' of conservative treatment. Patients were randomized in a 2:1 ratio to either the investigational arm (coflex® Interlaminar Stabilization Device following laminec-tomy/decompression) or to the control arm (posterolateral fusion with autograft and ped-icle screw fixation preceding or following laminectomy/decompression). The per protocol analysis for the trial included 215 patients in the coflex® arm and 107 patients in the con-trol arm. The primary endpoint evaluated for FDA approval was a composite clinical suc-cess (CCS) assessment that was comprised of the following components: an improvement of at least 15 points on the Oswestry Disability Index; no reoperations, revisions, or sup-plemental fixation; no lumbar epidural steroid injections; no major device-related com-plications and no new or worsening, persistent neurologic deficits. The two-year results showed that coflex® successfully met the non-inferiority endpoint as compared to instru-mented fusion (Bayesian posterior probability = 0.999 using a non-inferiority margin of 0.10). Three-year findings reflected clinical composite success with superiority of coflex after decompression versus decompression with instrumented spinal fusion. Results at four (Bae *et al.*, 2015) and five (Arega *et al.*, 2006) years showed similar trends.

To ensure the data from this study could not potentially be influenced by the spon-sor, data management was outsourced in its entirety to an independent Clinical Research Organization (CRO) with no financial ties to the study sponsor. Similarly, to minimize site-to-site reporting variability, all adverse events were adjudicated by an independent Clinical Events Committee (CEC) with the adjudication binding on the sponsor (Auer-bach *et al.*, 2013).

As part of the composite endpoint, the clinical trial included the Oswestry Disability Index (ODI), a patient-reported questionnaire completed by trial participants at every follow-up visit. Using a published algorithm, the ODI allowed for derivation of SF-6D utility scores (Carreon *et al.*, 2009). Scores were calculated at various time points for patients and reported for those who achieved clinical success or failure and among patients who experienced particular adverse events or complications.

Costs for the index procedure were derived from the Medicare Fee Schedule, as published by the Centers for Medicare and Medicaid Services, and included payment for physician services and inpatient hospital reimbursement for the index surgical procedure. The 2014 Medicare Physician Fee Schedule and applicable conversion factor were used to derive the reimbursement for physician services for each primary procedure. Physician services included the index procedure as well as certain follow-up services occurring up to 90 days post-operatively and thus covered as part of the global surgery package. The 2014 Inpatient Prospective Payment System (IPPS) Final Rule was used to estimate the Medicare national average for the applicable Medical Severity Diagnosis-Related Group (MS-DRG) to which each primary procedure would typically be assigned. The DRG reimbursement amounts represented the total payment provided to the hospital. Professional services billed by the surgeons, which are billed separately, were also included in the model. As the reimbursement for devices and medical supplies is included in the DRG reimbursement, no additional or separate reimbursement for implanted devices was considered. It was assumed that primary procedures were performed in an inpatient setting and would be coded using the appropriate CPT codes to report the implantation of coflex® following decompression or posterolateral fusion with pedicle screw fixation and autograft bone following decompressive laminectomy. Based on the clinical data from the IDE trial, the payment amount used in the model assumed that 68% of cases were 1-level procedures and the remainder was 2-level procedures. The costs for the procedure used as the base case in the model reflect this distribution of 1- versus 2-level procedures.

For both cohorts, expected treatment patterns through five years were derived from published sources (North America Spine Society, 2007), analysis of the Medicare Limited Data Set (LDS) 5% Sample (2005–2009) (Auerbach JD *et al.*, 2012) and expert opinion (a survey of six orthopedic practices in the United States). Treatment patterns from the IDE trial could not be used directly because of the various protocol-driven assessments, such as imaging requirements, as well as the number of follow-up visits (week 6, months 3, 6, 12, 18, and yearly thereafter), both of which exceed the normal standard of care. The expert opinion elicitation consisted of a survey, asking surgeons to provide details on expected follow up care for patients, including the specific Current Procedural Terminology (CPT) codes and the frequency of each encounter or procedure. Participants were given an initial list that included outpatient visits, imaging (X-ray, magnetic resonance imaging, and computed tomography), and physical and occupational therapy. Participants were also asked to include other encounters, and acupuncture and chiropractic care were added in this fashion. The reimbursement amount from the Medicare Fee Schedule (for the Medicare cost estimate) or the 75th percentile of a national average usual and customary rate (Practice Management Information Corporation, 2010) (for the private insurance cost estimate) was multiplied by the average cost per year for each category of care from the survey, taking into account the frequency and the specific amount for each CPT code.

Annual follow-up expenses were estimated by weighting costs for each of the resources identified by the expert panel by the proportion of patients who would be expected to use each type of resource. Thus, for example, if 20% of patients were expected to have a certain test, then the model applied 20% of the cost for the test to each patient. Using this approach, an average cost per patient was developed. Sensitivity analyses examined the robustness of the findings and identified the inputs that most strongly influenced the model. This was accomplished by varying multipliers for specific resources and utilities, i.e., increasing or decreasing them by a set amount. Threshold analyses were used to determine the point at which changes in key model inputs result in a reversal of study conclusions.

Complication rates were derived from the clinical trial, while costs associated with treating complications were derived from analysis of the Thomson Reuters MarketScan data (Auerbach J et al., 2012) and scaled down for the Medicare analysis. Commercial insurance rate was assumed to be 20% greater than the Medicare payment. This was a conservative (i.e., high) estimate of commercial payments to Medicare rates, as anecdotal evidence indicates that payments made by commercial insurance carriers are typically higher than 20% above Medicare rates.

As much as possible, data collected directly from the coflex® U.S. IDE clinical trial were used for the model. Interested readers are directed to these studies for more detailed clinical findings (Davis R et al., 2013; Davis RJ et al., 2013; Bae et al., 2015). Demographic, clinical, and health status characteristics from the trial are presented in Table 1.

| Characteristic | coflex® | Instrumented Fusion | P-value* |
|---|---|---|---|
| N | 215 | 107 | |
| Age, mean ± standard deviation | 62.1 ± 9.2 | 64.1 ± 9.0 | 0.089 |
| Gender, % female | 49.3% | 54.2% | 0.411 |
| Race, % white | 88.8% | 86.96% | 0.381 |
| Current smoker, % yes | 10.2% | 14.0% | 0.355 |
| 1 level decompression | 64.2% | 63.6% | 1.000 |
| BMI | 29.7 ± 4.5 | 29.6 ± 4.9 | 0.789 |
| Oswestry Disability Index | 60.8 ± 11.8 | 60.7 ± 11.5 | 0.911 |
| SF-12 PCS | 28.1 ± 6.6 | 28.2 ± 6.0 | 0.745 |
| SF-12 MCS | 45.5 ± 13.0 | 44.9 ± 12.2 | 0.706 |
| VAS back pain | 79.5 ± 15.0 | 79.2 ± 13.5 | 0.584 |
| Utilities | 0.468 | 0.468 | 1.000 |

**Table 1:** Baseline Demographic and Clinical Characteristics of Trial Participants. *All were not statistically significant, i.e., p > 0.05.

There were no significant differences in baseline or disease severity characteristics between the coflex® and instrumented fusion groups. Patients who reported complications were scored with mild decrements; e.g., those patients with component problems had a utility score of 0.637 while those reporting new or worsening pain reported a score of 0.604. Expert opinion was used to estimate the number of months over which each complication affected utilities. For example, a fracture was assumed to affect utility scores for 9 months while a wound problem decreased utilities for 1 month. After this decrement, patients bounced back to a pre-adverse event utility score. These values were also subjected to sensitivity analysis. The same utility values were used for both cohorts; that is, regardless of how the patient achieved clinical success, the same value was assigned. Similarly, regardless of the type of surgery that was followed by a wound infection, the utility value assigned for the wound infection was identical across cohorts. This approach is based on the assumption that the utility value should be guided by the current health state, not by prior surgical history.

# 3   Results

Clinical inputs to the model are presented in Table 2. These include the rates of clinical success and complications. Note that success and failure would sum to 100%; failure is the inverse of success and is not shown in the table. Patients could meet the criteria for clinical success but still experience a complication, and patients could experience more than one complication. Thus success and complications should not be summed together; nor should complications be summed. Complications were recorded as having occurred at least once during an interval; it was not reported whether patients had a single event of a complication or if a complication could have occurred twice during the assessment interval. Utilities are also presented in Table 2. Based on ODI scores measured before randomization, the pre-operative utility score was determined to be 0.468, reflecting patient-reported well-being in the immediate pre-procedure time period. Those who achieved overall clinical success had utility scores increase to 0.687, while those with failure had utility calculated at 0.583. Utility values for patients who had each type of complication, as measured at the assessment during which the complication was reported, also appear in Table 2.

Costs for complications used as inputs to the model appear in Table 3. Treatment costs associated with routine follow-up care and for selected complications are presented in Table 4. Costs presented in the table reflect the average payment per person, with a combination of physician expert opinion and reimbursement fee schedules used as source data. Rates of utilization of each health care resource or complication were multiplied by the listed cost per encounter or complication. For simplicity, the table presents only summary information, but it is important to note that the values in this table take into account a variety of costs and are designed not to include visits already covered as part of the global surgery payment amount. For example, based on input from an orthopedic expert panel regarding the first six weeks after surgery, all patients treated with coflex® would have an X-ray procedure (CPT 72100, reimbursed at $37 by Medi care), 30% would have

| Event | coflex® Rate (%) | | | | Fusion Rate (%) | | | | Utilities[1] |
|---|---|---|---|---|---|---|---|---|---|
| Year | 1 | 2 | 3 | 4 | 1 | 2 | 3 | 4 | n/a |
| Clinical success[2] | 74.8 | 66.2 | 62.8 | 54.9 | 71.2 | 57.7 | 47.4 | 46.7 | 0.687 |
| Complications — Component problems | 0.9 | 1.5 | 0.0 | 0.6 | 0.9 | 2.0 | 0.0 | 4.8 | 0.637 |
| Complications — Deep infection | 0.9 | 0.0 | 0.0 | 0.0 | 0.0 | 0.0 | 0.0 | 0.0 | 0.531 |
| Complications — Fracture | 4.7 | 0.5 | 1.1 | 0.0 | 2.8 | 0.0 | 0.0 | 0.0 | 0.531 |
| Complications — Wound problems | 13.5 | 0.0 | 0.0 | 0.0 | 9.3 | 0.0 | 0.0 | 0.0 | 0.614 |
| Complications — New or worsening pain | 28.8 | 14.4 | 9.4 | 9.8 | 26.2 | 18.0 | 14.9 | 7.1 | 0.604 |

[1] Computed from Oswestry Disability Index scores based on methods described in Carreon (Carreon *et al.*, 2009). Utilities were calculated based on scores reported from patients who had each event during the most recent interval, regardless of whether they achieved clinical success.

[2] The overall success endpoints over time were similarly defined except that the Month 12 endpoint did not include 'new or worsening, persistent neurological deficit'. This is because 'persistence' was not evaluable until Month 24 (and later).

[3] Patients could have had more than one complication.

**Table 2:** Clinical Inputs.

| Type of Cost | Medicare | Private Insurance | Source |
|---|---|---|---|
| Component problems | $13,090 | $15,708 | Auerbach J et al., 2012. |
| Deep infection | $9,995 | $11,994 | Auerbach J et al., 2012. |
| Fracture | $5,324 | $6,389 | Auerbach J et al., 2012. |
| Wound infection | $10,348 | $12,417 | Auerbach J et al., 2012. |
| New or worsening pain | $376 | $451 | Outpatient visit (CPT 99245) plus either X-ray (CPT 72110) or MRI (CPT 72148). |

**Table 3:** Complication Costs, Per Event. Abbrev.: CPT = Current Procedural Technology. MRI = Magnetic Resonance Imaging.

| Type of Cost | Medicare | | Private Insurance | |
|---|---|---|---|---|
| | coflex® | Fusion | coflex® | Fusion |
| Index hospitalization | $12,411 | $24,395 | $14,893 | $29,277 |
| Routine follow-up care through 12 months | $344 | $416 | $1,070 | $1,350 |
| — Evaluation and management (outpatient visits, CPT 99241-99245, 99212) | $124 | $149 | $155 | $186 |
| — Imaging (CPT 72100, 72110, 72114, 72120, 72131, 72148) | $134 | $160 | $180 | $216 |
| — Physical and/or occupational therapy (CPT 97001-97004, 97110-97140, 97535) | $80 | $96 | $70 | $84 |
| — Irrigation and debridement (CPT 10140) | $2 | $2 | $7 | $8 |
| — Alternative and complementary medicine (CPT 98940-98942, 97810-97814) | $1 | $6 | $5 | $6 |
| Complications through 12 months[1] | $1,963 | $1,328 | $2,356 | $1,593 |
| — Component problems | $117 | $118 | $141 | $141 |
| — Deep infection | $89 | $0 | $108 | $0 |
| — Fracture | $250 | $149 | $300 | $179 |
| — Wound infection | $1397 | $962 | $1676 | $1155 |
| — New or worsening pain | $108 | $98 | $130 | $118 |
| Follow-up care, total years 2-5 | $119 | $208 | $341 | $987 |
| — Evaluation and management (outpatient visits, CPT 99241-99245, 99212) | $94 | $60 | $223 | $137 |
| — Imaging (CPT 72100, 72110, 72114, 72120, 72131, 72148) | $15 | $131 | $94 | $809 |
| — Physical and/or occupational therapy (CPT 97001-97004, 97110-97140, 97535) | $10 | $17 | $25 | $41 |
| — Irrigation and debridement (CPT 10140) | $0 | $0 | $0 | $0 |
| — Alternative and complementary medicine (CPT 98940-98942, 97810-97814) | $4 | $0 | $0 | $0 |
| Complications, total years 2-5[1] | $407 | $970 | $489 | $1,164 |
| — Component problems | $262 | $827 | $315 | $992 |
| — Deep infection | $0 | $0 | $0 | $0 |
| — Fracture | $26 | $0 | $31 | $0 |
| — Wound infection | $0 | $0 | $0 | $0 |
| — New or worsening pain | $119 | $143 | $143 | $172 |

[1] Table 2 presents the proportion of patients experiencing each complication at each time period:
- Costs are expressed in 2014 US$. Numbers may not sum due to rounding. Values presented for years 2-5 have been discounted.
- Hospitalization costs were derived from published values for the Diagnosis-Related Group from the Inpatient Prospective Payment System Final Rule, and included the inpatient hospital reimbursement and payment for physician services.
- Routine follow-up care costs were based on applying CPT codes from the Medicare Physician Fee Schedule to survey data provided by orthopedic surgeons that estimated the number of outpatient visits, imaging, and physical and occupational therapy encounters.
- Complication rates were derived from the IDE trial with costs derived from analyses of Medicare and commercial data for patients with the CPT or ICD-9 codes for each relevant complication.

**Table 4:** Cost Inputs, Annual Average Per Patient.

an additional X-ray (CPT 72110, reimbursed at $51 by Medicare), 1% would have an MRI (CPT 74128, reimbursed at $246 by Medicare) and 9% would have a physical therapy evaluation (CPT 97001, reimbursed at $76 by Medicare). Similarly, among patients treated with instrumented fusion an X-ray procedure, 20% would have an additional X-ray, 2% would have a CT scan (CPT 72131, reimbursed at $177 by Medicare) and 2% would have a physical therapy evaluation. Over these initial six weeks, average Medicare reimbursements, excluding payment for the index event and follow-up services considered to be part of the global surgery package, were estimated to be $344 for coflex® patients and $416 for instrumented fusion patients. The plurality of follow-up costs was attributed to imaging in the first year; physical and occupational therapy were responsible for costs in the first year but tapered off afterwards. Alternative and complementary medicine was mentioned by survey participants; the small costs attributed to these encounters (chiropractic and acupuncture) are also included. Table 4 also presents the costs for routine follow-up care and complications (of which there were few reported) in years two through five after surgery. The table aggregates costs over those four years, with appropriate discounting (3% in the base case) conducted to arrive at the total cost. In the years after surgery, patients from both study cohorts attended similar rates of outpatient visits but the instrumented fusion patients were expected to have higher use of X-rays, in order to verify bony fusion success over time. Patients treated with instrumented fusion typically have more use of physical therapy, which is associated with increased annual costs, with the costs for years two through five being more than twice as high for patients who had undergone fusion compared to coflex® patients.

Initial costs were substantially greater for fusion compared to coflex® patients, as shown in Table 5. Expected costs for the initial procedure, as reimbursed by Medicare, were determined to be $14,617 for coflex® patients and $26,239 for fusion patients. Over the five-year follow-up horizon, expected costs were $15,244 and $27,316, respectively, for coflex® and fusion.

As five-year results have not yet been reported, the weighted utility values from 48 months, which took into account the success rates at that time period, were applied to the final year of the model and discounted from the 48-month value at the same 3% rate as other costs and outcomes. Quality-adjusted life years (QALYs) over a five-year period were estimated to be 2.99 for coflex®-treated patients and 2.98 for instrumented fusion patients. Because coflex® patients were determined to have both lower average costs and higher average utilities over five years than those patients treated with fusion, there was no need to consider the comparison in terms of trade-offs between the costs and benefits of the investigational device via calculation of an incremental cost-effectiveness ratio (ICER) ratio; for coflex® both the QALYs and the costs were better than the comparator (fusion). In the terms of health economics, coflex® was said to dominate fusion, since outcomes were favorable in terms of costs (lower) and outcomes (better).

Sensitivity analyses explored varying input parameters. Changing the discount rate had almost no effect because more than 75% of the cost for each cohort was attributed to the initial year, before any discounting would apply (Table 6). Sensitivity analyses showed no reasonable scenario in which coflex® would not be cost-effective compared to instrumented fusion.

|  | coflex® | Fusion |
|---|---|---|
| Total cost | $15,244 | $27,316 |
| Total utilities | 2.99 | 2.98 |
| Incremental cost-effectiveness ratio | Cannot be calculated: coflex® dominates | |

**Table 5:** Model Results: Base Case — Medicare.

| Assumptions | | coflex® | | Fusion | | ICER |
|---|---|---|---|---|---|---|
| | | Cost | QALYs | Cost | QALYs | |
| Base case – Medicare | | $15,244 | 2.99 | $27,316 | 2.98 | coflex® dominates |
| Sensitivity analyses | Discount 0% | $15,274 | 3.20 | $27,403 | 3.16 | coflex® dominates |
| | Discount 5% | $15,225 | 2.87 | $27,261 | 2.86 | coflex® dominates |
| | Increase costs by 25% | $19,055 | 2.99 | $34,145 | 2.98 | coflex® dominates |
| | Decrease costs by 25% | $11,433 | 2.99 | $20,487 | 2.98 | coflex® dominates |
| | Increase utilities by 25% | $15,244 | 3.74 | $27,316 | 3.72 | coflex® dominates |
| | Decrease utilities by 25% | $15,244 | 2.25 | $27,316 | 2.23 | coflex® dominates |

**Table 6:** Model Results and Selected Sensitivity Analyses Based on Medicare Base Case. Note: Only surgical costs and success and failure rates have been changed for the one and two level analyses. Complication rates and costs associated with complications have not been changed from the base case.

Assuming Medicare payment rates and 3% discounting, threshold analyses revealed that coflex® could cost as much as $24,482 ($12,071 more than the current cost) and still be no more costly than instrumented fusion over the observation period. Similarly, fusion payments would need to be decreased to $12,322 (from the current $24,395 cost) in order to achieve the same five-year costs as coflex®.

# 4    Discussion

The safety and clinical equivalence of coflex® interlaminar stabilization compared to fusion has now been established (Davis R *et al.*, 2013; Davis RJ *et al.*, 2013). Our previous study reported substantial advantage in cost-effectiveness with coflex® compared to fusion using data from the first two years of the IDE (Schmier *et al.*, 2014). The current study incorporated trial data for two additional years and found similar results. Over the five-year follow-up period, total costs were consistently lower for patients who received coflex® procedure than for those who underwent fusion and patient-reported utilities also consistently favored coflex® patients. Thus, coflex® is said to dominate fusion, with lower costs and better patient-reported outcomes.

This study has several limitations that should be considered when interpreting the results. The analysis is limited by the clinical input assumptions that were required in order to develop the model. Perhaps the most obvious clinical assumption is the metric of success: the composite clinical success (CCS) endpoint used in the IDE trial. The CCS was designed to incorporate multiple types of measures, and is likely a conservative measure of success. For example, use of one of the components of the CCS, a 15-point improvement on the ODI, alone would have favored coflex® more.

Other clinical inputs also are sources of uncertainty. For example, while the trial outcomes were essential to determining the cost-effectiveness of coflex®, a wider patient population might differ from a randomized clinical trial cohort. Further, the model used clinical data from a 48-month analysis and while only 12 months remained in the study, it is possible that there might be slight modifications of results once those data are available.

Utility values in this model were calculated based on patient-reported Oswestry Disability Index (ODI) scores using a published algorithm (Carreon et al., 2009), as there was no direct utility elicitation included in the IDE trial. A range of direct or estimated utility values have been reported in other studies using other tools such as the EQ-5D, Health Utilities Index, and the SF-6D (Suarez-Almazor et al., 2000; Tosteson et al., 2011). The utility values are similar to those found in our patient population although our sample sizes were smaller, but it is challenging to compare across studies because there is evidence that the choice of assessment tool can affect utility scores (Tosteson et al., 2011). In this model, which used a fairly narrow difference in utility values for success and failure, and relatively small variation in utility decrements associated with complications across the cohorts, there was no reasonable scenario in which patients treated with coflex® would have utilities that were not higher than fusion patients.

The difference in utilities over the five-year period in this study was small, with the base case favoring coflex by 0.01 units. This is on the low side of estimates for meaningful differences or change in utility assessments (Horsman et al., 2003). However it is perhaps more important that this gap persisted and that it only increased in the course of sensitivity analyses. Although there was never a large difference between QALYs in the coflex® and fusion cohorts, the difference always favored coflex®. The algorithm used to convert the ODI to utilities effectively constrains variation since the highest possible utility value is 0.78 (Carreon et al., 2009), thus even a highly effective intervention in an otherwise healthy population would limit the maximum number of QALYs, based on the ODI, to less than 3.9 over a five-year period. Considered in this context, smaller differences and the consistent direction of the model's findings should be valued more highly.

The cost differences determined in this study are subject to various other uncertainties. Although cost inputs to the model were based on standard and nationally-representative amounts, there is variation among these sources and other factors, such as hospital size or type, geography, and patient mix (Wasserman Medical Publishers, 2011; MAG Mutual Healthcare Solutions Inc., 2011; FAIR Health, 2016). Costs for spinal surgeries among Medicare beneficiaries have been found to vary substantially (Schoenfeld et al., 2014) and the applicability of findings may be limited; however the five-year reimbursements are similar to those estimated in another study of instrumented fusion (Glassman *et al.*, 2012). The panel of orthopedic experts that supplied guidance on treatment patterns suggested that patients may use a cane or walker for a period of time after surgery. Because these costs are highly variable due to differences in local coverage policies and rates, we did not include them. However, given that the use of these assistive devices was expected to be higher and/or for longer periods among fusion patients, the decision not to include them is conservative, that is, had they been included, they likely would have favored coflex® over fusion.

The use of reimbursed costs rather than submitted charges is another limitation that may affect how providers can use these data. Reimbursed amounts may cover costs for certain procedures at some facilities; in other cases, there may be substantial differentials between what proportion of actual costs are covered even among procedures that may seem similar. Also, certain facilities may find more intrinsic value in lower complication rates, either due to initiatives to reduce specific events or the increased availability of resources for other patients. Certain benefits may be more meaningful based on the circumstances at that site; however, the substantial advantages shown by coflex® are likely to be recognized widely.

# 5   Conclusion

Physicians and the health insurance communities each have vested interest in identifying treatment options for moderate to severe LSS with and without spondylolisthesis that are both clinically beneficial and cost-effective. Future risk sharing arrangements and bundled payment options for payors and providers will focus on value and comparative effectiveness for reform-based underwriting and overall cost savings. This study found that over five years, treatment with coflex® resulted in substantial reductions in health care costs accompanied by increases in patient-reported utilities compared to patients treated with fusion. This finding was robust and no reasonable sensitivity analysis scenario identified instrumented fusion as a cost-effective option compared to coflex®.

# Acknowledgement

We thank Edmund Lau, MS, of Exponent for his analytic contribution to this manuscript.

# Disclosure

Exponent has been paid fees for the consulting services related to this research by Paradigm Spine, LLC (New York, NY). Authors JS and KO are employees of Exponent; GM is the owner of Biomedical Statistical Consulting. The initial framework and problem statement was developed by JS and KO. JS developed the model with input from KO. GM provided analytic support for model inputs. JS drafted the manuscript; GM and KO provided critical input and approval of the final version. Results from an analysis with two-year data from the IDE have been published (Schmier *et al.*, 2014).

# References

Andersen, T., Bunger, C., & Sogaard, R. (2013). *Long-term health care utilization and costs after spinal fusion in elderly patients. European Spine Journal, 22(5), 977–984.*

Arega, A., Birkmeyer, N.J., Lurie, J.D., Tosteson, T., Gibson, J., Taylor, B.A., Morgan, T.S., & Weinstein, J.N. (2006). *Racial variation in treatment preferences and willingness to randomize in the Spine Patient Outcomes Research Trial (SPORT). Spine (Phila Pa 1976), 31(19), 2263–2269.*

Auerbach, J., Schmier, J., Ong, K., Lau, E., & Zigler, J. (2012). *Cost-effectiveness of coflex interlaminar stabilization compared with instrumental posterior spinal fusion for spinal stenosis and spondylolisthesis. Paper presented at: North American Spine Society 27ᵗʰ Annual Meeting; October 24–27, 2012; Dallas, TX.*

Auerbach, J.D., McGowan, K.B., Halevi, M., Gerling, M.C., Sharan, A.D., Whang, P.G., & Maislin, G. (2013). *Mitigating adverse event reporting bias in spine surgery. Journal of Bone & Joint Surgery Am., 95(16), 1450–1456.*

Auerbach, J.D., Ong, K.L., Lau, E., Ochoa, J., Schmier, J.K., & Zigler, J.D. (2012). *Perioperative outcomes, complications, and costs associated with lumbar spinal fusion in older patients with spinal stenosis and spondylolisthesis: analysis of the United States Medicare claims database. Value in Health, 15(4), A3.*

Bae, H.W., Lauryssen, C., Maislin, G., Leary, S., & Musacchio, M.J., Jr. (2015). *Therapeutic sustainability and durability of coflex interlaminar stabilization after decompression for lumbar spinal stenosis: a four year assessment. International Journal of Spine Surgery, 9, 15.*

Battie, M.C., Jones, C.A., Schopflocher, D.P., & Hu, R.W. (2012). *Health-related quality of life and comorbidities associated with lumbar spinal stenosis. The Spine Journal, 12(3), 189–195.*

Bono, C.M. & Vaccaro, A.R. (2007). *Interspinous process devices in the lumbar spine. Journal of Spinal Disorders & Techniques, 20(3), 255–261.*

Carreon, L.Y., Glassman, S.D., McDonough, C.M., Rampersaud, R., Berven, S., & Shainline, M. (2009). *Predicting SF-6D utility scores from the Oswestry disability index and numeric rating scales for back and leg pain. Spine (Phila PA 1976), 34(19), 2085–2089.*

Chen, E., Tong, K.B., & Laouri, M. (2010). *Surgical treatment patterns among Medicare beneficiaries newly diagnosed with lumbar spinal stenosis. The Spine Journal, 10(7), 588–594.*

Davis, R., Auerbach, J.D., Bae, H., & Errico, T.J. (2013). *Can low-grade spondylolisthesis be effectively treated by either coflex interlaminar stabilization or laminectomy and posterior spinal fusion? Two-year clinical and radiographic results from the randomized, prospective, multicenter US investigational device exemption trial: clinical article. Journal of Neurosurgery: Spine, 19(2), 174–184.*

Davis, R.J., Errico, T.J., Bae, H., & Auerbach, J.D. (2013). *Decompression and coflex interlaminar stabilization compared with decompression and instrumented spinal fusion for spinal stenosis and low-grade degenerative spondylolisthesis: two-year results from the prospective, randomized, multicenter, Food and Drug Administration Investigational Device Exemption trial. Spine (Phila PA 1976), 38(18), 1529–1539.*

Davis, R.J., Errico, T.J., Bae, H.W., Lauryssen, C., & Leary, S.P. (2014). *Decompression and implantation of an interlaminar stabilization implant for the minimally invasive treatment of lumbar spinal stenosis with back pain; operative and three year clinical and radiographic outcomes from a level 1 US IDE study. Society for Minimally Investive Spine Surgery Global Forum 2014. Miami, FL.*

Deyo, R.A., Mirza, S.K., Martin, B.I., Kreuter, W., Goodman, D.C., & Jarvik, J.G. (2010). *Trends, major medical complications, and charges associated with surgery for lumbar spinal stenosis in older adults. Journal of the American Medical Association, 303(13), 1259–1265.*

FAIR Health. *FH Benchmarks (description available at http://www.fairhealthus.org/DataSolution?sk= STANDARD%20PRODUCTS). Accessed March 2 2016.*

Fritzell, P., Hagg, O., Jonsson, D., Nordwall, A., & Swedish Lumbar Spine Study Group. (2004). *Cost-effectiveness of lumbar fusion and nonsurgical treatment for chronic low back pain in the Swedish Lumbar Spine Study: a multicenter, randomized, controlled trial from the Swedish Lumbar Spine Study Group. Spine (Phila Pa 1976), 29(4), 421–434, discussion Z423.*

Glassman, S.D., Polly, D.W., Dimar, J.R., & Carreon, L.Y. (2012). *The cost effectiveness of single-level instrumented posterolateral lumbar fusion at 5 years after surgery. Spine (Phila Pa 1976), 37(9), 769– 774.*

Harrop, J.S., Hilibrand, A., Mihalovich, K.E., Dettori, J.R., & Chapman, J. (2014). *Cost-effectiveness of surgical treatment for degenerative spondylolisthesis and spinal stenosis. Spine (Phila Pa 1976), 39(22 Suppl 1), S75–85.*

Horsman, J., Furlong, W., Feeny, D., & Torrance, G. (2003). *The Health Utilities Index (HUI): concepts, measurement properties and applications. Health and Quality of Life Outcomes, 1, 54.*

Kalichman, L., Cole, R., Kim, D.H., Li, L., Suri, P., Guermazi, A., & Hunter, D.J. (2009). *Spinal stenosis prevalence and association with symptoms: the Framingham Study. The Spine Journal, 9(7), 545–550.*

Katz, J.N., Lipson, S.J., Lew, R.A., Grobler, L.H., Weinstein, J.N., Brick, G.W., Fossel, A.H., & Liang, M.H. (1997). *Lumbar laminectomy alone or with instrumented or noninstrumented arthrodesis in degenerative lumbar spinal stenosis. Patient selection, costs, and surgical outcomes. Spine (Phila Pa 1976), 22(10), 1123–1131.*

Kumar, N., Shah, S.M., Ng, Y.H., Pannierselvam, V.K., Dasde, S., & Shen, L. (2014). *Role of coflex as an adjunct to decompression for symptomatic lumbar spinal stenosis. Asian Spine Journal, 8(2), 161–169.*

MAG Mutual Healthcare Solutions Inc. (2011). *Physicians Fee and Coding Guide. Augusta, GA: MAG Mutual Healthcare Solutions.*

North American Spine Society. (2011). *Evidence-based clinical guidelines for multidisciplinary spine care. Diagnosis and treatment of degenerative lumbar spinal stenosis 2011. Available at https://www.spine.org/Documents/ResearchClinicalCare/Guidelines/LumbarStenosis.pdf.*

Otani, K., Kikuchi, S., Yabuki, S., Igarashi, T., Nikaido, T., Watanabe, K., & Konno, S. (2013). *Lumbar spinal stenosis has a negative impact on quality of life compared with other comorbidities: an epidemiological cross-sectional study of 1862 community-dwelling individuals. The Scientific World Journal, Article ID 590652.*

Practice Management Information Corporation. (2010). *Medical Fees in the United States 2010.*

Roder, C., Baumgartner, B., Berlemann, U., & Aghayev, E. (2015). *Superior outcomes of decompression with an interlaminar dynamic device versus decompression alone in patients with lumbar spinal stenosis and back pain: a cross registry study. European Spine Journal, 24(10), 2228–2235.*

Schaefer, C., Mann, R., Sadosky, A., Daniel, S., Parsons, B., Nieshoff, E., Tuchman, M., Nalamachu, S., Anschel, A., & Stacey, B.R. (2014). *Burden of illness associated with peripheral and central neuropathic pain among adults seeking treatment in the United States: a patient-centered evaluation. Pain Medicine, 15(12), 2105–2119.*

Schmier, J.K., Halevi, M., Maislin, G., & Ong, K. (2014). Comparative cost effectiveness of Coflex® interlaminar stabilization versus instrumented posterolateral lumbar fusion for the treatment of lumbar spinal stenosis and spondylolisthesis. ClinicoEconomics and Outcomes Research, 6, 125–131.

Schoenfeld, A.J., Harris, M.B., Liu, H., & Birkmeyer, J.D. (2014). Variations in Medicare payments for episodes of spine surgery. The Spine Journal, 14(12), 2793–2798.

Sigmundsson, F.G., Jonsson, B., & Stromqvist, B. (2013). Impact of pain on function and health related quality of life in lumbar spinal stenosis. A register study of 14,821 patients. Spine (Phila Pa 1976), 38(15), E937–945.

Skolasky, R.L., Maggard, A.M., Thorpe, R.J., Jr., Wegener, S.T., & Riley, L.H., 3rd. (2013). United States hospital admissions for lumbar spinal stenosis: racial and ethnic differences, 2000 through 2009. Spine (Phila Pa 1976), 38(26), 2272–2278.

Suarez-Almazor, M.E., Kendall, C., Johnson, J.A., Skeith, K., & Vincent, D. (2000). Use of health status measures in patients with low back pain in clinical settings. Comparison of specific, generic and preference-based instruments. Rheumatology (Oxford), 39(7), 783–790.

Tosteson, A.N., Skinner, J.S., Tosteson, T.D., Lurie, J.D., Andersson, G.B., Berven, S., Grove, M.R., Hanscom, B., Blood, E.A., & Weinstein, J.N. (2008). The cost effectiveness of surgical versus nonoperative treatment for lumbar disc herniation over two years: evidence from the Spine Patient Outcomes Research Trial (SPORT). Spine (Phila Pa 1976), 33(19), 2108–2115.

Tosteson, A.N., Tosteson, T.D., Lurie, J.D., Abdu, W., Herkowitz, H., Andersson, G., Albert, T., Bridwell, K., Zhao, W., Grove, M.R., Weinstein, M.C., & Weinstein, J.N. (2011). Comparative effectiveness evidence from the spine patient outcomes research trail: surgical verses nonoperative care for spinal stenosis, degenerative spondylolisthesis, and intervertebral disc herniation. Spine (Phila Pa 1976), 36(24), 2061–2068.

Wasserman Medical Publishers. (2011). Physicians' Fee Reference: Wasserman Medical Publishers.

# Chapter 5

# Posterior Reversible Encephalopathy Syndrome

Yashpal Singh[1], Bikram K Gupta[1] and Ram Badan Singh[1]

## 1  Introduction

Posterior reversible encephalopathy syndrome (PRES) is a neurotoxic state with a unique imaging appearance on CT or MRI, initially described in 1996 by Hinchey and co-workers (Hinchey J et al., 1996). This condition has been designated by a variety of names- reversible posterior leukoencephalopathy syndrome, reversible posterior cerebral edema syndrome, and reversible occipital parietal encephalopathy. The term PRES is misnomer as the syndrome involves or extends beyond the posterior cerebrum. It is a clinical-neuroradiological entity characterized by headache, visual disturbances, seizures, altered mental status and radiological findings of edema in the white matter of the brain, perfused by the posterior brain circulation (Lim MH et al., 2008; Kozak OS et al., 2007). If timely recognized and treated, clinical syndrome resolves within a week but MRI changes resolve over days to week.

PRES is commonly recognized in patients with eclampsia, organ transplantation, autoimmune disease, nonspecific renal inflammatory conditions (glomerulonephritis, hepatorenal syndrome), hypertension, and post chemotherapy (Bartynski WS et al., 2001; Schwartz RB et al., 2000; Lin JT et al., 2003). Renal failure (chronic or acute) is a classic disorder associated with PRES, and is present in more than half of cases. Nearly half of patients with PRES have a history of autoimmune disorder (Fugate et al., 2015). It is therefore important to consider PRES in the differential diagnosis of patients with renal disease and rapidly progressive neurologic symptoms.

---

[1]  Department of Anaesthesiology, Institute of Medical Sciences, Banaras Hindu University, Varanasi, India

The mechanism of its development is not well understood but altered integrity of the blood brain barrier is the basic pathology. Hyperperfusion with endothelial damage or hypoperfusion with cerebral ischemia leads to development of vasogenic edema in occipital and parietal regions, relating to the posterior cerebral artery supply but also found within the frontal, inferior temporal, cerebellar and brainstem regions. Both cortical and subcortical locations are affected. Differential diagnosis of PRES includes vasculitis, infectious encephalitis, ischemic stroke (posterior cerebral artery territory), ictal or post-ictal state (with or without status epilepticus), progressive multifocal leukoencephalopathy (PML), acute disseminated encephalomyelitis, Creutzfeldt-Jakob disease and cerebral venous sinus thrombosis (Lamy C et al., 2001; Legriel S et al., 2008).

Diagnostic strategy includes careful history and thorough physical examination; investigation should be performed step wise as necessary for diagnosis. Most commonly used diagnostic modality is computed tomography (CT), magnetic resonance imaging (MRI), electroencephalography (EEG) and Cerebrospinal fluid (CSF) analysis (Lee VH et al., 2008; Bartynski WS et al., 2007; Covarrubias DJ et al., 2002). Management strategy includes symptomatic measures, early recognition and resolution of the underlying cause. A symptomatic measure includes hemodynamics, airway control, antiepileptic treatment and glycemic control usually taken in the intensive care unit (ICU). Persistence of the cause carries a risk of ischemia, bleeding, and death.

# 2   Epidemiology

Worldwide incidence of PRES is unknown and epidemiological data come from retrospective studies of patients seen between 1988-2008 (Hinchey J et al., 1996; Bartynski WS et al., 2007). Majority of case reported in young to middle-aged adult (mean age 39-47 year) with marked female predominance. Many patients have underlying comorbidities such as chronic renal failure, chronic hypertension and bone marrow or solid organ transplantation. Patient may require ICU admission for status epilepticus or mechanical ventilation. Mean hospital length of stay was 20 days (Lee VH et al., 2008).

# 3   Pathophysiology

The cerebral blood perfusion abnormalities and blood brain barrier dysfunction with cerebral vasogenic edema is the key factor in the pathogenesis of PRES. There are two hypotheses which contradict each other. One hypothesis involves increased cerebral blood flow due to impaired cerebral auto regulation while other involves cerebral hypo perfusion due to endothelial dysfunction.

## 3.1   Cerebral Hyperperfusion and Vasogenic Edema

Cerebral autoregulation is maintained between mean arterial blood pressure (MAP) of 60–120 mmHg range via various auto regulatory mechanisms (vasodilation or vasoconstriction). When mean arterial blood pressure increases above 150-170 mmHg, auto regulatory mechanism fails resulting in cascade of events that leads to blood brain barrier dysfunction. Vasodilator agent such as nitric oxide (NO) and prostacyclin (PGI2) are produced under the action of substances P, acetylcholine and noradrenaline released from endothelial cells due to cerebral hyperperfusion and consequently, there is overproduction of catecholamine's, vasopressin, thromboxane, and endothelin 1. These substances increases vasoreactivity and activate the renin-angiotensin-aldosterone system, which activates the gene expression of pro-inflammatory cytokines such as interleukin (IL-6) and the transcription of nuclear factor-kappa B (NF-κB), leading to direct cytotoxic effects on the blood vessel wall. This damage to the vascular endothelium causes blood-brain barrier dysfunction and cerebral vasogenic edema (Vaughan CJ et al., 2000). Hypertension is a feature in 67 % to 80 % of cases of PRESS supporting the hyperperfusion hypothesis. In addition, regional hyperperfusion in the occipital lobe and cerebellum is shown by single photon emission CT (SPECT) 99mTc-HMPAO imaging also (Schwartz RB et al., 1992).

## 3.2   Cerebral Hypoperfusion and Vasogenic Edema

In non-hypertensive PRES patient cytotoxicity has been hypothesized to be the mechanism underlying the brain edema. Causes of PRES without hypertension include cyclosporine toxicity, wegener granulomatosis, systemic lupus erythematosus (SLE), and infection/sepsis/septic shock. Release of various inflammatory mediators such as histamine, free radicals, NO, bradykynin, and arachidonic acid from endothelial cells due to immune system activation. These inflammatory mediators activate production of pro-inflammatory cytokines (e.g., tumor necrosis factor [TNF-α], IL-1, IL-6, and interferon [IFN-γ]) (Ferrara JL., 2000; Schots R et al., 2003; de Vries HE et al., 1997). Vascular tone alteration occurs due to upregulation of endothelial surface antigens and the release of endothelin (Narushima I et al., 2003). All these changes lead to vascular instability with vasoconstriction, hypoperfusion with blood-brain barrier dysfunction, leads to vasogenic cerebral edema (Wijdicks EF., 2001). This hypothesis is supported by studies involving catheter angiography, MRA, and MR perfusion imaging, which show cerebral hypoperfusion (Bartynski WS et al., 2008; Brubaker LM et al., 2005). Hydropic axonal swelling and myelin edema are seen on histopathological examination of PRES. This is shown as myelin pallor without tissue destruction (Okeda R et al., 2007).

# 4   Conditions Most Commonly Associated With PRES

Various etiological factor involved in pathogenesis of PRES is increasing steadily. Common causes are listed in Table 1.

## 4.1   Hypertension induced PRES

Whenever there is sudden increase in systemic blood pressure, compensatory mecha-

```
┌─────────────────────────┐          ┌─────────────────────────┐
│ Precipitating factors   │          │ Genetic Predisposition  │
│ Vasoactive substances,  │          │ (Val66 BDNF genes)      │
│ Pregnancy/postpartum,   │          │ Female gender           │
│ Other triggers          │          │                         │
└─────────────────────────┘          └─────────────────────────┘
```

Catecholamines,
Preinflammatory cytokines
Proangiogenic factors
Prostaglandins

**Endothelial Dysfunction**

Sympathetic overactivity ──────►◄────── Oxidative stress

**Cerebral vascular
tone dysregulation**

Autoregulation failure │ BBB Breakdown

**PRES**

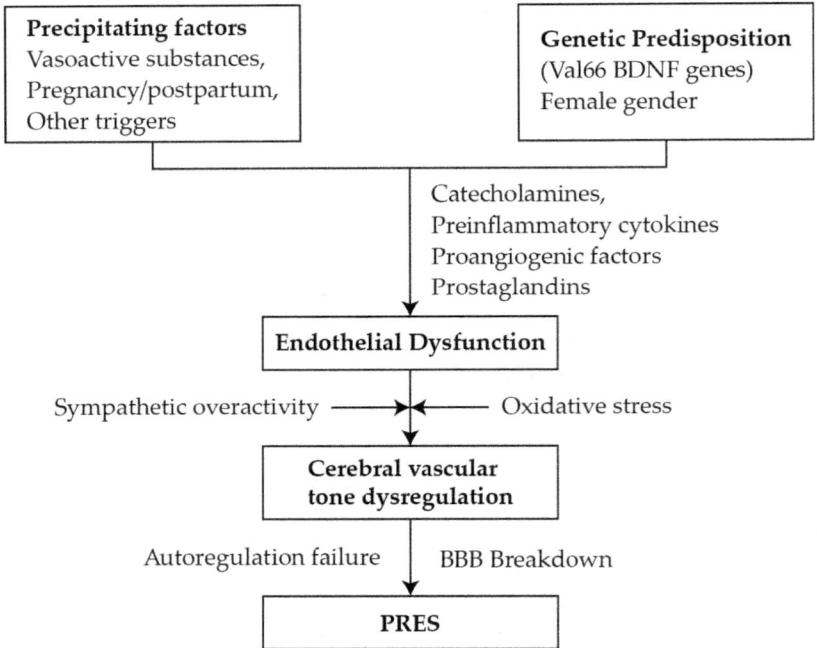

**Figure 1:** Flow chart depicting pathophysiology of PRES (BBB: Blood Brain Barier).

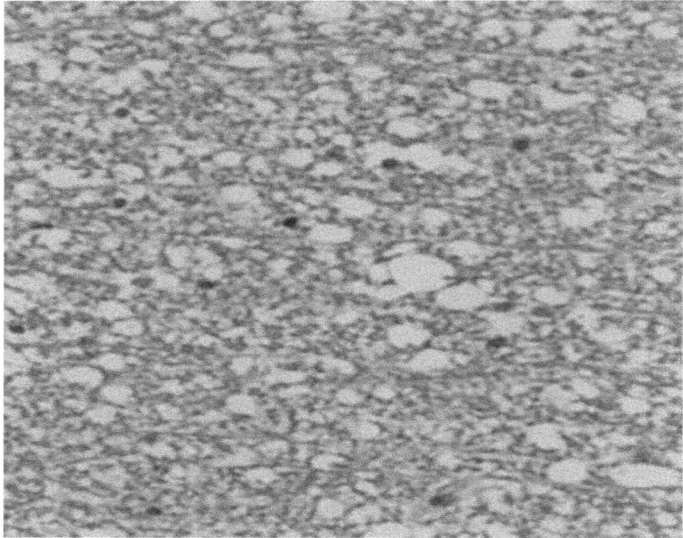

**Figure 2:** Marked oedema in the white matter, giving it a "vacuolar "appearance. No sign of inflammation (Autopsy from affected area of brain).

| Chemotherapy Agent | Cytokines and Immunoglobulin's | Medications | Others |
|---|---|---|---|
| Cisplatin | Interferon-alpha | Antiretroviral | Hypertension |
| Carboplatin | Interleukin-2 | Erythropoietin | Pre-eclampsia |
| Cyclosporine | Infliximab | Carbamazepine | Eclampsia |
| Methotrexate | Etanarcept | Corticosteroids | Sepsis |
| Vincristine | Tacrolimbus | Cocaine | Autoimmune disease |
| Cytarbine | Sirolimbus | Lysergic acid | Blood Transfusion |
| Gemcitabine | | Linezolid | Tumor lysis syndrome |
| Irenotecan | | | |
| Bevazicumab | | | Renal Failure |

**Table 1:** Common causes of PRES.

nisms in the body limits the blood flow and avoiding fluid leakage from the intravascular space to the interstitium. In PRES, this compensatory mechanism becomes abnormal resulting in disruption of normal blood brain barrier (BBB) and resulting in vasogenic brain edema. (Cipolla MJ., 2007; Kontos HA et al., 1978). Due to partial lack of sympathetic innervation of the vasculature in posterior CNS area particularly that originates from the basilar artery, edema usually occurs in the posterior CNS areas in the occiptoparietal areas. (Hinchey J et al., 1996; Vaughan CJ et al., 2000).

Endothelial dysfunction is the common pathway in pathogenesis of PRES, regardless of cause because it also reported in non-hypertensive patients. Diabetes mellitus, dyslipidemia, and smoking may indirectly play a role in pathogenesis of PRES by causing endothelial dysfunction. (Yano Y et al., 2005) The cytotoxic theory postulates that an acute rise in blood pressure produces hypoperfusion leading to hypoxia resulting in endothelial damage with subsequent edema. Edema can compromise the circulation of that particular area producing hypoxia with subsequently adenosine triphosphate (ATP) depletion resulting in sodium-potassium pump failure leads intracellular swelling. (Doelken M et al., 2007).

## 4.2   Pregnancy-induced PRES

Pre-eclampsia or eclampsia was present in up to 20% of patients with PRES and outcome was usually favorable (Lee VH et al., 2008; Servillo G et al., 2008). Hypertension was usually associated with it, occurs from 28 weeks 'gestational age to day 13 postpartum. In pregnancy-induced HTN, it is believed that pregnancy predisposes the brain to edema formation (Cipolla MJ., 2008). In animal model, due to unknown reason, there is a vasoconstriction activity in late-pregnancy in cerebral arteries in response to serotonin exposure, while the contrary occurs in non-pregnant specimens, in which the response results in vasodilatation (Cipolla MJ et al., 2004).

## 4.3   Drugs Related in the Development of PRES

Toxic agents are most commonly associated with PRES ranging from11 % to 61 % of cases but exact mechanism are not known (Lee VH et al., 2008; McKinney AM et al., 2007). Various hypotheses for development of PRES include drug-induced endothelial damage, nephrotoxicity, neurotoxicity and HTN (Rajasekhar A et al., 2007; Yokobori S et al., 2006). Common drugs associated with development of PRES are cisplatin, oxaliplatin, carboplatin, gemcitabine, cytarabine, methotrexate, mitotic inhibitors, vincristine, L-asparagine, interferon-alpha, interleukin-2, rituximab (anti-CD20), infliximab (anti-TNF-$\alpha$), intravenous immunoglobulin, anti-TNF-$\alpha$ protein, etanercept , cyclosporine A , tacrolimus (FK 506), sirolimus, High-dose corticosteroid therapy (e.g., dexamethasone and methylprednisolone), Blood transfusion and many other drugs (Kwon EJ et al., 2009; Vieillot S et al., 2007; Saito B et al.,2007; Dicuonzo F et al., 2009; Hualde Olascoaga J et al., 2008; Cumurciuc R et al., 2008 ).

Cyclosporine by increasing the efferent sympathetic activity with possible acute HTN development and also by direct activation of the central sympathetic neurons it is able to cross the BBB. It has been linked more frequently with PRES when administered via intravenous (IV) access (Lyson T et al., 1994). Sirolimus causes altered astrocytes metabolism with secondary changes leading to brain edema (Bodkin CL et al., 2007). Neurotoxic effect caused by gemcitabine, a synthetic pyrimidine nucleoside analogue antineoplastic agent has recently been associated with PRES development (Rajasekhar A et al., 2007). Oxaliplatin has been stated as a possible cause of PRES by crossing BBB; it causes cerebral edema due to secondary fluid transudation (Pinedo DM et al., 2007). Moreover, glucocorticoids such as dexamethasone have been shown to induce PRES, although it is an uncommon steroids-use complication, and thought to be related to HTN secondary to its mineralocorticoid effects (Irvin W et al., 2007).

## 4.4   Miscellaneous Conditions

PRES has also been reported in patients with bloodstream infection, often with hypertension at diagnosis (Bartynski WS et al., 2006). Sepsis and septic shock leads to endothelial damage and altered microcirculation leads to exaggerated immune response (Mutunga M et al., 2001). Microcirculation alterations seen in sepsis are due to micro vessel blockade by leukocytes reducing tissue perfusion that lead to edema formation.

Autoimmune disease has been encountered in 8 % to 10 % of cases. PRES has been reported in patients with wegener's granulomatosis, systemic lupus erythematosus, polyarteritis nodosa, takayasu arteritis, hashimoto encephalopathy and crohn's disease (Nishio M et al., 2009; Yong PF et al., 2003, Burrus TM et al., 2010; Fujita M et al., 2008; Zipper SG et al., 2006). Other condition associated with PRES includes sickle cell disease, tumor lysis syndrome, guillain-barr'e syndrome, porphyria, porphyria and cushing syndrome (Greenwood MJ et al., 2003; Fugate JE et al., 2009; Kang SY et al., 2010).

# 5    Clinical Features

The clinical feature of PRES includes headache, altered consciousness, visual disturbances, seizure activity, nausea/vomiting, and focal neurological signs (Hinchey J et al., 1996). Headache is the most common symptoms but not present in all patients. Consciousness alteration seen in 13%-90% of cases and spectrum of severity ranges from confusion, somnolence, and lethargy to encephalopathy or coma. (Burnett MM et al., 2010). Visual disturbances consist of blurred vision, hemianopia, visual hallucination, permanent visual field defects and cortical blindness (Kwon Set al., 2001). Isolated generalized seizures are rare but secondary seizures are common in 53-62% cases. Continuous seizure activity for more than 5 minutes (Status epilepticus) without full recovery of consciousness reported in 3-13% of cases (Lee VH et al., 2008; Kozak OS et al., 2007). Motor dysfunction like hemiparesis, dystonia, dysmetria and pyramidal tract signs such as babinski's reflex, hyper or hyporeflexia are possible but uncommon findings (Pinedo DM et al., 2007; Irvin W et al., 2007). Sluggish pupillary reflexes can be part of the clinical picture and brain stem involvement leads to dysphasia, dysarthria and dyspnea. Papilledema and hemorrhages can be noted on funduscopic examination if HTN is the part of PRES. Recurrence is another clinical situation that could be present in few patients (Sweany JM et al., 2007).

| Features |
| --- |
| Impaired consciousness |
| Headache |
| Visual disturbances |
| Seizure activity |
| Focal neurological sign |
| Acute hypertension |
| Nausea / Vomiting |

**Table 2:** Clinical features of PRES.

# 6    Diagnostic Studies

Computed tomography (CT) is usually normal or nonspecific and if hypodensities are present then it is difficult to distinguish between PRES and acute stroke. Magnetic resonance imaging (MRI) is therefore investigation of choice in PRES (Bartynski WS et al., 2007; Okeda R et al., 2007). Proton-density and T2-weighted images show regions of high signal indicating edema. Fluid-attenuated inversion recovery (FLAIR) sequences also visualize the lesions. The use of FLAIR has been shown to improve the diagnosis of PRES and the detection of subcortical and cortical lesions in PRES (Casey SO et al., 2000). T1-weighted images show low-intensity foci. Diffusion-weighted imaging (DWI) is normal but the apparent diffusion coefficient is increased (Covarrubias DJ et al.,

2002). The most common findings in MRI studies are bilateral and symmetric regions of edema typically located in the white matter and predominating in the posterior parietal and occipital lobes. However, different distribution has been reported, postfrontal cortical, subcortical white matter, cortex, brainstem, basal ganglia and cerebellum.

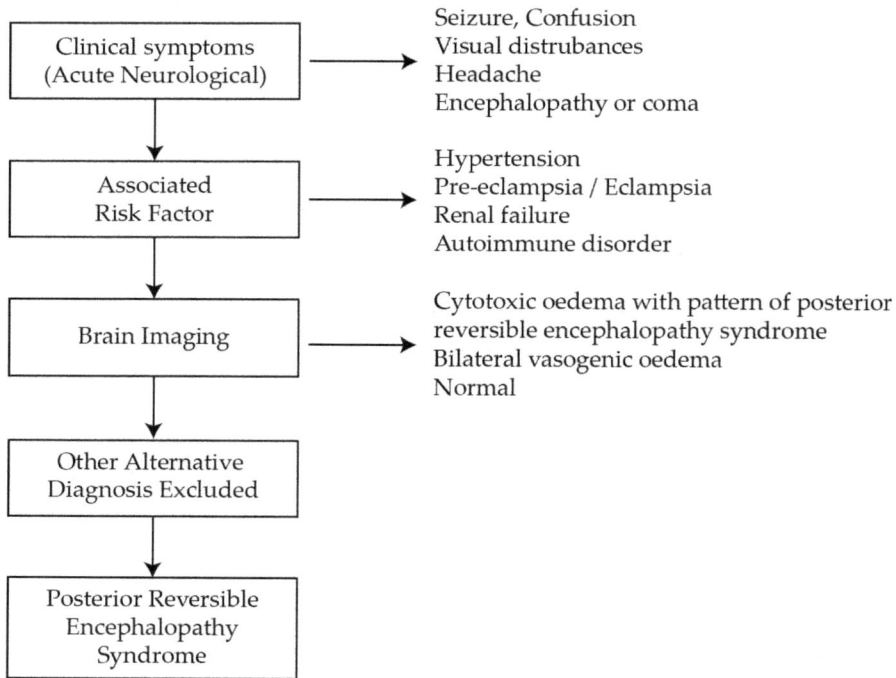

```
┌─────────────────────┐        Seizure, Confusion
│  Clinical symptoms   │ ─────▶ Visual distrubances
│ (Acute Neurological) │        Headache
└─────────────────────┘        Encephalopathy or coma
          │
          ▼
┌─────────────────────┐        Hypertension
│     Associated       │ ─────▶ Pre-eclampsia / Eclampsia
│     Risk Factor      │        Renal failure
└─────────────────────┘        Autoimmune disorder
          │
          ▼
┌─────────────────────┐        Cytotoxic oedema with pattern of posterior
│    Brain Imaging     │ ─────▶ reversible encephalopathy syndrome
└─────────────────────┘        Bilateral vasogenic oedema
          │                     Normal
          ▼
┌─────────────────────┐
│  Other Alternative   │
│  Diagnosis Excluded  │
└─────────────────────┘
          │
          ▼
┌─────────────────────┐
│ Posterior Reversible │
│    Encephalopathy    │
│      Syndrome        │
└─────────────────────┘
```

**Figure 3:** Algorithm for the diagnosis of posterior reversible encephalopathy syndrome.

Four radiological patterns were found on imaging includes (Bartynski et al., 2007):

- **Superior frontal sulcus pattern-** Bilateral vasogenic edema in a non-confluent pattern involving the frontal sulcus area and, to a lesser degree, the white matter of the parietal, occipital, and temporal lobes on Fluid-attenuated inversion recovery (FLAIR) sequences. The frontal abnormality appeared linear and was located along the mid to posterior aspect of the superior frontal sulcus. This was similar to the appearance in the holohemispheric watershed pattern, with more isolated superior frontal sulci involvement and no frontal pole extension. Intermediate expression of this pattern was also noted, with either nonconfluent areas of cortical vasogenic edema along the superior frontal sulcus or regions of focal or patchy white matter vasogenic edema.

- **Holohemispheric watershed pattern-** Fluid-attenuated inversion recovery (FLAIR) sequences showing bilateral vasogenic edema in a linear pattern involving the white matter of the cerebellum, brainstem, and occipital, parietal, frontal, and temporal lobes . This linear vasogenic edema seemed to be present at the junction between the medial hemispheric (anterior cerebral [ACA] and posterior cerebral arteries [PCA]) and lateral hemispheric branches (middle cerebral artery [MCA]) consistent with the watershed or anastomotic border zone. Reduced involvement in the cortex or deep white matter typically appeared as nonconfluent cortical vasogenic edema, which was most commonly identified along the superior frontal sulcus or a "string-of-pearl" pattern of linearly arranged, disconnected white matter edema.

- **Dominant parietal-occipital pattern-** Fluid-attenuated inversion recovery (FLAIR) sequences showing bilateral vasogenic edema in the white matter of the occipital and parietal lobes. Extensive as well as lesser degrees of severity of this pattern were identified.

- **Partial or asymmetric expression of the primary patterns-** Bilateral absence of edema in either the parietal or the occipital lobes and frontal lobes are often involved (Figure 4). The asymmetric form is characterized by unilateral absence of edema in either a parietal or an occipital lobe.

Complication of PRES like cerebral ischemia, hemorrhage and cerebral herniation can be diagnosed radiologically. The non-specific clinical manifestations and diversity of radiological patterns raise diagnostic challenges. Differential diagnosis of PRES includes ictal or post-ictal state (with or without status epilepticus), progressive multifocal leukoencephalopathy (PML), severe leukoaraiosis, neoplasms, encephalitis, cerebral autosomal dominant arteriopathy with subcortical infarcts and leukoencephalopathy (CADASIL), vasculitis, Creutzfeldt-Jakob disease, cerebral venous sinus thrombosis, and ischemic stroke (Lamy C et al., 2001; Legriel S et al., 2008).

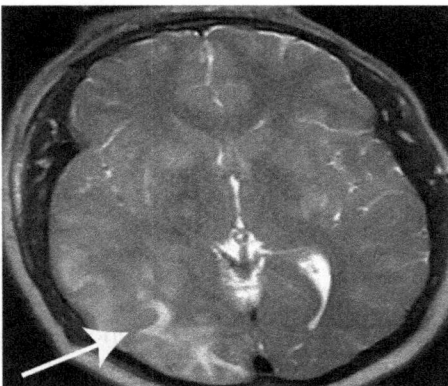

**Figure 4:** Posterior reversible encephalopathy syndrome – MRI of the brain shows edema in the occipital lobe, which appears as white.

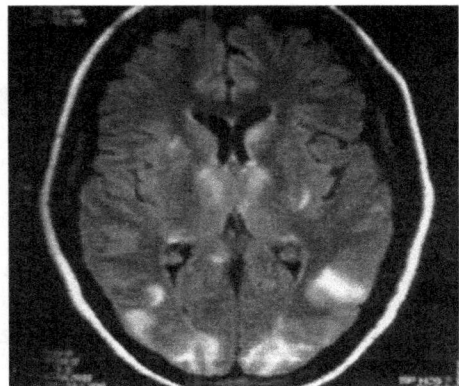

**Figure 5:** Hyperintense lesions mainly in posterior parieto-occipital area on both sides seen on MRI T2 FLAIR.

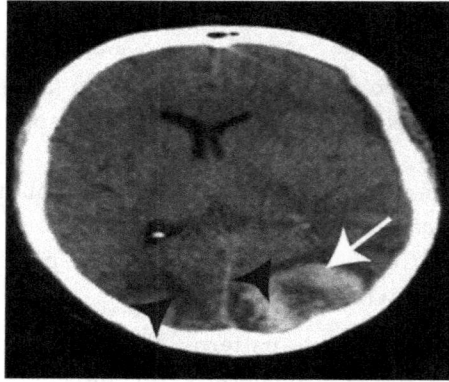

**Figure 6:** CT scan shows vasogenic edema in the parietal region bilaterally (arrowheads), along with an acute hematoma in the left parietal lobe (arrow).

# 7 Management

The treatment consists of general measures and withdrawal of the triggering factors as soon as possible to avoid risk of irreversible damage (Mak A et al., 2008). A general measure includes airway protection, seizure control, hemodynamic stability and glycemic control. Precipitating factors like eclampsia, hypertension, sepsis and various drugs should be managed.

## 7.1 General Measures

### 7.1.1 Airway protection

Symptomatic measures started immediately preferably in setting of intensive care unit or high dependency unit. Upper airway protection is the top priority in patient with altered sensorium or seizure activity. If airway is compromised then endotracheal intubation is performed, rapid-sequence induction with Etomidate /Thiopentone / Propofol and succinylcholine should be used and ventilatory support if needed.

### 7.1.2 Seizure Control

Antiepileptic treatment should be initiated on an emergency basis and according to guidelines. Patients with continuous seizure activity should receive intravenous benzodiazepines either before ICU admission or in the ICU. The dose can be repeated up to three times if necessary. If seizure activity persists despite intravenous benzodiazepines then patient should receive intravenous anticonvulsant drugs (phenobarbital 10 to 15 mg/kg, phenytoin 18 mg/kg, or equivalent dose of fosphenytoin). Intravenous midazolam, propofol, or thiopental in titrated doses is given in patients with refractory status epilepticus till remission of the clinical seizure activity (Meierkord H et al., 2010).

### 7.1.3    Glycemic Control

Hyper and hypoglycemia both have adverse neurological outcome, so should be managed promptly according to ICU protocols. Hypoglycemia should be watched regularly and corrected. If glucose is given, 100 mg of thiamine should be administered concomitantly, most notably when there is evidence of vitamin B1 deficiency. Hyperglycemia should be managed with intravenous insulin. Patients should be regularly evaluated for hyperthermia and metabolic disturbances, in particular hypomagnesaemia, which require prompt correction. Aspiration pneumonia may complicate the initial consciousness disorders.

### 7.1.4    Control of Blood Pressure

In case of hypertensive emergency the aim is to decrease the MAP by 20–25 % within the first 2 hours and to bring the blood pressure down to 160/100 mmHg within the first 6 hours (Ramsay LE et al; 1999). Rapid decrease in blood pressure is not recommended because this leads to cerebral ischemia by alteration in cerebral perfusion pressure. Thus IV drugs having short half-life permit easy titration would be the good pharmacological therapy. An intravenous antihypertensive drug includes labetalol, nicardipine, or fenoldopam should be used as required (Varon J et al., 2003).

### 7.1.5    Anti-edema Measure

Brain edema can develop due recurrent seizure or high blood pressure or due to metabolic disturbances. It should be treated according to hospital protocol. Mannitol, diuretics and steroids are commonly used drugs for control of brain edema as required. External ventricular drain or ventriculoperitoneal shunt may be required in cases of obstructive hydrocephalous, which is the rare complication of PRES due to cerebrospinal fluid obstruction. Neurological status improved within three days of successful procedure (Lee SY et al., 2008).

## 7.2    Correction of the Underlying Cause of PRES

Timely correction of the cause is crucial to decrease the risk of ischemia or bleeding and therefore to avoid permanent disability or death (Hinchey J et al., 1996). Correction of underlying cause includes blood pressure control, esarean section, withdrawal of cancer chemotherapy or immunosuppressive agents, control of sepsis or other intervention as required.

# 8    Conclusions

After initial description of PRES in 1996, many cases are reported till date and various etiological factors have been identified which helps in understanding the pathophysiol-

```
                    ┌──────────────────────────────────────┐
                    │  Clinical Feature Suggestive of PRES   │
                    └──────────────────────────────────────┘
                         │                          │
                         ▼                          ▼
              ┌─────────────────┐        ┌─────────────────┐
              │  CT with contrast │        │       MRI        │
              └─────────────────┘        └─────────────────┘
                         │                          │
                         ▼                          
                    ┌──────────────────────────────────┐
                    │     Definite Diagnosis of PRES     │
                    └──────────────────────────────────┘
         ┌──────────────────┐        │        ┌──────────────────┐
         │   Search for      │        │        │  Evaluation of    │
         │ PRES associated   │◄──────────────►│  Organ Failure    │
         │   Conditions      │        │        └──────────────────┘
         └──────────────────┘        │
                  │          ┌──────────────────────────────┐
                  │          │ Electroencephalogram (EEG)    │
                  │          │      Laboratory tests          │
                  │          │      Topological inv.          │
                  │          │      Lumber puncture?          │     ┌──────────────────────┐
                  │          └──────────────────────────────┘     │ Orotracheal intubation │
                  │                      │                          └──────────────────────┘
         ┌──────────────────┐            │              ┌──────────────────────────────┐
         │ Correction of     │◄───────────────────────►│       Symptomatic m/m           │
         │ underlying cause  │                          └──────────────────────────────┘
         │    of PRES        │
         └──────────────────┘            ┌────────────────┬──────────────────────┐
         ┌──────────────────┐            │ Anticonvulsant  │   Intravenous         │
         │ If required toxic │            │                 │ anti-hypertensive     │
         │ agent withdrawal  │            ├────────────────┼──────────────────────┤
         │ - Blook pressure  │            │ Midazolam       │ Labetalol             │
         │   control         │            │ Phenytoin       │ Nicardipine           │
         │ - Cesarean section│            │ Propofol        │ Fenoldopam            │
         │ - Dialysis        │            │ Thiopental      │ Urapidil              │
         │ - Nimodipine      │            └────────────────┴──────────────────────┘
         └──────────────────┘
```

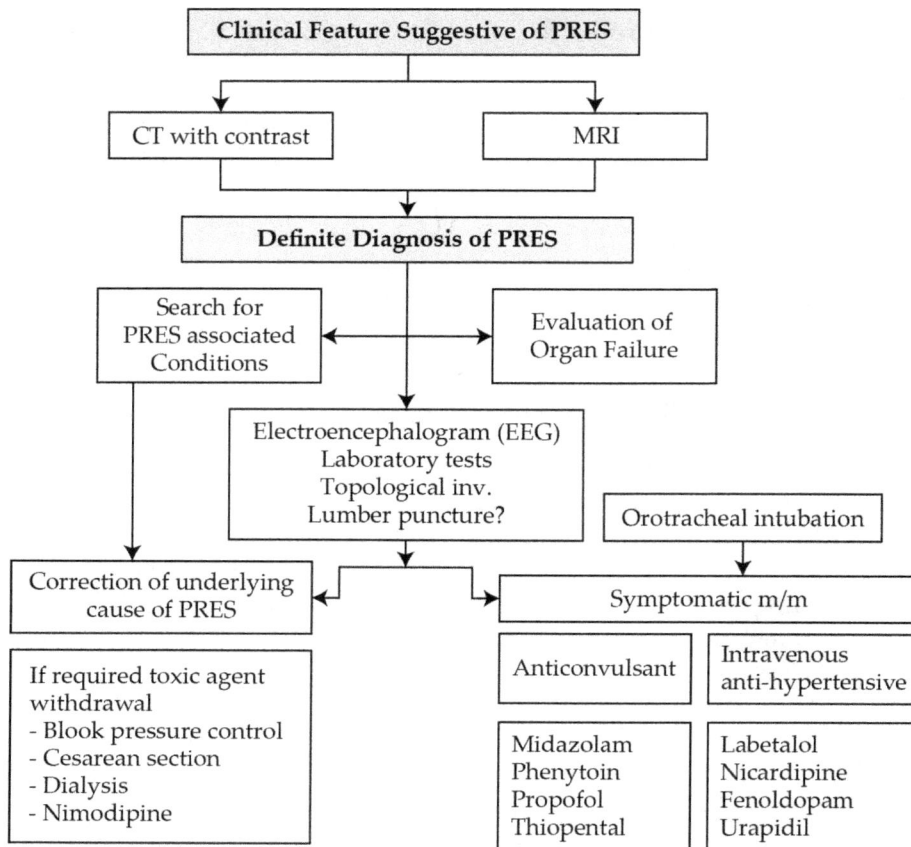

**Figure 7:** Treatment Algorithm of PRES.

ogy behind it but still numerous aspects are yet to be elucidated. The clinical presentation is non-specific; most of patients have spectrum of symptoms from mild headache to deep comma or unconsciousness. It is essential to recognize the condition and possible causative factor as soon as possible to avoid irreversible brain damage. Early identification of this syndrome is achieved by MRI specifically with DWI which is crucial for diagnosing, monitoring the course, and assessing treatment. Invasive procedure like lumber puncture is usually not required. The main features obtained with MRI are high density areas suggestive of CNS edema mostly in the posterior white matter of the brain, although anterior structures and gray matter may also be involved. The list of conditions known to be associated with PRES is increasing since its initial report however pathophysiology of PRES remains controversial since then. However, the early recognition of the condition and treatment or withdrawal of the underlying cause is the keystone of management. Persistence of the cause carries a risk of ischemia, bleeding, and death. Finally, studies are needed to identify factors of adverse prognostic significance and to develop neuroprotective strategies.

# References

Bartynski, W.S. & Boardman, J.F. (2007). *Distinct imaging patterns and lesion distribution in posterior reversible encephalopathy syndrome. AJNR Am J Neuroradiol, 28, 1320–1327.*

Bartynski, W.S. & Boardman, J.F. (2008). *Catheter angiography, MR angiography, and MR perfusion in posterior reversible encephalopathy syndrome. AJNR Am J Neuroradiol, 29, 447–455.*

Bartynski, W.S., Boardman, J.F., Zeigler, Z.R., Shadduck, R.K. & Lister, J. (2006). *Posterior reversible encephalopathy syndrome in infection, sepsis, and shock. AJNR Am J Neuroradiol, 27, 2179–2190.*

Bartynski, W.S., Zeigler, Z., Spearman, M.P., Lin, L., Shadduck, R.K. & Lister, J. (2001). *Etiology of cortical and white matter lesions in cyclosporin-A and FK-506 neurotoxicity. AJNR Am J Neuroradiol, 22, 1901–1914.*

Brubaker, L.M., Smith, J.K., Lee, Y.Z., Lin, W. & Castillo, M. (2005). *Hemodynamic and permeability changes in posterior reversible encephalopathy syndrome measured by dynamic susceptibility perfusion-weighted MR imaging. AJNR Am J Neuroradiol, 26, 825–830.*

Burrus, T.M., Mandrekar, J., Wijdicks, E.F. & Rabinstein, A.A. (2010). *Renal failure and posterior reversible encephalopathy syndrome in patients with thrombotic thrombocytopenic purpura. Arch Neurol, 67, 831–834.*

Burnett, M.M., Hess, C.P., Roberts, J.P., Bass, N.M., Douglas, V.C. & Josephson, S.A. (2010). *Presentation of reversible posterior leukoencephalopathy syndrome in patients on calcineurin inhibitors. Clin Neurol Neurosurg, 112, 886–889.*

Casey, S.O., Sampaio, R.C., Michel, E., & Truwit, C.L. (2000). *Posterior reversible encephalopathy syndrome: utility of fluid-attenuated inversion recovery MR imaging in the detection of cortical and subcortical lesions. AJNR Am J Neuroradiol, 21, 1199–1206.*

Cipolla, M.J. (2007). *Cerebrovascular function in pregnancy and eclampsia. Hypertension, 50, 14–24.*

Cipolla, M.J., Vitullo, L., & McKinnon, J. (2004). *Cerebral artery reactivity changes during pregnancy and the postpartum period: a role in eclampsia? Am J Physiol Heart Circ Physiol, 286, H2127–2132.*

Covarrubias, D.J., Luetmer, P.H. & Campeau, N.G. (2002). *Posterior reversible encephalopathy syndrome: prognostic utility of quantitative diffusion-weighted MR images. AJNR Am J Neuroradiol, 23, 1038–1048.*

Cumurciuc, R., Martinez-Almoyna, L., Bodkin, C.L. & Eidelman, B.H. (2007). *Sirolimus induced posterior reversible encephalopathy. Neurology, 68, 2039–2040.*

de Vries, H.E., Kuiper, J., de Boer, A.G., Van Berkel, T.J. & Breimer, D.D. (1997). *The blood- brain barrier in neuroinflammatory diseases. Pharmacol Rev, 49, 143–155.*

Dicuonzo, F., Salvati, A., Palma, M., Lefons, V., Lasalandra, G., De Leonardis, F., & Santoro, N. (2009). *Posterior reversible encephalopathy syndrome associated with methotrexate neurotoxicity: conventional magnetic resonance and diffusion-weighted imaging findings. J Child Neurol, 24, 1013–1018.*

Doelken, M., Lanz, S., Rennert, J., Alibek, S., Richter, G., & Doerfler, A. (2007). *Differentiation of cytotoxic and vasogenic edema in a patient with reversible posterior leukoencephalopathy syndrome using diffusion-weighted MRI. Diagn Interv Radiol, 13, 125–128.*

Ferrara, J.L. (2000). *Pathogenesis of acute graft-versus-host disease: cytokines and cellular effectors. J Hematother Stem Cell Res, 9, 299–306.*

Fugate, J.E. &, Rabinstein, A.A. (2015). *Posterior reversible encephalopathy syndrome: clinical and radiological manifestations, pathophysiology, and outstanding questions.* Lancet Neurol, 14, 914–925.

Fugate, J.E., Wijdicks, E.F., Kumar, G., & Rabinstein, A.A. (2009). *One Thing Leads to Another: GBS Complicated by PRES and Takotsubo Cardiomyopathy.* Neurocrit Care, 11, 395–397.

Fujita, M., Komatsu, K., Hatachi, S., & Yagita, M. (2008). *Reversible posterior leukoencephalopathy syndrome in a patient with Takayasu arteritis.* Mod Rheumatol,18, 623–629.

Greenwood, M.J., Dodds, A.J., Garricik, R., & Rodriguez, M. (2003). *Posterior leukoencephalopathy in association with the tumour lysis syndrome in acut lymphoblastic leukaemia — a case with clinico-pathological correlation.* Leuk Lymphoma, 44, 719–721.

Henry, C., Husson, H., & de Broucker, T. (2008). *Posterior reversible encephalopathy syndrome during sunitinib therapy.* Rev Neurol (Paris), 164, 605–607.

Hinchey, J., Chaves, C., Appignani, B., Breen, J., Pao, L., Wang, A., Pessin, M.S., Lamy, C., Mas, J.L. & Caplan, L.R. (1996). *A reversible posterior leukoencephalopathy syndrome.* N Engl J Med, 334, 494–500.

Hualde Olascoaga, J., Molins Castiella, T., Souto Hernandez, S., Becerril Moreno, F., Yoldi Petri, M.E., Sagaseta de Ilurdoz, M., & Molina Garicano, J. (2008). *[Reversible posterior leukoencephalopathy: report of two cases after vincristine treatment].* A Pediatr (Barc), 68, 282–285.

Irvin, W., MacDonald, G., Smith, J.K. & Kim, W.Y. (2007). *Dexamethasone-induced posterior reversible encephalopathy syndrome.* J Clin Oncol, 25, 2484–2486.

Kang, S.Y., Kang, J.H., Choi, J.C. & Lee, J.S. (2010). *Posterior reversible encephalopathy syndrome in a patient with acute intermittent porphyria.* J Neurol, 257, 663–664.

Kontos, H.A., Wei, E.P., Navari, R.M., Levasseur, J.E., Rosenblum, W.I. & Patterson, J.L. (1978). *Responses of cerebral arteries and arterioles to acute hypotension and hypertension.* Am J Physiol, 234, H371–383.

Kozak, O.S., Wijdicks, E.F., Manno, E.M., Miley, J.T. & Rabinstein, A.A. (2007). *Status epilepticus as initial manifestation of posterior reversible encephalopathy syndrome.* Neurology, 69, 894–897.

Kwon, E.J., Kim, S.W., Kim, K.K., Seo, H.S. & Kim, do. Y. (2009). *A case of gemcitabine and cisplatin associated posterior reversible encephalopathy syndrome.* Cancer Res Treat, 41, 53–55.

Kwon, S., Koo, J., & Lee, S. (2001). *Clinical spectrum of reversible posterior leukoencephalopathy syndrome.* Pediatr Neurol, 24, 361–364.

Lamy, C., & Mas, J.L. (2001). *[Reversible posterior leukoencephalopathy. A new syndrome or a new name for an old syndrome?].* Presse Med, 30, 915–920.

Lee, S.Y., Dinesh, S.K. & Thomas, J. (2008). *Hypertension-induced reversible posterior leukoencephalo-pathy syndrome causing obstructive hydrocephalus.* J Clin Neurosci, 15, 457-459.

Lee, V.H., Wijdicks, E.F., Manno, E.M. & Rabinstein, A.A. (2008). *Clinical spectrum of reversible posterior leukoencephalopathy syndrome.* Arch Neurol, 65, 205–210.

Legriel, S., Bruneel, F., Spreux-Varoquaux, O., Birenbaum, A., Chadenat, M.L. & Mignon, F. (2008). *Lysergic acid amide-induced posterior reversible encephalopathy syndrome with status epilepticus.* Neurocrit Care, 9, 247–252.

Lim, M.H., Kim, D.W., Cho, H.S., Lee, H.J., Kim, H.J., & Park, K.J. (2008). *Isolated cerebellar reversible leukoencephalopathy syndrome in a patient with end stage renal disease.* Intern Med, 47, 43–45.

Lin, J.T., Wang, S.J., Fuh, J.L. Hsiao, L.T., Lirng, J.F. & Chen, P.M. (2003). Prolonged reversible vasospasm in cyclosporin A-induced encephalopathy. AJNR Am J Neuroradiol, 24, 102–104.

Lyson, T., McMullan, D.M., Ermel, L.D., Morgan, B.J. & Victor, R.G. (1994). Mechanism of cyclosporine-induced sympathetic activation and acute hypertension in rats. Hypertension, 23, 667–675.

Mak, A., Chan, B.P., Yeh, I.B., Ho, R.C., Boey, M.L., Feng, P.H., Koh, D.R. & Ong, B.K. (2008). Neuropsychiatric lupus and reversible posterior leucoencephalopathy syndrome: a challenging clinical dilemma. Rheumatology (Oxford), 47, 256–262.

McKinney, A.M., Short, J., Truwit, C.L., McKinney, Z.J., Kozak, O.S., SantaCruz, K.S. & Teksam, M. (2007). Posterior reversible encephalopathy syndrome: incidence of atypical regions of involvement and imaging findings. AJR Am J Roentgenol, 189, 904–912.

Meierkord, H., Boon, P., Engelsen B., Gocke, K., Shorvon, S., Tinuper, P., & Holtkamp, M. (2010). EFNS guideline on the management of status epilepticus in adults. Eur J Neurol, 17, 348–355.

Mutunga, M., Fulton, B., Bullock, R., Batchelor, A., Gascoigne, A., Gillespie, J.I. & Baudouin S.V. (2001). Circulating endothelial cells in patients with septic shock. Am J Respir Crit Care Med, 163, 195–200.

Narushima, I., Kita, T., Kubo, K., Yonetani, Y., Momochi, C., & Yoshikawa, I. (2003). Highly enhanced permeability of blood-brain barrier induced by repeated administration of endothelin-1 in dogs and rats. Pharmacol Toxicol, 92, 21–26.

Nishio, M., Yoshioka, K., Yamagami, K., Morikawa, T., Konishi, Y., & Hayashi, N. (2008). Reversible posterior leukoencephalopathy syndrome: a possible manifestation of Wegener's granulomatosis-mediated endothelial injury. Mod Rheumatol, 18, 309–314.

Okeda, R., Kawamoto, T., Tanaka, E., & Shimizu, H. (2007). An autopsy case of drug-induced diffuse cerebral axonopathic leukoencephalopathy: the pathogenesis in relation to reversible posterior leuko-encephalopathy syndrome. Neuropathology, 27, 364–370.

Pinedo, D.M., Shah-Khan, F., & Shah, P.C. (2007). Reversible posterior leukoencephalopathy syndrome associated with oxaliplatin. J Clin Oncol, 25, 5320–5321.

Rajasekhar. A., & George, T.J. Jr (2007). Gemcitabine-induced reversible posterior leukoencephalopathy syndrome: a case report and review of the literature. Oncologist, 12, 1332–1335.

Ramsay, L.E., Williams, B., Johnston, G.D., MacGregor, G.A., Poston, L., Potter, N.R. & Russell, G. (1999). British Hypertension Society guidelines for hypertension management. BMJ, 319, 630–635.

Saito, B., Nakamaki, T., Nakashima, H., Usui, T., Hattori, N., Kawakami K., & Tomoyasu, S. (2007). Reversible posterior leukoencephalopathy syndrome after repeat intermediate- dose cytarabine chemotherapy in a patient with acute myeloid leukemia. Am J Hematol, 82, 304–306.

Schwartz, R.B., Feske, S.K., Polack, J.F, DeGirolami, U., Iaia, A., Beckner, K.M., Bravo, S.M., Klufas, R.A. & Chai, R.Y. (2000). Preeclampsia-eclampsia: clinical and neuroradiographic correlates and insights into the pathogenesis of hypertensive encephalopathy. Radiology, 217, 371–376.

Schots, R., Kaufman, L., Van, Riet. I., Ben Othman, T., De Waele, M., Van Camp, B., & Demanet, C. (2003). Proinflammatory cytokines and their role in the development of major transplant-related complications in the early phase after allogeneic bone marrow transplantation. Leukemia, 17, 1150–1156.

Schwartz, R.B., Jones, K.M., Kalina, P., Bajakian, R.L., Mantello, M.T., Garada, B., & Holman, B.L. (1992). Hypertensive encephalopathy: findings on CT, MR imaging, and SPECT imaging in 14 cases. AJR Am J Roentgenol, 159, 379–383.

Servillo, G., Apicella, E., & Striano, P. (2008). Posterior reversible encephalopathy syndrome (PRES) in the parturient with preeclampsia after inadvertent dural puncture. Int J Obstet Anesth, 17, 88–89.

Sweany, J.M., Bartynski, W.S. & Boardman, J.F. (2007). "Recurrent" posterior reversible encephalopathy syndrome: report of 3 cases —PRES can strike twice! J Comput Assist Tomogr2007, 31, 148-156.

Varon, J., & Marik, P.E. (2003). Clinical review: the management of hypertensive crises. Crit Care, 7, 374–384.

Vaughan, C.J. & Delanty, N. (2000). Hypertensive emergencies. Lancet, 356, 411–417.

Vieillot, S., Pouessel, D., de Champfleur, N.M., Bech,t C., & Culine, S. (2007). Reversible posterior leuko-encephalopathy syndrome after carboplatin therapy. Ann Oncol, 18, 608–609.

Wijdicks, E.F. (2001). Neurotoxicity of immunosuppressive drugs. Liver Transpl, 7, 937–942.

Yano, Y., Kario, K., Fukunaga, T., Ohshita, T., Himeji, D., Yano, M., Nakagawa, S., Sakata, Y., & Shimada, K. (2005). A case of reversible posterior leukoencephalopathy syndrome caused by transient hypercoagulable state induced by infection. Hypertens Res, 8, 619–623.

Yokobori, S., Yokota, H., & Yamamoto, Y. (2006). Pediatric posterior reversible leukoencephalopathy syndrome and NSAID-induced acute tubular interstitial nephritis. Pediatr Neurol, 34, 245-247.

Yong, P.F., Hamour, S.M. & Burns, A. (2003). Reversible posterior leukoencephalopathy in a patient with systemic sclerosis/systemic lupus erythematosus overlap syndrome. Nephrol Dial Transplant, 18, 2660–2662.

# Chapter 6

# Fluoride: It's Biphasic Behavior

Patricia Vázquez-Alvarado[1], Alejandra Hernández-Ceruelos[2],
Sergio Muñoz-Juárez[2], Jesús Ruvalcaba-Ledezma[2], Julieta Macías-Ortega[1],
Juan Carlos Paz-Bautista[2], Josefina Reynoso-Vázquez[3],
Alejandro Chehue-Romero[3]

## 1 Introduction

Fluorine comes from the latin word *fluere* that means to flow. It is a pale green-yellow gas that is slightly heavier than air, reactive and poisonous. It belongs to the halogen group (VII A; molecular weight 17 g/mol), with the lowest atomic number. Its atom has very small distance between the nucleus and the valence electrons (Dingrano et al., 2003). As this element is highly electronegative and chemically reactive, except with the noble gases, it combines indirectly with nitrogen, chloride, calcium, hydrogen and oxygen to form fluorides (Dingrano et., al 2003; Lehninger et al., 1993).

Fluorine is the 13th more abundant element on the earth's crust. Human beings are exposed to it naturally in the water sources, with levels ranging from 0.1 to more than 25 mg/L in fresh water, and from 1.2 to 1.5 mg/L in sea water (WHO, 1984; WHO, 2002). Fluorine is not found as a free element, nevertheless, it can be found in rocks and the ground in a huge variety of minerals such as calcium fluoride, ($CaF_2$), cryolite ($Na_3AlF_6$), apatite [$Ca_5 (PO_4)_3F$] and topaz [$Al_2SiO_4 (FOH)_2$]. During the formation of some minerals in the presence of fluoride ions, the hydroxyl ion can be substituted in some of them such

[1] Dentistry School, Instituto de Ciencias de la Salud, Universidad Autónoma del Estado de Hidalgo, México.
[2] Medical School, Instituto de Ciencias de la Salud, Universidad Autónoma del Estado de Hidalgo, México.
[3] Pharmacy School, Instituto de Ciencias de la Salud, Universidad Autónoma del Estado de Hidalgo, México.

as muscovite $(K_2Al_4)(Si_6Al_2O_{20})(OH,F)_4$, that is a kind of mica, and in amphiboles like amosite $(FeMg)_7(Si_4O_{11})_2$-$(OH)_4$, and also in horns of animals $(Ca,Na)_{2-3}Mg,Fe,Al)_5$-$(Si,Al)_8O_{22}OH)_2$. Fluoride can also be found in andosols of volcanoes and as a subproduct of phosphate fertilizer production (Delmelle et al., 2003; Msonda et al., 2007; Mirlean and Rosenberg, 2007). $CaF_2$ is found in limestone and sand and it is present in hydrothermal deposits in contact with carbonated rocks. $CaF_2$ $(PO_4)_6$ is part of dolomites and limestone (Hernández, 1997).

Natural products of $F^-$ vary in function by the geology of the region, particularly considering the water source (Department of Health and Human Service, 1991), by height above sea level, and by geothermal activity (Sánchez et al., 2004; Hurtado and Gardea, 2005). Fluorides are liberated into the environment in a natural way through the weathering and dissolution of minerals, through volcanic emissions, and through sea aerosols. Anthropogenic activities, such as charcoal combustion; the production of iron, aluminum, copper and nickel; and the manufacture of glass, bricks and ceramics, also contribute to the release of F- to the air. Flouride is also used in the glue industry. Hexafluorosilicic acid $(H_2SiF_6)$ and disodium hexafluorosilicate $(Na_2SiF_6)$ are used in the fluorination of tap water (Hernández 1997). Human detritus can increase $F^-$ concentration in the environment (WHO, 2002).

$F^-$ in contact with the environment cannot be destroyed, only transformed. It can be found as a gas or in small particles that are transported by wind and atmospheric turbulences. Its presence in water depends on pH, water hardness and the presence of materials like clay that have the capacity to interchange ions, transported through the hydrologic cycle. The presence of $F^-$ in the ground depends on a slightly acidic pH (5.5-6.5) and a chemical complex formation, especially with aluminum and calcium. It is not easy to leach into the ground (ATSDR 2003).

## 1.1   Dynamic of F- *in vivo*

In humans and animals, $F^-$ absorption occurs mainly in the stomach and the intestine. This process depends of the solubility of the ingested fluorinated compound. In the presence of aluminum, phosphate, magnesium and calcium, it the absorption can decrease. The fluoride is quickly distributed through systemic circulation, both intracellularly and extracellularly. In humans and laboratory animals, 99 % of $F^-$ is retained in bones and teeth (Whitford, 1990; WHO, 2002). It is able to cross the placental barrier to the fetus, where the levels are lower than those observed in the mother (Caldera et al., 2004). In children, nearly 80 to 90% of $F^-$ is retained, compared to approximately 60% in adults. The highest concentrations are is in calcified tissues bone, dentine and enamel. $F^-$ is eliminated from the body in urine, sweat, tears and feces (WHO 2002).

## 1.2   Structure and Synthesis of Dental Enamel

The process of formation of dental enamel requires the participation of diverse agents including cells, proteins, enzymes and inorganic minerals. The most important cell in this process is the ameloblast that synthesizes a variety of proteins, the essential one being amelogenin, which assembles it into nanosphere deposits on the substrate dentine. The mineral called hydroxyapatite (HA), a special kind of calcium phosphate, forms in that matrix. In the absence of amelogenin, hydroxyapatite can crystalize on the dentine substrate, and grow homogeneously, without preferential orientation. In the presence of amelogenin, growth takes a very special form. Amelogenin nanoparticles act as scaffolding and guide for hydroxyapatite to grow into long fibrous crystals as a part of tooth enamel. As the crystals grow longer and wider, the protein amelogenin is digested by enzymes and takes up less space in the developing tooth enamel (Habelitz and Serry, 2005).

## 1.3   Incorporation of F⁻ into Dental Enamel

A number of hypotheses exist to explain the mechanism of $F^-$ metabolism. Many studies have been conducted to focus on the effects of fluoride, apatite nucleation and crystal growth (Browne, 2005). Dental enamel is formed mainly as a prismatic structural unit with a high content of hydroxyapatite $Ca_{10}(PO_4)_6(OH)_2$. Enamel has a porous structure that allows the diffusion and interchange of ions of a specific size and charge with the exterior media, permitting the process of mineralization or demineralization (Limeback, 1994). $F^-$ can be incorporated into dental tissue by:

### (a) Tissue concentration
$F^-$ incorporated into apatite crystals during tooth development, decreases the solubility forming crystals of apatite, transforming the HA into fluorapatite (FA) and making enamel more resistant to the attack of the acid-producing bacteria (Irigoyen and Sánchez, 2000).

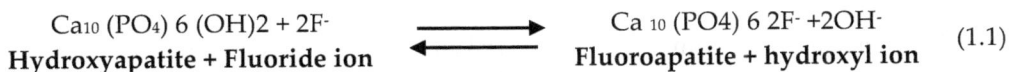

$$Ca_{10}(PO_4)6(OH)2 + 2F^- \rightleftarrows Ca_{10}(PO_4)6\ 2F^- + 2OH^- \tag{1.1}$$

**Hydroxyapatite + Fluoride ion**     **Fluoroapatite + hydroxyl ion**

### (b) Re-mineralizing effect
Occurs when the tooth is calcified by incorporation of $F^-$ in high concentrations, and then the loss of minerals from the hydroxyapatite crystal surface can be minimized, further allowing re-mineralization through the inclusion of calcium and phosphate salts (Irigoyen and Sánchez 2000).

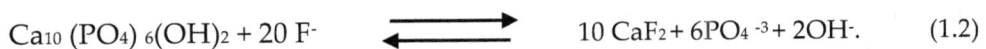

$$Ca_{10}(PO_4)_6(OH)_2 + 20\ F^- \rightleftarrows 10\ CaF_2 + 6PO_4^{-3} + 2OH^-. \tag{1.2}$$

However, if the concentration of $F^-$ during the enamel development is toxic, there can be an alteration in cellular function, inhibition of synthesis, cyst formation on tooth germs or an enamel abnormality (Ling and Jian, 2006; Wang et al., 2004; Limeback, 1994).

Histologically, in dental fluorosis there are two identified zones: surface and subsurface layers. The first one is translucent and hypermineralized, containing high amounts of $F^-$ and small aberrations on the enamel crystals. The subsurface is opaque and hypomineralized, with great numbers of pores. Enamel crystals with a low content of F⁻

are eroded. The effect of F- in the enamel crystals is completed with the formation of the molecular unit of hydroxyapatite

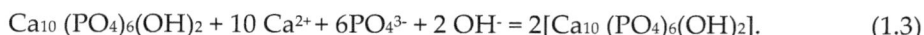

$$Ca_{10} (PO_4)_6(OH)_2 + 10\ Ca^{2+} + 6PO_4^{3-} + 2\ OH^- = 2[Ca_{10} (PO_4)_6(OH)_2]. \tag{1.3}$$

In presence of high concentrations of F- in the fluid phase of enamel, a large quantity of mineral is turned into FA. This reaction releases the hydroxyl groups, limiting the drop in the acidity level that is normally observed during fast growth of the crystal.

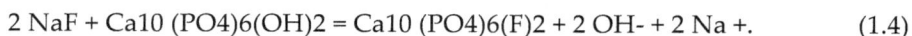

$$2\ NaF + Ca10\ (PO4)6(OH)2 = Ca10\ (PO4)6(F)2 + 2\ OH- + 2\ Na +. \tag{1.4}$$

This change in pH can produce abnormal amelogenesis and prevent diffusion of the protein out of the mature enamel. Proteins of enamel are more soluble in acid conditions, but they form insoluble aggregates in neutral conditions. The surface of the crystals of HA also can be affected by local changes in pH. A secondary effect of the presence of F- in the enamel crystals is that FA grows more in thickness than in length (Limeback, 1994).

F- has been shown to have the following effects: an increase in the size of apatite crystals, an improvement in the crystallinity of apatite and an to increase in the driving force towards apatite nucleation and growth (Legeros and Tung, 1983). Scanning and electron micrographic studies of fluorotic enamel have revealed alterations in morphology and crystal defects. (Yanagisawa et al., 1989) These collective–studies suggest that excessive concentrations of F- in developing enamel partially inhibit proteinases that split larger molecular weight amelogenins (Bawden et al., 1995). Inhibition at the critical stage of enamel formation could have major effects in structural appearance of fully formed enamel. It is important to assess the calcification and eruption dates of primary and permanent teeth in order to identify when developing teeth are at the most risk of enamel fluorosis (Browne, 2005).

With the aim of minimizing fluorosis risk, it is important to identify the age of susceptibility for the developmental alteration in children, the critical period or "window of maximum susceptibility for fluorosis" (Rippa y Clark 2001; Baden, 1996). It has been learned that the susceptibility period for complete permanent dentition is from 11 months to 7 years of age. After age seven, an excess in F- ingestion does not represent a risk for dental fluorosis, since by this age all permanent teeth except third molars have developed their crowns (Ishii and Suckling, 1991).

The first year of life is considered as a crucial period for fluorosis development (Ismail and Messer, 1996). Other studies have concluded that the critical time is between 15 and 30 months of age (Baden, 1991; Evans and Darvel, 1995; Evans and Stamm, 1991). Dental fluorosis becomes is evident when a child has consumed an excessive amount of F- during enamel development (Ripa and Clark, 2001).

## 2   Benefits of F-

F- is considered as a trace element. In low concentrations it is essential for bones and tooth formation in animals and human beings (Eckabaram and Paul, 2001). The use of F- for the promotion of bucodental health is still valid, mainly for the decrease of the prevalence and incidence of dental decay worldwide (Gutiérrez and Morales, 2006). Approximately 210 million people consume tap water with optimal concentrations of F- to prevent dental decay and 500 million use fluoridated toothpaste (WHO, 2002).

Bacteria in the oral cavity are subjected to many environmental stresses, including recurrent cycles of low pH, resulting from the production of organic acids by the bacteria that are exposed to dietary carbohydrates (Carlsson and Hamilton, 1994). Some bacteria, such as lactobacillus, are acid tolerant; others can, in response to sub-lethal values, initiate an acid tolerance response (ATR). The ATR thereby allows the bacteria to survive and continue producing acids at low pH values (Hamilton and Buckley, 1991; Marsh, 2003; Matsui and Cvitkovitch, 2010). *Streptocuccus mutants* biofilm-grown cells have been shown to express a more acid tolerant phenotype. This characteristic disappears if the biofilm cells are dispersed, indicating that acid tolerance is phenotypic and not genotypic in nature. An acid tolerant microflora can cause prolonged periods of low pH in plaque, with demineralization in enamel and development of dental caries (Bowden, 1991).

Fluoride's primary anti-caries effect is thought to be the conversion of HA to FA, which resists acid dissolution. However, another important property of F- is its effect on bacterial physiology. F- inhibits bacterial carbohydrate metabolism by affecting the enzyme enolase in the glycolytic pathway (Hamilton, 1990; Hamilton and Ellwood, 1978). It has also been shown to affect a range of other enzymes such as catalase, urease, and the F-ATPases (Thibodeau and Keefe 1990; Marquis 1977). A more recently discovered property of is that it can inhibit the induction of an ATR in *S. mutants* and it has been shown in plaque biofilms *in vivo* (Welin-Neilands and Svensater, 2007; Neilands et al., 2012).

In recent years there has been an increase in dental caries, and there is a need for new preventive strategies (Bagramian et al., 2009). One strategy could be the prevention of acid-tolerant oral bacteria. F- is an important factor in caries prevention; however, in high doses, it can result in the development of fluorosis (Moller; 1982).

Low concentrations of delmopinol in combination with low concentrations of F- inhibited acid adaptation in plaque biofilms *in vitro,* and the combination of both also prevents pH decrease in plaque biofilms after glucose pulsing at levels where F- or delmopinol alone had no effect (Neilands et al., 2014).

Erosion and erosive tooth wear refers to the chemical-mechanical process that has become prevalent in 11 to 16-year-old children (Shellis et al., 2011; Huysmans et al., 2011). As dental caries disease tooth erosion is a multifactorial condition (patient-related and nutritional factors), overtime, the interaction of all these factors may lead to progression. Different methods, such as the use of topical fluorides, have been indicated to prevent or slow the progression of dental erosion (Magalhaes et al., 2009).

Fluoride therapy has been suggested as a preventive measure against tooth erosion, and its effects are reported to be better when applied at high concentrations (Sorvari et al., 1994; Magalhaes et al., 2009; Manarelli et al., 2013). Despite the fact that gel is a more affordable vehicle (lower cost), with high concentrations of F-, there are few studies in which compounds are added to improve its effect against erosion (Bueno and Marsicano,

2010). Utilization of sodium trimetaphosphate (TMP) and F- association has shown decreased enamel demineralization and dental erosion (Manarelli et al., 2013; Moretto et al., 2010; Takeshita et al., 2009; Takeshita et al., 2011; Manarrelli et al., 2011). In addition, F- topical gel with 4500 ppm, associated with TMP, presented the same ability to produce enamel re-mineralization as gel with 12300 ppm (Danelon et al., 2013). Nevertheless, the erosive challenge is a process that occurs at a pH < 4.0 and it is the pH of the dissolution of calcium fluoride. (Fushida and Cury 1999; Barbour et al., 2011).

The addition of TMP in the fluoride gel gave a superior result, not related to calcium fluoride deposition on enamel. As observed in a recent study the use of a topical gel with 4500 ppm F-, the TMP did not influence the absorption of calcium fluoride, and neither enhanced nor reduced precipitation (Danelon et al., 2013; Souza et al., 2013). Based in previous studies, TMP has been shown to interact with enamel, producing a protective layer on the enamel surface, and thereby hindering acid diffusion (Takeshita et al., 2011; Van Dijk et al., 1980, Pancote et.al. 2014).

# 3   Risk Factors for Developing Enamel Fluorosis

A certain degree of enamel fluorosis is inevitable with water fluoridation. Dean (Dean et al., 1950) regarded an increase prevalence of enamel fluorosis as an acceptable risk when compared to the benefits to oral health that would result from the introduction of this public health measure. However, other fluoride-containing products, such as toothpastes have become available to the public for consumption since the time of Dean, and now there is clear evidence that fluorosis is increasing in the USA and worldwide. As F- level in water has remained relatively stable, the increase in fluorosis is likely to be related to increased consumption of F- containing products in on children under six years old (Browne, 2005).

Fluoridated toothpaste, since its introduction into the European market in the 1970s, now occupies over 95 % of the toothpaste market. It has led to a marked decreased in caries in all countries. The European Union guidelines stated that fluoridated toothpaste sold over the counter should contain no more than 1500 ppm. An increasing number of infants and very young children have tended to swallow toothpaste, and this is likely to be contributing to the increasing level on enamel fluorosis. An excess of F- can be ingested if children inadvertently swallow too much toothpaste (Center for Disease Control and Prevention, 2001).

Fluoride supplements are a risk factor for fluorosis in young children when used inappropriately and not conforming to appropriate dosing schedules. The non-observed adverse effect limit (NOAEL) is defined as the highest dose of a chemical in a single study, found by experiment or observation, which causes non detectable adverse health effects (Deparment of health and children, 2002). The NOAEL is based on long-term studies, preferably of ingested drinking water, for F- is 0.05 mg/kg/body weight in the case of enamel fluorosis. This level, for children under 8 years, will not produce mild fluorosis in permanent teeth. The lowest observed adverse effect limit (LOAEL) is the lowest dose of a chemical in a single study that causes a detectable adverse health effect. In the context of enamel fluorosis, the LOAEL is 0.1 mg F-/kg body weight. (Browne, 2005).

Children (< 6 years) should not use fluoridated toothpaste and mouth rinse without prior consultation with a dentist, as fluorosis could occur if both are swallowed. Fluoride supplements can be prescribed for children at high risk of dental caries. For children aged < 6 years, dentists should weigh the risk for caries without fluoride supplements, the caries prevention offered by supplements, and the potential for enamel caries when considering the use of F- mouth rinses (Centers for Disease Control and Prevention, 2001). Children aged between 2 and 7 years of age should be supervised when brushing, and only a pea-size amount of toothpaste should be used. The use of pediatric toothpaste with low concentrations of F- requires further research before it can be recommended. (Department of health and children, 2002). The child should also be encouraged to spit out excess toothpaste. When use appropriately, F- is a safe and effective method of reducing dental caries. It is needed throughout life to prevent and control dental decay (Browne, 2005)

## 3.1   Defining and Measuring Enamel Fluorosis

Enamel fluorosis is a hypomineralization of enamel characterized by greater surface and subsurface porosity that in normal enamel as a result of excess of F- intake during the period of enamel formation (Burt and Eklund, 1992). It has also been defined as being a dose response effect caused by F- ingestion during the pre-eruptive development of teeth. This change in the enamel is characterized by altered appearance of the tooth ranging from fine white lines to pitting or staining of enamel. (Browne, 2005).

Dean found that the maximum caries reduction in a community served with naturally occurring fluoride in domestic water supplies was observed at 1 ppm. At this level, however, it was reported that one would expect to see 1% with mild, 19 % with very mild and 31 % with questionable fluorosis. This gives a cumulative total of 51 % with some degree of fluorosis and 49 % with no change in the appearance of the tooth enamel. At the time of Dean, it was decided that this level of risk (fluorosis) was acceptable; taking into account the reduced caries levels (Dean, 1934).

There are two main methods for recording enamel fluorosis. The first are the etiological indices. Dean observed a correlation between F- in the drinking water and mottled enamel, and from this, he devised Dean's Index of Fluorosis (Dean, 1934). These indices score the two teeth that are most affected. The first index grades fluorosis as very mild, mild, moderate or severe, and notes the percentage of the labial surface that is affected by fluorosis (Thylstup and Fejerskov, 1978) Dean's index has proven to be a robust classification and is recommended for the use by the WHO in its publication *Oral Health Survey-Basic Method* (WHO, 1994).

Thylstup and Fejerskov (1978) proposed a modification of Dean's index known as the TF index. This classifies clinical features of fluorosis that reflect histopathological changes following histological examination of affected enamel using ordinary and polarized light. The index requires that the teeth be dried before examination.

The Tooth Surface Index of Fluorosis (TSIF) described by Horowitz et al., (1984) provides an analysis based on an esthetic concern and examines teeth when wet. The

Fluorosis Risk Index (FRI), developed by Pendrys (1990), is designed to produce an accurate association between age-specific exposures to F- and the development of fluorosis. It divides the enamel surface of the permanent teeth into two developmentally related groups of surface zones. Code one began formation during the first year of life, and code two occurred during the third to sixth years of life. Scores are recorded for each zone.

The second methods for recording fluorosis are the descriptive indices. The descriptive index developed by Young (1973) formed the basis of several indices that were to be developed later. He used three features to define the clinical characteristics of enamel defects: location, color, and hypoplasia. He also attempted to ascribe an esthetic severity to the opacities within his index. The indices used by Al-Alousi et al., (1975) Jackson et al., (1975) and Murray and Shaw (1974) were all modifications of the descriptive method proposed by Young (1973). Differences included the tooth surface recorded and condensing category groups. The Developmental Defects of Enamel (DDE) were developed in 1982 by the Federation Dentaire Internationale (FDI 1992), and has since been modified (Clarckson, 1992). It divides defects into three types: demarcated, diffuse and hypoplasia. The modified version of DDE index suggested that the extent of the defect should be recorded in thirds of the tooth surface area and that a limit in size of greater than 1 mm in diameter should be used to distinguish between normal and abnormal enamel.

# 4   Fluoride Levels in the Environment and Human Exposure

Since the first reports of Dean and collaborators in the 1930's and 1940's, (Dean and Elvove, 1935; Dean, 1938; Dean et al., 1939 and Dean, 1942) the maximum concentration of F- in the tap water has changed with time, according to the government of each country. In the 1950's it was determined that a 1 ppm of F- in drinking water, providing the maximum protection against dental cavities and a minimum level of fluorosis (Ismail and Messer, 1996). In 1969, after 30 years of research, WHO implemented the massive fluoridation of drinking water internationally. In Europe, the countries that applied this measure were Ireland, East Germany, The Czech Republic, Hungary, Russia and the Netherlands. Denmark and France supplemented with F- and salt respectively (Gale, 2006).

The EPA (United States Environmental Protection Agency), established the maximum permitted level of F- concentration in drinking water in the US as 4.0 mg/L. At the same time, for natural water, a second law marked the maximum level as 2.0 mg/L, but it did not require residents of the area to be informed about the risk of development dental fluorosis when the level was exceeded. (United States Environmental Protection Agency, http://water.epa.gov/drink/contaminants/).

In Mexico, a maximum level of 1.5 mg/L has been established in tap water (NMX-AA-077-SCFI-2001) and a maximum concentration of 0.7 mg/L for bottled water (NOM-041-SSA1-1995). Nevertheless, there is a national program for salt fluorination, as a specific massive protection against dental decay (NMX-040-SSA1-1996), but with restricted distribution of this product in places where the concentration of F- in water for human consumption is over 0.7 ppm.

## 4.1  F⁻ Levels in Endibles

All edibles contain small amounts of F⁻, ranging from 2 to 100 ɫg/L, as well as, breast milk with levels from 5 to 10 g/L (WHO, 2002). Tea leaves are particularly rich in F⁻, depending of the quantity of F⁻ in water for the preparation of the infusion, the time of boiling, the kind of tea, the amount of tea, the frequency of ingestion, and the size of the cup (Duckworth and Duckworth, 1978; Lung et al., 2008).

The aquatic and terrestrial biota bioaccumulate soluble F⁻ depending on the route of the exposition and its bioavailability (Enger and Smith, 2006). Edible plants can accumulate F⁻ through the deposition of airborne particles, absorption of F- on the ground and contact with phosphate fertilizers that contain high amounts of F⁻ (1-3 %). Water for plant irrigation that can contain over 3.1 mg/L, can increase F⁻ concentration in edibles for human consumption (WHO, 1970).

# 5  F⁻ Toxicity

Even when F⁻ has beneficial effects, there is evidence of toxicity in humans, such as dental and skeletal fluorosis (Choubisa, 2001). In addition, liver, kidney, parotid glands and brain damage have been observed (Shan et al., 2004; Shantakumari 2004; Wang et al., 2004). There is also a higher risk of brain damage and IQ reduction in children (Wang et al., 2007).

An acute toxic dose of 5 mg/kg can provoke a variety of effects such as nausea, vomit, abdominal pain, diarrhea, fatigue, somnolence, convulsions, cardiac arrhythmia, coma, respiratory arrest and death. For a human, it has been estimated that a lethal dose for NaF is between 5 and 10 g (32-64 mg/Kg) (ATSDR, 2003; Zeiger et al., 1993). Toxicity of F⁻ depends on the compound ingested. One of the more soluble salts of inorganic F⁻ is NaF, which is more toxic than the less soluble F⁻ salts, such as $CaF_2$ (WHO, 2002).

The acute ingestion of toxic amounts of F⁻ can provoke a corrosive gastric mucosal injury through the action of hydrofluoric acid, which is produced when the F⁻ salt interacts with the acid media of the stomach. Gastric damage leads to bleeding and loss of epithelial cells. In the oral cavity it can cause a hypersensitivity reaction, presenting with ulcerations, after topic treatment with stannous fluoride (Whitford, 1990).

Respiratory effects of F⁻ such as bleeding, pulmonary edema and apnea have been observed in persons after the inhalation of hydrofluoric acid (ASTDR 2003). Other clinical signs described in intoxicated persons are, labial paralysis, vertigo, limb spasticity and general disorientation (Machalinska et al., 2001).

Exposure to F⁻ affects cells of hard tissues like teeth and bones, as well as soft tissues such as reproductive organs, kidneys and the endothelium (National Research Council, 2006). Exposure to F⁻ increases the production of superoxide as a consequence of hydrogen peroxide metabolism inducing eroxinitrate, hydroxyl radicals, and increasing oxidative stress (Barbier et al., 2010; Garcia-Montalvo et al., 2009; Chinoy, 2003) and inducing lypoperoxidation of membranes, apoptosis and DNA damage (Wang et al., 2007). The clinical application of NaF induced genotoxicity on the oral epithelium in acute exposition according to Zeiger et al., (1993). Tiwari and Rao (2010) considered F- as a mutagenic agent that even in low concentrations can increase the induction of chromosomal aberrations. In a previous study, a community exposed to F- presented dental fluorosis and a positive correlation with the high concentration of F- in the well water (Vazquez-Alvarado et al., 2010).

However, the high concentration of F- also affected DNA of epithelial cells, making them susceptible to mutations, transformation and the development of neoplasia. Evidence that cytogenetic biomarkers are correlated with cancer risk has been strongly validated (Guachalla and Ascarrunz, 2003). In recent results from both cohort and nested case-control studies, showing that Comet assay is a marker of cancer risk, reflecting both, the genotoxic effects of carcinogens and individual cancer susceptibility as showed in many studies (Bonassi et al., 2007; Smerhovsky et al., 2001; Rekhadevi et al., 2007). The increase in DNA damage of epithelial cells when they were in contact with NaF (2 %) made evident the high genotoxic potential of F-, since most of the cells of this group were classified with the maximum degree of damage (45%). Considering that the samples were taken from the same students used for negative control, the topical appliance of fluoride gel on teeth is able to induce a very significant DNA damage on the oral epithelial cells in an acute exposure. In a community with water concentration for human consumption of 1.67 mg/L, severe genotoxic damage was observed in oral epithelial cells with the comet assay, similar to that observed after the clinical appliance for NaF (Vázquez-Alvarado et al., 2012).

Chronic fluoride exposure can induce oxidative stress (Bouaziz et al., 2007), while oxidative stress is closely related to inflammation and endothelial cell activation. The excess fluoride promotes atherosclerosis by inducing oxidative stress and endothelial activation. Experimental studies in animals have demonstrated that the atherogenic effect and inflammatory responses are due to fluoride, and not lipid metabolic disorder, which plays a crucial role in the cardiovascular toxicity of fluoride (Flora et al., 2011; Gamkrelidze, et al., 2008). A positive closed relationship between fluoride exposure and the prevalence of carotid artery atherosclerosis was found using cross-sectional study. It is also noted that elevated inter cellular adhesion molecule 1 (ICAM-1) and decreased glutatine peroxidase (GPx) were associated with carotid atherosclerosis in fluoride endemic areas (Liu et al., 2014).

Epidemiological evidence supports that fluoride may impair children's learning and memory ability. Children's intelligence quotient (IQ) scores are significantly lower in high-level fluoride areas of Shanxi Province compared to those of children in non-endemic areas (Wang et al., 2007). Calderon et al., (2000) found that 6–8-year-old children showed lower reaction rates and reduced abstract thinking ability in the city of San Luis Potosi (Mexico), which is probably due to long-term excessive intake of fluoride through drinking water.

Previous studies have investigated the mechanisms of the effect of fluoride on cognition and found that excess fluoride can pass through the blood brain barrier and exert a negative impact on the brain tissue. Fluoride may affect the content of monoamine neurotransmitters, such as noradrenaline (NA), dopamine (DA) and serotonin (5-HT), which could lead to impaired neurotransmission. Pereira et al., (2011) found that NaF-induced memory impairment was associated with NA and 5- HT increases in discrete rat brain regions. In addition, fluoride may affect the activity of some enzymes in the brain. Bharti et al. (2012) confirmed that F- significantly reduces acetylcholine esterase (AchE) content in rat brain. Degroot et al., (2002) found that AchE can inhibit the formation of physostigmine in either the dorsal or the ventral hippocampus, resulting in increased exploratory behavior in the open arm elevated-plus maze, which was in accordance with the findings of Liu et al, (2014.) The learning and memory deficits are the result of interaction of fluoride with the activity of the enzyme acetylcholine esterase. Exposure to fluoride also results in a decrease of the nicotinic acetylcholine receptors (Shan et al., 2004). Fluoride exposed rats showed inhibition of spontaneous motor activity, due to alterations in the function of neurotransmitters, their structure and cholinergic mechanisms (Paul et al., 1998; Raghu et al., 2013)

Essential hypertension is the most common type of hypertension (HTN) in 90% of patients. Although the root causes of HTN are still being explored, endocrine system components such as the renin–angiotensin system, mineralocorticoids, catecholamines, endothelins (ET), and nitric oxide (Carey, 2011) have been demonstrated to play an important role in essential HTN.

In recent years, the role of ET in HTN has received more attention. As the principal member of the ET family, Endothelin-1 (ET-1) was originally isolated and characterized from the culture media of aortic endothelial cells (Yanagisawa et al., 1988). ET-1 carries out a variety of physiological and pathophysiological functions in vascular biology, and its main action is to increase blood pressure (BP) and vascular tone (Agapitov and Haynes, 2002; Kawanabe and Nauli, 2011). Moreover, ET-1 was suggested to play a crucial role in several cardiovascular diseases, including congestive heart failure (CHF), HTN, atherosclerosis (AS), renal disease and many others (Masaki, 2004; Khimji and Rockey, 2010).

There is a significant relationship between an excess of F- exposure from drinking water and essential HTN in adults living in fluoride endemic areas; although, the underlying mechanisms were somewhat unclears, the ET-1 might be related with this phenomenon (Sun et al., 2013). Vascular oxidative stress could contribute to vascular stiffness (Delles et al., 2008; Noma et al., 2007). With an increase of fluoride concentrations in drinking water, vascular compliance decreased and stiffness increased (Varol et al., 2010; Varol and Varol, 2012).

Occurrence of F- bone injury is a complex process that involves both exogenous and endogenous factors. Except for F- burden, F- bone injury is also associated with the genetic background (Cooper et al. 2006). F- enters the body primarily through respiratory or digestive tract and accumulates in bone and soft tissue via blood circulation. By stimulating osteoblasts, F- promotes bone formation in both cortical and trabecular bone, but its effect on trabecular bone is greater, occurs earlier, and leads to a more pronounced increase in spine density on x-ray films (Baylink et al., 1983). Increased risk was due to the excessive F- burden, which could lead to the accumulation of fluorapatite in bone (Jun et al., 2011). Fluorapatite is difficult to absorb, can destroy the dynamic balance of bone resorption and formation, and finally leads to bone metabolic disorders depending on the genotype effects where the polymorphic forms TC, TT and CC genotypes for the calcitonin receptor (CTR) gene are able to develop more bone injury (Jun, et al., 2011). Flourosis results in an osteocondensation by altering bone mass through effects on skeletal mineralization, impaired bone resorption and ion induced decreased bone strength (Assefa et al., 2004; Kleerekoper, 1996). These are all contradictory effects leading to a combination of osteosclerosis, stress fractures, ligamentous calcification, ossification and a radiculomyelopathy owing to mechanical compressive effects (Haettich et al., 1991; Tamer et al., 2007; Reddy, 2009). A high concentration of F- in Pakistan is related to vertebral sclerosis, a combination of premature degeneration with anterior disc herniation and an unusual high frequency of vertebral hemangioma. These formed the spectrum of magnetic resonances image findings in subjects with spinal flourosis having backache but no neurological findings. (Ahmed et al., 2013; Sang et al., 2010).

Reproductive function of female rats was markedly damaged when they were exposed to NaF (100, 150 and 200 mg/L). The endometrial cells became larger, and the endometrial glands became hypertrophic. The total number of each type of follicle was changed in NaF groups: the number of small follicles increased and the large follicle number decreased. This indicates that sufficiently high fluoride intake through drinking water may reduce female reproductive function by affecting steroidogenesis and steroid hormone receptor expression, underlying poor reproduction in females that have been exposed to sodium fluoride (Zhou et al., 2013; Del Raso et al., 1993 ) .

Fluorine compounds also act on the organic part of supporting tissues, including proteins. Fluoride increases the mass of non-collagen proteins such as proteoglycans and glucosaminoglycans, accelerating skin aging even though protein biosynthesis is generally suppressed. Final outcome includes progressive vascular lesions (Machoy-Mokrzynska 2004). Excessive exposure to fluoride may lead to acute poisoning, hyperemia, cerebral edema, and liver degeneration. Fluoride can increase the rate of DNA damage, and induce apoptosis and expression of p53 in human embryo hepatocytes. Furthermore, for both apoptosis and the level of p53 expression, there exists a rising tendency with the increasing concentration of fluoride (Jha et al., 2012). Reduction in liver protein content in mice induced by NaF, observed by Chang (1978), might be due to either increased proteolysis or decreased protein synthesis or fluoride induced osmotic imbalance caused by lipid peroxidation. The reduction in protein content of NaF-treated animals supports the view that fluoride inhibits oxidative decarboxylation of branched chain amino acids and simultaneously promotes protein breakdown. This reduction or loss of enzymatic activity could be due to fluoride-generated free radicals ultimately causing inactivation of enzymes. Kathpalia and Susheela (1978) have observed that administration of large doses of NaF to rabbits caused a 10 to 46% reduction in protein content in most body tissue (Jha et al., 2012).

Apoptosis plays an important role in F- toxicity in several cell types, including pancreatic cells (Loweth et al., 1996), possibly because of the involvement of oxidative stress, as reported for HL-60 cells exposed to 2 mM NaF (Anuradha et al., 2001) or primary cultured hippocampal neurons exposed to 0.476, 0.952 and 1.904 mM NaF (Zhang et al., 2007). The effects of F- on glucose metabolism have been examined in both *in vivo* and *in vitro* studies. Trivedi et al., (1993) reported impaired glucose tolerance in 10 of 25 residents of an area with endemic fluorosis. An increase of 17% in serum glucose was observed in rabbits administered with F- in drinking water at 100 mg/L for 6 months (Turner et al., 1997). Additionally, Rigalli et al., (1992; 1995) reported a decreased in insulin levels, an increased in plasma glucose and a disturbance of the glucose tolerance test in rats after an oral dose of a solution 40 M NaF per 100 g body weight. *In vitro* studies have been controversial, for example, Komatsu et al., (1995) found that, in rat insulinoma (RINm5F) cells exposed to 5–15 mM NaF increased insulin release for up to 60 minutes in a dose-dependent manner. Studies done in Langerhans islets isolated from rats showed a relationship between F- exposure and decreased insulin secretion. However, Menoyo et al. (2005) found an inhibitory effect on insulin secretion at micromolar concentrations (5–20 M).

Decreased expression of insulin mRNA in pancreatic TC-6 cells could be associated with oxidative stress induced by F- exposure. Sakai et al., (2003) reported that hydrogen peroxide in murine pancreatic cells (MIN6) induced mitochondrial ROS, which suppressed first-phase Glucose-stimulated insulin secretion (GSIS), at least, in part through the suppression of Glyceraldhyde-3-phosphatedehydrogenase (GAPDH) activity. Some authors propose that mitochondrial overwork may be a potential mechanism through which first-phase GSIS becomes impaired in the early stages of diabetes mellitus. Furthermore, Kaneto et al., (2005) reported that when oxidative stress was induced in cells in vitro, insulin gene promoter activity and mRNA levels were suppressed. They were accompanied by a reduced activity of pancreatic and duodenal homeobox factor-1 (PDX-1), which is an important transcription factor for the insulin gene. Moreover, diabetic individuals may have higher F- intake and retention than healthy individuals (Lantz et al., 1987; Torra et al., 1998), due to increased water intake and decreased renal clearance. Also, there is increased retention of F- in the body for patients with kidney damage, or those with compromised renal clearance, such as the elderly, and those whose diets are deficient of $Ca^{2+}$ (Guggenheim et al., 1976). Therefore, in these conditions, the severity of the diabetes could increase as the F- exposure increases (García-Montalvo et al., 2009).

The liver is the most effective organ of the body in synthesizing cholesterol (Yu et al., 1991). There are significantly adverse changes in the lipid and lipoprotein profiles, total cholesterol, high-density lipoprotein (HDL), low-density lipoprotein (LDL) and triglycerides in postmenopausal women (Oral and Ozbasar 2003) and fluorotic patients (Shashi and Kumar 2008; Juganmohan et al., 2010). Fluorides reduce lipoprotein lipase (LPL) activity and cause a diminished peripheral removal of lipoproteins in plasma (Kokotos et al., 2010). Theoretically, the reduction in LPL activity could result from the direct inhibition of the enzyme by fluorides, or from the decreased levels of plasma apoprotein CII, known as an activator of LPL. The decline in the cholesterol content may be due to inhibition of lipid synthesis by fluoride as well as increased utilization of stored lipids as a source of energy to conduct regular metabolic functions. Fluoride is a well-known inhibitor of lipases, phosphatases, esterases, and acetyl Co-A synthetase. It interferes with fatty acid oxidation which results in decreased synthesis of cholesterol from Acetyl Co-. Fluoride reduces the absorption of cholesterol and bile salt from plasma and intestine, which could result in an increased conversion of bile acids in the liver. Bile acids are known to inhibit cholesterol synthesis in the intestine. This is indicative of hepato-biliary disturbances in fluoride intoxication (Bennis et al., 1993).

A study showed hypocholestrolemia and hypolipidemia, and hypertriglycer-idemia, and revealed a significantly increased TC/HDL, and LDL/HDL ratio in fluorotic patients. High fluoride levels in drinking water may prevent atherosclerosis. Hypocho-lesterolemia was observed in patients affected with fluorosis due to high fluoride intake through drinking water. Fluoride may cause disturbances in lipid metabolism (Bhardwaj and Sashi 2013). The decline in the cholesterol content may be due to inhibition of lipid synthesis by fluoride as well as increased utilization of stored lipids as a source of energy to conduct regular metabolic functions. Flavonoids reduce the levels of cholesterol in plasma and thus slow down the process of atherosclerosis in blood vessels. Biochemical work on lipid metabolism and endemic fluorosis is limited and results are conflicting. Earlier workers demonstrated decreased levels of cholesterol in the patients with skeletal fluorosis (Chinoy et al., 1992). Michael et al., (1996) observed normal levels of serum cho-lesterol among fluorotic individuals at 6.53 ppm fluoride in drinking water.

F- ingestion is associated with hypoplastic enamel (in healty patients), and in severe cases, can present itself as a pitted enamel surface ( Fejerskov et al., 1977; Denbesten 1999). During tooth formation, renal insufficiency is also associated with defective tooth struc-ture and in particular, enamels hypoplasia (Farge et al., 2006; Koch, 1999). In patients with renal insufficiency, the decreased ability to excrete F- leads to increased retention of this anion. Indeed, the serum levels of F- are elevated in children (Spack et al., 1985) and adults (Schiff and Binswanger 1980) with impaired renal function. Donacian et al., (2008) tested that uremia aggravates the F-, inducing changes in developing teeth of rats incisors. This tooth model continuously erupts and contains all stages of dentine and enamel formation in a single tooth. There are series of retrospective clinical studies in children or adults with chronic renal failure, end-stage renal disease, or following kidney transplantation that have associated poor renal function with enamel developmental defects in primary (mainly canines) (Koch et al., 1999) and permanent dentition (Lucas and Roberts 2005; Nunn et al., 2000; Al Nowaiser et al., 2003).

Moreover, the severity of the renal- failure induced pathology in dentition is cor-related with age at disease onset. Most teeth are affected if renal insufficiency occurs dur-ing the first four years of childhood (Nunn et al., 2000). The enamel defects described in these studies, included demarcated and diffuse enamel opacities and the more serious enamel hypoplasia (pits) (Wysocky et al., 1983; Nasstrom et al., 1993).

The transitional-stage ameloblast appears to be particularly sensitive to both the effects of uremia and F- (Lyaruu et al., 2006). The effects of uremia are primarily in the dentine but also occur in enamel, resulting in hyperplasia and pitting of the enamel sur-face. The crown portion of human central incisors (the most aesthetically visible teeth) forms up to approximately five years of age, with the second permanent molars forming by about eight year of age. Therefore, children who present with renal insufficiency be-fore the age of eight years are at risk for tooth defects. These effects will be more severe with an increased ingestion of F- by young children with renal failure. F- supplements or swallowing F- containing toothpaste is contraindicated as suggested previously (Lucas and Roberts 2005). Further studies to determine the specific stage of uremia and F- on tooth formation may result in a better understanding of the overall effects of uremia on mineralized tissues such as dentine, enamel and bone (Donacian et al., 2008).

There is not a specific treatment for the many toxic effects of F-. Symptoms and signs of provoked for the damage of this toxic to a particular organ are normally controlled as a part of the standard procedure of the disease, for example, hypertension, renal or liver falure, are treated according to standard procedures, not focused on the toxicity of F- (Shantakumari et al., 2004; Wang et al., 2004). For dental fluorosis, there is only the use of prosthetic rehabilitation, to cover the aesthetic problem, but not acting over the damaged enamel (Rakow and Ligth, 1986). As a measure of protection against the oxidative stress induced by F-, an increase in the consumption of antioxidants, fruit and vegetables may decreased the oxidative damage. Several researchers had tested different natural compounds like curcumin, *Aloe vera, Oscimum sanctum, Ginkgo biloba* and ascorbic acid, for their efficacy against fluoride toxicity (Raghu et al., 2013).

# 6   Defluoridation

Remedial measures have to be considered for the prevention of fluorosis, if a F- concentration in a water source exceeds the permissible level, these can be broadly divided into three categories: precipitation, adsorption and membrane based. Precipitation methods involve the addition of soluble chemicals to water. F-is removed either by precipitation, co-precipitation or adsorption onto the formed precipitate (Culp and Stoltenberg, 1958; Nawlakhe et al., 1975; Saha, 1993). The adsorption process involves the passage of raw water through an adsorbent bed, where F- is removed by physical-exchange or surface chemical reactions with the solid matrix. A wide range of adsorbents such as activated alumina, bone chart clay, zeolites, yash, brick, tricalcic phosphate, sea fossils treated with aluminum sulfate and specific ion exchange resins have been reported for F- removal (Maier, 1953; Bhargaba and Killedar 1992; Chaturvedi et al., 1990; Chauhan et al., 2007).

Other defluoridation methods include membrane based reverse osmosis and nanofiltration as well as electrodialysis and electrocoagulation (Chauhan et al., 2007), flocculation with mud of phosphate alumina, silica gel or decantation (Diawara et al., 2003; NOM 127 SSA1-1994),

Activated alumina (AA) seems to be better suited for a large-scale defluoridation due to its specificity and affinity towards F- chemical-physical properties and bulk availability. Adsorption of F- onto AA depends of various factors such as raw water characteristics, as well as AA grade, particle size, low rate and adsorbent depth. If the bed depth is decreased, even though the other conditions are maintained constant, concentration of the solute in treated water will rise sharply from the time that effluent is first discharged from the adsorbent (Weber, 1972).

Thus there exists a critical minimum depth that needs to be maintained. A cylindrical column unit is considered as the best shape for adsorption. Activated alumina exhibited a maximum F- uptake capacity of 254 mg/L from groundwater matrix under the experimental conditions used by Chauhan et al., (2007). Some of these processes do not permit ground level under 2 ppm of F- ions (Astel et al., 2000; Dernaucourt, 1980; Mazounie and Mouchet, 1984; Belle and Jersale, 1984; Dieye et al., 1994). One of the main differences between nanofiltration (NF) and electrodialysis (ED) is that the solvent phases through the membrane with more or less selective solute retention in NF, whereas the solutes passes through the membrane with more or less selective transfer in ED. There are also no ion-exchange resins or specific membranes for F-, there are nitrates and borates. Reverse osmosis cannot be used for partial or selective demineralization. NF and ED are more suitable for producing drinking water directly without the need of re-mineralization (Diawara et al., 2003). In NF a synergism between both can be observed but varies, depending upon operating conditions such a pH, ionic strength, flow rate and transmembrane pressure and also on the kind of membrane materials displayed (Pontie et al., 2003).

The mechanism of removal F- ions by calcinated Mg/ Al, Co3-LDH as adsorbent of F- from aqueous solution, where F- is removed much faster at low pH than at high pH to incorporate anions into its structure by means of the so-called memory effect. (Lv, 2006).

Point of use (POU technologies) has been proposed as solutions for meeting the Millennium Development Goal (MDG) for safe water. Their goal is to reduce the risk of contaminations between the water source and the home, by providing treatment at the household level. These technologies have not been rigorously tested to see if they meet WHO drinking water guidelines. Murphy et al., (2010) evaluated POU biosand arena and ceramic filters in terms of microbiological and chemical quality of the treated water. The F- levels measured for source water from both ceramic and biosand filters rarely exceeded the WHO guidelines. Consequently the results regarding F- removal were somewhat inconclusive; the filter provided some or not F- removal in all cases, treated water values never came close to the WHO guideline value of 1.5 mg/L. It appears there may be F- in the claypot mixtures that are being released into the treated water as it passes through the filter. This result was unexpected given that clay has been identified as a potential treatment for F- in water supplies (Hauge et al., 2007).

To determine the equilibrium between fluorination of water or defluorination, hydrogeological and geochemical studies of groundwater quality and monitoring in aquifers can help to identify safe zones of water for human consumption. The results would indicate if F- level is optimal, but when it is found that the water source has levels over the permissible limit, it is advisable changing to a well with lower levels of F- or using defluorination methods to warranty the quality (Váquez et al., 2010).

# 7   Conclusions

1.  Because of the universal presence of fluorides in the earths's crust, it is found in rivers, lakes, oceans and underground water. Also in rocks, sediments, andandosols volcanoes, in air biota, dead organic matter and anthropogenic sources.
2.  F- is absorbed by living things, and it can have beneficial effects in low amounts, but it is very toxic when ingested in amounts over 0.05 mg/kg/day for a chronic oral exposure.
3.  Prevention of dental decay is the main use of F- products. Its capacity to modify the

carbohydrate metabolism in plaque bacteria such as *Streptocuccus mutants* and *Lactobacillus spp* may be related to the reduction of caries.

4.  In case of dental fluorosis, there are two types of abnormal enamel; in one, the surface is translusent and hypermineralized, and it contains high amounts of F- and aberrations on enamel crystals. In the other, the subsurface is opaque and hypo-mineralized, with low concentrations of F- and erosion of the crystals.

5.  In calcified teeth, the incorporation of F- in high concentrations, as in professional applications, minimized the loss of minerals from hydroxyapatite crystal.

6.  The ingestion of F- by humans depends on its concentration in water and edible products. International regulations indicate a maximum level of 1.5 mg/L in tap water and 0.7 mg/L in bottled water.

7.  The lethal dose for NaF varies between 32 to 64 mg/Kg. In acute intoxication, the symptoms include nausea, vomiting, abdominal pain, diarrhea, fatigue, somnolence, convulsions, cardiac arrhythmia, coma, respiratory arrest and death.

8.  Chronic toxic effects in hard tissues include dental fluorosis, skeletal fluorosis, bone deformation and hips fractures. F- toxicity is also related to gastrointestinal dysfunction some types of neoplasias and damage to soft tissues like kidney, liver, parotid glands and the brain. It is also related to premature aging.

9.  To prevent the development of dental and skeletal fluorosis in endemic areas with F- concentrations in water above the permitted level, defluorination through different methods have been tried. Nevertheless, the results regarding F- removal were somewhat inconclusive

10. Future researchers should be done, in order to determine what other measures besides prevention can avoid the damaging potential of F-.

## Acknowledgement

We thank MPH, Kenneth Clark for his contribution to this chapter.

## References

Agapitov, A.V., Haynes, W.G. (2002). *Role of endothelin in cardiovascular disease. J. Renin. Angiotensin. Aldosterone. Syst. 3: 1–15.*

Ahmed, I., Sohail, S., Hussain, M., Khan, N., Khan, M.H. (2013). *MRI features of spinal Fluorosis: Results of an endemic community screening. Pak J Med Sci 29(1): 177–180. http://dx.doi.org/10.12669/pjms.291.3200*

Al –Alousi, W., Jackson, D., Crompton, G., Jenkins, O.C. (1975). *Enamel mottling in a fluoride and in a non-fluoride community. Brit.Dent. J. 138(9–15): 56–60.*

Al Nowaiser, A., Roberts, G.J., Trompeter, R.S., Wilson, M., Lucas, V.S. (2003). *Oral health in children with chronic renal failure. Pediatr Nephrol 18: 39–45.*

Anuradha, C.D., Kanno, S., Hirano, S. (2001). *Oxidative damage to mitochondria is a preliminary step to caspase-3 activation in fluoride –induced apoptosis in HL-60 cell. Free Radical Biol. Med. 31: 367–373.*

*Assefa, G., Sheifera, G., Melaku, Z., Haimanot, R.T. (2004). Clinical and radiological prevalence of skeletal fluorosis among retired employees of Wonji-Shoa sugar estate in Ethiopia. East Afr. Med. J. 81(12): 638–640.*

*Astel, C., Schweizer, M., Simonot, M.O., Sardin, M. (2000). Selective removal of fluoride ions by a two-way ion-exchange cyclic process. Chem. Engineer Sci. 55: 3341.*

*ATSDR. (Agency for Toxic Substances and Disease Registry). (2003). Toxicological Profile for Fluorine, Hydrogen Fluoride and Fluorides, Atlanta, GA, US. Department of Health and Human Services, Public Health Services.*

*Baden, J.W. (1996). Changing patterns of fluoride intake. Proceedings of the workshop at the University of North Carolina. J. Dent. Res. 70: 952–956.*

*Barbier, O., Arreola-Mendoza, L., Del Razo, L.M. (2010). Molecular mechanisms of fluoride toxicity. Chemico-Biologic Interact. 188: 319–333.*

*Barbour, M.E., Lussi, A., Shellis, R.P. (2011). Screening and prediction of erosive potential. Caries Res. 45(1): 24–32.*

*Bawden, J.W., Crenshaw, M.A., Wright, J.T., LeGeros, R.Z. (1995). Considerations of possible biologic mechanisms of fluorosis. J. Dent. Res. 74: 1349–52.*

*Baylink, D.J., Duane, P,B,, Farley, S,M,, Farley, J.R. (1983). Monofluorophosphate physiology: the effects of fluoride in bone. Caries Res. 17(1): 56–76.*

*Belle, J.P., Jersale. C. (1984). Elimination des fluorures par adsorption-echange sur alumina active. T.S.M. 1'eau 2: 79–87.*

*Bennis, A., Kessabi, M., Hamliri, A., Farge. FL, Braun, J.P. (1993). Plasma biochemistry of adult goats with chronic fluoride poisoning in Morocco. Fluoride 26: 241–6.*

*Bhardwaj, A., Shashi, D. (2013). Dose effect relationship between high fluoride Intake and biomarkers of lipid metabolism in endemic fluorosis. Biomedicine and Preventive Nutrition. 3: 121–127.*

*Bhargava, D.S., Killedar, D.J. (1992). Fluoride adsorptionon fishbone charcoal through a moving media adsorber. Water Res. 26: 188–781.*

*Bharti, V.K., Srivastava, R., Anand, A.K., Kusum, K. (2012). Buffalo (Bubalus bubalis) epiphyseal proteins give protection from arsenic and fluoride-induced adverse changes in acetylcholinesterase activity in rats. J. Biochem. Mol. Toxicol. 26: 10–5.*

*Bonassi, S., Znaor, A., Ceppi, M., et al. (2007). An increased micronucleus frequency in peripheral blood limphocytes predicts the risk of cancer in humans. Carcinogenesis. 28: 625–63.*

*Bouaziz, H., Boudawara, F., Soleihavoup, J.P., Zeghal, N. (2007). Oxidative stress induced by fluoride in adult mice and their suckling pups. Exp. Toxicol. Pathol. 58: 339–349.*

*Bowden, G. (1991). Which bacteria are cariogenic in humans? In: Johnson NM, Editor. 54.*

*Bragamian, R.A., García-Godoy, F., Volpe, A.R. (2009). The global increase in dental caries. Apending public health crisis. Am. J. Dent. 22: 3–8.*

*Browne, D., Whelton, H., O´Mullane. (2004). Fluoride metabolism and fluorosis. J. Dentistry. 33: 177–186. doi:10.1016/j.jdent.2004.10.003.*

*Bueno, M.G., Marsicano, J.A., Sales-Peres, S.H.C. (2010). Preventive effect of iron gel with or without fluoride on bovine enamelerosion in vitro. Aust. Dent. J. 55(2): 177–80*

Burt, B.A., Eklund, S.A. (1992). Dentristy, dental practice and the community. 4th ed. Philadelphia: WB Saunders, pp 147.

Caldera, R., Chavinie, J., Fermanian, J., Tortrat, D., Laurent, A.M. (2004). Maternal-fetal transfer of fluoride in pregnant woman. Biology Neonate. 54: 263–269.

Calderon, J., Machado, B., Navarro, M., Carrizales, L., Ortiz, M., Díaz-Barriga, F. (2000). Influence of fluoride exposure on reaction time and visuospatial orcanization in children. Epidemiology. 11: 5153.

Cao, J., Chen, J., Wang, J., Klerks, P., Xie, Lingtian. (2014). Effects of sodium fluoride on MAPKs signaling pathway in the gills of a freshwater teleost, Cyprinus carpio. Aquatic Toxicol. 152: 164–172. http://dx.doi.org/10.1016/j.aquatox.(2014).04.007.

Carey, R.M. (2011). Overview of endocrine systems in primary hypertension. Endocrinol. Metab. Clin. North Am. 40: 265–77.

Carlsson, J., Hamilton, I. (1994). Metabolic activities of oral bacteria In: Thylstrup A, Fejerskov O, Editors, Textbook of clinical cariology. 2nd ed. Copenhagen: Munksgaard pp 71–88.

Center for Disease Control and Prevention. (2001). Record for using fluoride to prevent and crontol dental caries in the U.S. Morbidity and Mortality Weekly Report 50: 1–4259.

Chang, T.W., Goldberg, A.L. (1978). The origin of alanine produced in skeletal muscle. J. Biol. Chem. 10: 3677–84.

Chaturvedi, A.K., Yadav, K.C., Pathak, K.C., Singh, V.N. (1990). Defluoridation of water by adsorption on clay ash, water, air, soil. Pollution. 49: 51–56.

Chauhan, V.S., Dwivedi, P.K., Lyengar, L. (2007). Investigations on activated alumina based domestic defluoridation units. J. Haz. Mat. 139: 103–107.doi:10.1016/j.jhazmat.2006.06.014.

Chinoy, N.J., Narayana, M.V., Sequeria, E., Joshi, S.M., Barot, J.M., Purohit, R.M., Parikh, D.J., Ghodasara, N.B. (1992). Studies on effects of fluoride in 36 villages of Mehsana district, North Gujarat. Fluoride. 25: 63–71.

Chinoy N.J. (2003). Fluoride stress on antioxidant defence systems. Fluoride. 36: 138–141.

Choubisa, S.L. (2001). Endemic fluorosis in southern Rajasthan, India. Fluoride 34: 61–70.

Clarkson J. (1992). A review of the developmental Defects of Enamel Index (DDE Index). Inter. Dent. J. 42: 411–26.

Cooper, L.F., Zhou, Y., Takebe, J., Guo, J., Abron, A., Holmén, A., Ellingsen, J.E. (2006). Fluoride modification effects on osteoblast behavior and bone formation at TiO2 grit-blasted c.p. titanium endosseous implants. Biomaterials 27(6): 926–936.

Culp, R.L., Stotlenberg, H.A. (1958). Fluoride reduction at La cross, Kansas. J. Am. Water Works Assoc. 50: 423–443.

Danelon, M., Takeshita, E.M., Sassaki, K.T., Delbem, A.C.B. (2013). In situ evaluation of a low fluoride concentration gel with sodium trimetaphosphate in enamel remineralization. Am. J. Dent. 26(1): 15–20.

Dean, H.T. (1934). Classification of mottled enamel diagnosis. J. Am. Dent. Asso. 21: 1421–6.

Dean, H.T., Elvove E. (1935). Studies en the minimal threshold of the dental signs of chronic endemic fluorosis (mottled enamel). Pub. Health Report. 50: 1719–1729.

Dean, H.T.1938. Endemic fluorosis and its relation to dental caries. Pub. Health Report. 53: 1443–1729.

Dean, H.T., Jay, P., Arnold, F.A. Jr., McClure, F.J., Elvove, E. (1939). Domestic water and dental caries, *including certain epidemiological aspects of oral L acidophilus. Pub. Health Res. 54: 862–888.*

Dean, H.T. (1942). *The investigation of physiological effects by the epidemiological method. In: Moulton RF editors. Fluorine and dental health, Washington, DC, American Association for the Advancement of Science.*

Dean, H.T., Arnold, F.A. Jr., Jay, P., Knutson, J.W. (1950). *Studies on mass control of dental caries through fluoridation of the public water supply. Pub. Health Resp. 65 1403–1408.*

Degroot, A., Treit, D. (2002). *Dorsal and ventral hippocampal cholinergic systems modulate anxiety in the plus-maze and shock-probe tests. Brain Res. 949: 60–70.*

Del Razo, L.M., Corona, J.C., García-Vargas, G., Albores, A., Cebrian, M.E. (1993). *Fluoride levels in well-water from a chronic arsenicism area of Northern Mexico. Environ. Pollut. 80: 91–94.*

Delles, C., Zimmerli, L., McGrane, D.J., Koh-Tan, C.H., Pathi, V.L., McKay, A.J. et al. (2008). *Vascular stiffness is related to superoxide generation in the vessel wall. J. Hypertens. 26: 946–55.*

Delmelle, P., Delfosse, T., Delvaux, B. (2003). *Sulfate, chloride and fluorosis retention in Andosols exposed to volcanic acid emissions. Environ. Pollut. 126: 445–457.*

Denbesten, P.K. (1999). *Biological mechanisms of dental fluorosis relevant to the use of fluoride supplements. Commun. Den. Oral Epidemiol. 27: 41–47.*

Department of Health and Children, Ireland. (2002). *Forum on Fluoridation. Stationary Office Dublin. [www.fluoridationforum.ie]*

DHHS (Department of Health and Human Services).1991. *A review of Fluoride, Risks and benefits, Public, Health Service. Department of Health and Human Services.*

Dernaucourt, J.C. (1980). *La defluoruration des eaux potables. T.S.M. 1' eau 3: 138.*

Diawara, C., Lo, S.M., Rumeau, M., Pontie, M., Sarr, O. (2003). *A phenomenolological mass transfer approach in nanofiltration of halide ions for a selective defluorination of brackish drinking water. J. Membrane Sci. 219: 103–112. doi: 10.1016/S0376-7388(03)00189-3*

Dieye, A., Mar, C., Rumeau, M. (1994). *Les procedes de defluoruration des eaux de biosson. Tribune de 1'eau 8: 568.*

Dingrano, L., Gregg, K., Hainen, N., Wistrom, C. (2003). *Química, Editorial McGraw Hill, Colombia.*

Donacian, M., Lyaruu, A., Bronckers, L.J.J., Santos, F., Mathias, R., DenBesten, P. (2008). *The effect of fluoride on enamel and dentin formation in the uremic rat incisor. Pediatr. Nephrol. 23: 1973–1979. doi:10.1007/s00467-008-0890-2.*

Duckworth, S., Duckworth, R. (1978). *The ingestion of fluoride in tea. British. Dent. J. 145: 368.*

Eckambaram, P., Paul, V. (2001). *Calcium preventing locomotor behavioral and dental toxicities of fluoride by decreasing serum fluoride level in rats. Environ. Toxicol. Pharmac. 9: 141–146.*

Enger, E., Smith, B. (2006). *Un estudio de interrelaciones. Ciencia Ambiental. McGraw-Hill, Interamericana Editores, S.A. de C.V. 82: 368–370.*

EPA (United States Environmental Protection Agency) *http://water.epa.gov/drink/contaminants.*

Evans, R.W., Darvell. (1995). *Refinbding estimate of the critical period for susceptibility to enamel fluorosis in human maxillary central incisors. J. Public Health Dent. 55: 238–249.*

Evans, R.W., Stamm, J.W. (1991). *An epidemiologic estimate of the critical period during which human maxillary central incisors are most susceptible to fluorosis. J. Public Health Dent. 51: 251–259.*

*Farge, P., Ranchin, B., Cochat, P. (2006). Four-year follow-up of oral health surveillance in renal transplant children. Pediatr. Nephrol. 21: 851–855.*

*FDI. (1992). An epidemiological index of Development Defects of Enamel (DDE Index) Inter. Dent. J. 42: 411–26.*

*Fejerskov, O., Thylstrup, A., Larsen, M.J. (1977). Clinical and structural features and possible pathogenic mechanisms of dental fluorosis. Scand. J. Dent. Res. 85: 510–534.*

*Flora,S.J., Pachauri, V., Mittal, M., Kumar, D. (2011). Interactive effect of arsenic and fluoride on cardio-respiratory disorders in male rats: posible role of reactive oxygen species. Biometals 24: 615–628.*

*Fushida, C.E., Cury, J.A. (1999). In situ evaluation of enamel-dentin erosion by beverage and recovery by saliva. Rev. Odontol. Univ. Sao Paulo 12(2): 127–34.*

*Galé, H. (2006).Fluor. Lexique, Francia.*

*Gamkrelidze, M., Mamamtavrishvili, N., Bejitashvili, N., Sanikidze, T., Ratiani, L. (2008). Role of oxidative stress in pathogenesis of atherosclerosis. Georgian Med. News. 54–57.*

*García-Montalvo, E.A., Reyes-Pérez, H., Del razo, L.M. (2009). Fluoride exposure in pairs glucose tolerance via decreased insulin expression and oxidative stress. Toxicol. 263: 75–83. doi:10.1016/j.tox. 2009.06.008*

*Gutierrez-Salinas, J., Morales-González, J.A. (2006). La ingesta de fluoruro de sodio produce estrés oxidativo en la mucosa bucal de la rata. Revista Mexicana de Ciencias Farmacéuticas 3: 11–22.*

*Guachalla, L., Ascarrunz, M. (2003). Genetic Toxicology: a science in constant development. Biofarbo. XI: 75–82.*

*Guggenheim, K., Simkin, A., Wolinsky. (1976). The effect of fluoride on bone of rats fed diets deficient in calcium or phosphorus. Alcif. Tissue Res. 22: 9–17.*

*Habelitz, S., Serry, M. (2005). Atomic force microscope study of dental enamel structure and synthesis. http://www.veeco.com*

*Haettich, B., Lebreton, C., Prier, Kaplan, G. (1991). Magnetic resonance imaging of Fluorosis and stress fractures due to fluoride. Rev. Rheum. Mal. Osteoartic. 58: 803–808.*

*Hamilton, I.R., Buckley, N.D. (1991). Adaptation by Streptococcus mutans to acid tolerance. Oral Microbiol. Inmunol. 6(2): 65–71.*

*Hauge, S., Osterberg, R., Bjorvatn, K., Selvig, K.A. (2007). Defluoridation nof drinking water with pottery: effect of firing temperature. Eur.J. Oral Sci. 102(6): 329–333.*

*Hernández, A. (1997). El flúor y el Abastecimiento del Agua. Tecnología Internacional del agua, Madrid, España, pp 26–239.*

*Horowitz, H.S. (1984). A new method for assessing the prevalence of dental fluorosis-the tooth surface index of fluorosis. J. Am. Dent. Asso. 109: 37–4164.*

*Hurtado, R., Gardea-Torresdey, J. (2005). Estimation of exposure to fluorides in the highlands of Jalisco, México. Pub. Health Mex. ISSN 0036-3634, 47: 58–63.*

*Huysmans, M.C., Chew, H.P., Ellwood, R.P. (2011). Clinical studies of dental erosion and erosive wear. Caries Res. 45: 60–8.*

*Irigoyen, M.A., Sánchez, G. (2000). Changes in dental caries prevalence 12 year old students in the state of México after 9 years of salt fluoridation, Caries Res 34: 303–307.*

*Jackson D, James PMC, Wolfe WB. (1975). Fluoridation in Anglesey: a clinical study. Brit. Dent. J. 138:*

165–71.

Ishii, T. and Suckling, G. (1991). *The severity in dental fluorosis in children exposed to water with a high fluoride content for various periods of time, J Dent Res, 70: 952–956.*

Ismail, A.I. and Messer, J.G.1996. *The risk of fluorosis in students exposed to a higher than optimal concentration of fluoride in well water, J Public Health Dent, 56: 22–27*

Jha, A., Shah, K., Verma, R.J. (2012). *Effects of sodium fluoride on DNA, RNA and protein contents in liver of mice and its amelioration by Camellia sinensis. Acta Polon. Pharmaceut. 69: 551–555.*

Juganmohan, P., Rao, S.V.L.N., Rao, K.R.S.S. (2010). *Lipid abnormalities in fluoride induced renal failure patients of Nellore District, Andhra Pradesh, India. Afr. J. Basic Appl. Sci. 2: 94–8.*

Jun, T., Liu, K., Song, Y., Zhang, Y., Cui, C., Lu, C. (2011). *Interactive effect of fluoride burden with calcitonin receptor gene polymorphisms on the risk of F bone injury. Int. Arch. Occup. Environ. Health 84: 533–538.*

Kaneto, H., Kawamori, D., Matsuoka, T., Kajimoto, Y., Yamasaki, Y. (2005). *Oxidative stress and pancreatic β-Cel dysfunction. Am. J. Ther. 12: 529–533.*

Kathpalia, A., Susheela, A.K. (1978). *Effect of sodium fluoride on tissue protein in rabbit. Fluoride; 11(3):125–9.*

Kawanabe, Y., Nauli, S.M. (2011). *Endothelin. Cell. Mol. Life Sci. 68: 195–203.*

Khimji, A.K., Rockey, D.C. (2010). *Endothelin-biology and disease. Cell Signal 22: 1615–25.*

Kleerekoper, M. (1996). *Fluoride and the skeleton. Crit. Rev. Clin. Lab. Sci. 33(2): 136–139.*

Koch, M.J., Buhrer, R., Pioch, T., Scharer. K. (1999). *Enamel hypoplasia of primary teeth in chronic renal failure. Pediatr. Nephrol. 13: 68–72.*

Kokotos, G., Kotsovolou, S., Constatinou, Kokotou, V., Wu, G., Olivecrona. G. (2010). *Inhibition of lipoproteins lipase by alkanesulfonyl fluorides. Bioorg. Med. Chem. Lett. 24: 2803–6.*

Komatsu, M., McDermott, A.M., Sharp, G.W. (1995). *Sodium fluoride stimulates exocytosis at a late site of calcium interaction in stimulus-secretion coupling: studies with the RINm5F beta cell line. Mol. Pharmacol. 47: 496–508.*

Lantz, O., Jouvin, M.H., DeVernejoul, Druet, M.C.1987. *Fluoride-induced chronic renal failure. Am. J. Kidney Dis. 10: 136–139.*

LeGeros, R.Z., Tung, M.S. (1983). *Chemical stability of carbonate and fluoride containing apatites. Caries Res. 17: 419–29.*

Lehninger, A.L., Nelson, D.L., Cox, M.M.1993). *Principles of Biochemistry, Worth Publishers, New York, NY USA.*

Limeback, H. (1994). *Enamel formation and the effects of fluoride. Commun. Dent. Oral Epidemiol. 22: 144–7.*

Ling, F.H., Jian, G.C. (2006). *DNA damage, apoptosis and cell cycle changes induced by fluoride in rat oral mucosal cells and hepatocytes. World J. of Gastroenterol. 12: 1144–1148.*

Liu, F., Ma, J., Zhang, H., Liu, P., Liu, Y-P., Xing, B., Dang, Y-H. (2014). *Fluoride exposure during development affects both cognition and emotion in mice. Physiol. & Behaivor 124: 1–7.*

Loweth, A.C., Williams, G.T., Scarpello, J.H., Morgan, N.G. (1996). *Heterotrimetric G-proteins are implicated in the regulation of apoptosis in prancreatic beta-cells. Exp. Cell. Res. 229: 69–76.*

Lucas, V.S., Roberts, G.J. (2005). Oro-dental health in children with chronic renal failure and after renal transplantation: a clinical review. Pediatr. Nephrol. 20: 1388–1394.

Lung, S-C., Cheng, H-W., Fu, C.B. (2008). Potencial exposure and risk of fluoride intakes from tea drinks produced in Taiwan. J. of Exposure Sci. and Environ. Epidem. 18: 158–166.

Lv, L., He, J., Wei, M., Evans, D.G., Duan, X. (2006). Factors influencing the removal of fluoride from aqueous solution by calcined Mg layered double hydroxides. J. Haz. Mat. 133: 119–128. doi:10.1016/j.jhazmat.2005.10.012

Lyaruu, D.M., Bervoets, T.J., Bronckers, A.L. (2006). Short exposure to high levels of fluoride induces stage-dependent structural changes in ameloblasts and enamel mineralization. Eur. J. Oral Sci. 114: 111–115.

Machalinska, A., Machoy-Mokrzynska, A., Marlicz, W., Stecewicz, I., Machalinski, B. (2001). NaF-induced apoptosis in human bone marrow and cord blood CD34 positive cells. Fluoride 34: 258–263.

Machoy-Mokrzyńska, A. (2004). Ann. Acd. Med. Stetin 50: 1–9.

Magalhaes, A.C., Wiegand, A., Ríos, D., Honório, H.M., Buzalaf, M.A.R. (2009). Insights into preventive measures for dental erosion. J. Appl. Oral Sci. 17: 75–86.

Maier FJ. (1953). Defluoration of municipal water supplies. J. Am. Water Works Assoc. 45: 879–888.

Manarelli, M.M., Moretto, M.J., Sassakiu, K.T., Martinhon, C.R., Pessan, J.P., Delbem, A.C. (2013). Effect of fluoride varnish supplemented with sodium trimetaphosphate on enamel erosion and abrasion in vitro study. Am. J. Dent. 26: 307–12.

Manarelli, M.M., Vieira, A.E.M., Matheus, A.A., Sassaki, K.T., Delbem, A.C.B. (2011). Effect of mouth rinses with fluoride and trimetaphosphate on enamel erosion: an in vitro study. Caries Res. 45(6): 506–9.

Marquis, R. E. (1977). Inhibition of streotococcal adenosine triphosphatase by fluoride. J. Dent. Res. 56: 704.

Marsh, P.D. (2003). Are dental diseases examples of ecological catastrophes? Microbiology 2: 279–94.

Masaki, T.2004. Historical review: endothelin. Trends Pharmacol. Sci. 25: 219–24.

Matsui, R., Cvitkovitch, D. (2010). Acid tolerance mechanisms utilized by Streptococcus mutans. Future Microbiol. 3: 403–17.

Mazounie, P., Mouchet, P. (1984). Available processes for fluoride removal from drinking waters. Revue Francaise des Sciences de 1'Eau 3: 29.

Menoyo, I., Rigall,i A., Puche, R.C. (2005). Effect of fluoride on the secretion of insulin in the rat. Arzneimittelforschun. 55: 455–460.

Mexican Official Norm: NMX-AA-077-SCFI-2001. Water analysis; Determination of natural, residual and residual water fluorides treated. Official newspaper of the Nation (it cancels to NMX-AA-077-1982).

Michael, M., Barot, V.V., Chinoy, N.J. (1996). Investigations of soft tissue functions in fluorotic individuals of north Gujarat. Fluoride. 29: 63–71.

Mirlean, N., Roisenberg, A. (2007). Fluoride distribution in the environment along the gradient of a phosphate-fertilizer production emission (southern Brazil). Environ. Geochem. Health. 29:179–187.

Moller, I.J. (1982). Fluorides and dental fluorosis. Int. Dent. J. 32 (2): 135–147.

Moretto, M.J., Magalhaes, A.C., Sassaki, K.T., Delbem. A.C., Martinhon, C.C. (2010). Effect of different fluoride concentrations of experimental dentifrices on enamel erosion and abrasion. Caries Res. 44(2): 135–40.

Msonda, K.W.M., Masamba, W.R.L., Fabiano, E. (2007). A study fluoride groundwater occurrence in Nathenje. Physics & Chemistry of the Earth 32:1178–1184.

Murphy, H.M., McBean, E.A., Farahbakhsh, K. (2010). A critical evaluation of two point-of-use water treatment technologies: can they provide water that meets WHO drinking water guidelines? J. of Water and Health. 8(4): 611– 628. doi:10.2166/wh.2010.156

Murray, J.J., Shaw, L. (1974). Classification and prevalence of enamel opacities in the human deciduous and permanent dentitions. Arch. Oral Biol. 24: 7–13.

Nasstrom, K., Moller, B., Petersson, A. (1993). Effect on human teeth of renal transplantation: a postmortem study. Scand. J. Den. Res. 101: 202–209.

Nawlakhe, W.G., Kulkarni, D.N., Pathak, B.N., Bulusu, K.R. (1957). Defluoridation of water by Nalgonda technique. Ind. J. Environ. Health. 17: 26–65.

Neilands, J., Peterson, L.G., Beighton, D., Svensater, G. (2012). Fluoride supplemented milk inhibits acid tolerance in root caries biofilms. Caries Res. 46: 156–60.

Neilands, J., Troedsson, U., Sjödin, T., Davies, J.R. (2014). The effect of delmepinol and fluoride on acid adaptation and acid production in dental plaque biofilms. Arch. Oral Biol. 59: 318–323.http://dx.doi.org/10.1016/j.archoralbio.2013.12.008

NOM-040-SSA1-1996. Iodized salt and fluoridated salt. List whereby disclosed by state areas where "no" must be marketed iodized salt fluoridated water have water for human consumption increased natural fluoride concentration 0.7mg / L.

NOM-041-SSA1-1995. Goods and services. Purified and bottled water. Sanitary specifications.

Noma, K., Goto, C., Nishioka, K., Jitsuiki, D., Umemura, T., Ueda, K., et al. (2007). Roles of rho-associated kinase and oxidative stress in the pathogenesis of aortic stiffness. J. Am. Coll. Cardiol. 49: 698–705.

NRC (National Research Council). (2006). Fluoride in drinking-water, a scientific review of EPA´s standards. Washington DC.

Nunn, J.H., Sahrp, J., Lamber,t H.J., Plant, N.D., Coulthard, M.G. (2000). Oral health in children with renal disease. Pediatr. Nephrol. 14: 997–1001.

Oral, B., Ozbasar, D. (2003). The effect of sodium monofluorophosphate therapy on lipid and lipopotrein metabolism in postmenopausal women. Eur. J.Obstet. Gynecol. Reprod. Biol. 2: 180–4.

Pancote, L.P., Manarelli, M.M., Danelon, M., Delbem, A.C.B. (2014). Effect of fluoride gels supplemented with sodium trimetaphosphate on enamel erosion and abrasion: in vitro study. Arch. Oral Biol. 59: 336–340. http://dx.doi.org/10.1016/j.archoralbio.(2013).12.008.

Paul, V., Ekambaram, P., Jayakumar, A.R. (1998). Effects of sodium fluoride on locomotor behavior and a few biochemical parameters in rats. Environ. Toxicol. Pharmacol. 6: 187–191.

Pendrys, D.G. (1990). The fluorosis risk index: a method for investigating risk factors. J. Pub. Health Dent. 50: 291–8.

Pereira, M., Dombrowski, P.A., Losso, E.M., Chioca, L.R., Cunha, C., Andreatini, R. (2011). Memory impairment induced by sodium fluoride is associated with changes in brain monoamine levels. Neurotox. Res. 19: 55–62.

Pontie, M., Rumeau, M., Letellier, P., Sarrade, S., Schrive, L., Mandin, P., Weck, V, Audions. 85.

Raghu, J., Raghuveer, V.C., Rao, M.C., Somayaji, N.S., Babu, P.B. (2013). The ameliorative effect of ascorbic acid and Ginkgo biloba on learning and memory deficits associated with fluoride exposure. Interdiscip.

*Toxicol. 6: 217–221.*

Rakow, B., Ligth, E. (1986). Evaluation of the acid etch technique in concealing discoloration. Quintessence Int. Rep. 21–31

Reddy, D.R. (2009). Neurology of endemic skeletal fluorosis. Neurol. India. 57: 7–12.

Rekhadevi, P.V., Sailaja. N., Chandrasekhar. M., Mahboob, M., Rahman, F., Paramjit, G. (2007). Genotoxicity assessment in oncology nurses handling anti-neoplastic drugs. Mutagenesis. 22: 395–401.

Rigalli, A., Alloati, R., Menoyo, I., Puche, R.C. (1995). Comparative study of the effect of sodium fluoride and sodium monofluorophosphate on glucose homeostasis in the rat. Arzneimittelforschung. 45: 289–292.

Rigalli, A., Ballina, J.C., Puche, R.C. (1992). Bone mass increase and glucose tolerance in rats chronically treated with sodium fluoride. Bone Miner. 16: 101–108.

Ripa, L., Clark, C. (2001).Water fluoridation. In: Primary Preventive Dentistry, Editorial El Manual Moderno, México, pp.135–136.

Saha, S. (1993). Treatment of aqueous effluent for fluoride removal, Water Res. 27: 1347–1350.

Sakai, K., Matsumoto, K., Nishikawa, T., Suefuji, M., Nakamuru, K., Hirashima, Y., Kawashima, J., Shirotani, T., Ichinose, K., Brownlee, M., Araki, E. (2003). Mitochondrial reactive oxygen species reduce insulin secretion by pancreatic beta-cells. Biochem. Biophys. Res. Commun. 300: 216–222.

Sánchez, S., Pontigo, A.P., Heredia, E., Ugalde, J.A. (2004). Fluorosis dental en adolescentes de tres comunidades del estado de Querétaro. Revista Mexicana de Pediatría. 71: 5–9.

Sang, Z.C., Zhou, W., Zhang, Z.J., Wu, G.N., Guo, P.H., Wang, E.M. et al. (2010). X-ray analysis on patients with moderate endemic skeletal fluorosis by treatment of Guo´s Chinese herbal. Zhongguo Gu Shang. 23(5): 379–382.

Schiff, H.H., Binswanger, U. (1980). Human urinary fluoride excretion as influenced by renal functional impairment. Nephron. 26: 69–72.

Shan, K.R., Qi, X.L., Long, Y.G., Nordberg, A., Guan, Z.Z. (2004). Decreased nicotinic receptors in PC12 cells and rat brains influenced by fluoride toxicity-a mechanism relatin to a damage at the level in post-transcription of the receptor genes. Toxicol. 200: 169–177. 94.

Shanthakumari, D., Srinivasalu, S., Subramanian, S. (2004). Effect of fluoride intoxication on lipidperoxidation and antioxidant status in experimental rats. Toxicol. 204: 219–228.

Shashi, A., Kumar, M. (2008). Age specific fluoride exposure in drinking water a clinical multiparametric study. Asian J. Microbiol. Biotech. Environ. Sci. 3: 145–50.

Shellis, R.P., Ganss, C., Ren, Y., Zero, D.T., Lussi, A. (2011). Methodology and models in erosion research: discussion and conclusions. Caries Res. 45: 69–77.

Smerhovsky, Z., Landa, K., Rossner, P., Brabec, M., Zudova, Z., Hola, N., Pokorna, Z., Mareckova, J., Hurychova, D. (2001). Risk of cancer in an occupationally exposed cohort with increased level of chromosomal aberrations. Environ. Health Perspect. 109: 41–45.

Sorvari, R., Meurman, J.H., Alakuijala, P., Frank, R.M. (1994). Effect of fluoride varnish and solution on enamel erosion in vitro. Caries Res. 28: 227–232.

Souza, J.A.S., Amaral, J.G., Moraes, L.C.S., Sassaki, K.T., Delbem, A.C.B. (2013). In vitro effect of sodium trimetaphosphate on hydroxyapatite solubility. Braz. Dent. J 2: 4. http://dx.doi.org/10.1590/0103-6440201302000.

Spak, C.J., Berg, U., Ekstrand, J. (1985). Renal clearance of fluoride in children and adolescents. Pediatrics. 75: 575–579.

Sun, L., Gao, Y., Liu, H., Zhang, W., Ding, Y., Li, B., Li M., Sun, D. (2013). An assessment of the relationship between excess fluoride intake from drinking water and essential hypertension in adults residing in fluoride endemic áreas. Sci. of the Total Environment 443: 864–869. http://dx.doi.org/ 10.1016/j.scitotenv.2012.11.021

Takeshita, E.M., Castro, L.P., Sassaki, K.T., Delbem, A.C.B. (2009). In vitro evaluation of dentifrice with low fluoride content supplemented with trimetaphosphate. Caries Res. 43(1): 50–6.

Takeshita, E.M., Exterkate, R.A.M., Delbem, A.C., Ten Cate, J.M. (2011). Evaluation of different fluorides concentrations supplemented with trimetaphosphate on enamel de- and remineralization in vitro. Caries Res. 45(5): 494–7.

Tamer, M.N., Kale, K.B., Arsalan, C., Akdogan, M., Koroglu, M., Cam, H. et al. (2007). Osteosclerosis due to endemic fluorosis. Sci. Total. Environ. 373: 43–48.

Thibodeau, E.A., Keefe, T.F. (1990). pH-dependent fluoride inhibition of catalase activity. Oral Microbio. Inmunol. 5: 328–31.

Thylstup, A., Fejerskoy, O. (1978). Clinical appearances of dental fluorosis in permanent teeth in relation to histological changes. Com. Dentist Oral Epidemiol. 6: 315–28.

Tiwari, H., Rao, M.V. (2010). Curcumin supplementation protects from genotoxic effects of arsenic and fluoride. Food Chem. Toxicol. 48: 1234–1238.

Torra, M., Rodamilans. M., Corbella, J. (1998). Serum and urine fluoride concentration: relantionships to age, sex and renal function in a nonfluoridated population. Sci. Total Environ. 220: 81–85.

Trivedi, N., Mithal, A., Gupta, S.K., Godbole, M.M. (1993). Reversible impairment of glucose tolerance in patients with endemic fluorosis. Fluoride Collaborative Study Group. Diabetología 36: 826–828.

Turner, C.H., Garetto, L.P., Dunipace, A.J., Zhang, W., Wilson, M.E., Grynpaqs, M.D., Chachra, D., McClintock, R., Peacock, M., Stookey, G.K. (1997). Fluoride treatment increased serum IGH-1, bone turn over and bone mass, but not bone strength in rabbits. Calcif. Tissue Int. 61: 77–83.

Van Dijk, J.W., Borggreven, J.M., Driessens, F.C.1980. The effect of some phosphates and phosphonate on the electrochemical properties of bovine enamel. Arch. Oral Biol. 25(8–9): 591–5.

Varol, E., Akcay, S., Ersoy, I.H., Ozaydin, M., Koroglu, B.K,, Varol, S. (2010). Aortic elasticity is impaired in patients with endemic fluorosis. Biol. Trace Elem. Res. 133: 121–7.

Varol, E., Varol, S. (2012). Effect of fluoride toxicity on cardiovascular systems: role of oxidative stress. Arch. Toxicol. 86: 1627, http://dx.doi.org/10.1007/s00204-012-0862-y.

Vázquez-Alvarado, P., Meléndez-Ocampo, A., Ortiz-Espinosa, R., Muñoz-Juárez, S., Hernández-Ceruelos, A. (2012). Genotoxic damage in oral epithelial cells induced by fluoride in drinking-water on students of Tula de Allende. Hidalgo, Mexico. J. Toxicol. and Environ. Health Sci. 4: 123–129.

Vázquez-Alvarado, P., Prieto-García, F., Coronel-Olivares, C., Gordillo–Martínez, A., Ortiz-Espinosa, R., Hernández-Ceruelos, A. (2010). Fluorides and dental fluorosis in students from Tula de Allende, Hidalgo, México. J. Toxicol. and Environ. Health Sci. 2: 24–3191.

Wang, A.G., Xia, T., Chu, Q.L., Zhang, M., Liu, F., Chen, X.M., Yang, K.D. (2004). Effects of fluoride on lipid peroxidation. DNA damage and apotosis in human embryo hepatocytes. Biomedic. Environ. Sci. 17: 217–222.

Wang, S.X., Wang, Z.H., Cheng, X.T., Li, J., Sang, Z.P., Zhang, X.D., Han, L.L., Qiao, S.Y., Wu, Z.M.,

Wang. Z.Q. (2007). Arsenic and fluoride exposure in drinking water: children´s IQ and growth in Shanyin County, Shanxi, China. Environ. Health Perspec. 115: 643–647.

Weber, W.J. (1972). Adsorption, physicochemical Process for Water Quality Control. Wiley Interscience, pp 199–259.

Welin-Neilands, J., Svensater, G. (2007). Acid tolerance of biofilm cells of Streptococcus mutans. Appl. Environ. Microbiol. 73: 5633–8.

Whitford, G.M. (1990). The physiological and toxicological characteristics of fluoride. J. Dent. Res. 69 (Spec Iss): 539–549.

World Health Organization, Fluorides. (2002). Environmental Health Criteria 227- Geneva.

World Health Organization. (1970). Fluorides and human health. Monograph Series N° 59. Geneva.

World Health Organization, Fluorine and Fluorides (1984). Environmen. Health Criteria, Geneva. WHO, 1: 25–36.

World Health Organization. (1994) Fluorides and oral health. Technical report series, Geneva: WHO, 846–71.

Wysocki, G.P., Daley, T.D., Ulan, R.A. (1983). Predentin changes in patients with chronic renal failure. Oral Surg. Oral Med. Oral Pathol. 56: 167–173.

Yanagisawa, M., Kunihara, H., Kimura, S., Tomobe, Y., Kobayashi, M., Mitsui, Y. et al. (1988). A novel potent vasoconstrictor peptide produced by vascular endothelial cells. Nature. 332: 411–5.

Yanagisawa, T., Takuma, S., Fejerskov, O. (1989). Ultraestructure and composition of enamel in human dental fluorosis. Advances in Dental Res. 3: 203–10.

Young, M.A. (1973). An epidemiological study of enamel opacities in temperate and sub-tropical climates. PhD Thesis, University of London.

Yu, Y.N., Chao, X.M., Xiao, K.Q. (1991). Morphometic study of the damaged liver rats with chronic fluorosis. Chiniese J. Endemiol. 1: 1–3.

Zeiger, E., Shelby, M., Witt, K.E. (1993). Genetic toxicity of fluoride. Environ. Mol. Mutagen. 21: 309–318.

Zhang, M., Wang, A., He, W., He, P., Xu, B., Xia, T., Chen, X., Yan, K. (2007). Effects of fluoride on the expression of NCAM, oxidative stress, and apoptosis in primary cultured hippocampal neurons. Toxicol. 236: 208–216.

Zhou, Y., Qiu, Y., He, J., Chen, X., Ding, Y., Wang, Y., Liu, X. (2013). The toxicity mechanism of sodium fluoride on fertility in female rats. Food Chemi. Toxicol. 62: 566–572. http://dx.doi.org/10.1016/fct.(2013).09.023

# Chapter 7

# Bacteria and Fungi Involved in the Diarrheic and Respiratory Diseases in Workers Tanning Process

Diana Carolina Castellanos Arévalo[1], Andrea Paola Castellanos Arévalo[2], David Alfonso Camarena Pozos[2], Juan Colli[3], Bertha Isabel Arévalo Rivas[4], Juan Jose Peña-Cabriales[5], María Maldonado-vega[6]

## 1   Introduction

### 1.1   Industrialization of Animal Hide

The tanning process has as its objective the preservation of the hide of the animal and having it as the raw material for diverse articles. The industrialization of animal skins or hides corresponds in its great majority to the skin of bovines. The tanning process includes six main steps: ribera, curing, re-curing, tanning and greasing (RTG), and finishing (Manual de Procedimientos para el Manejo Adecuado de los Residuos de la Curtiduría, 1999).

In the ribera stage of the process, the clearing of the animal skin is carried out, eliminating all of the components that cannot be transformed into leather, such as hair, sodium salts, and protein material. In the tanning stage, chemical stability is achieved to

[1]  Faculty Biology Medical Molecular, University of Buenos Aires, Argentia.
[2]  Department of Biotechnology, Centro de Investigacion y Estudios Avanzados – IPN, Mexico.
[3]  Faculty Biology, Instituto Tecnologico de Irapuata, Mexico.
[4]  Faculty of Medicine, University of Guanajuato, Mexico.
[5]  CINVESTAV – IPN, Unidad Irapuato, Mexico.
[6]  Department of Research, Hospital Regional de Alta Especialidad del Bajio, Mexico.

avoid pu-trefaction of the hide, this employing material of vegetal origin or inorganic salts that contain metals such as chromium, iron, and aluminum, among others. In the RTE stage, the hide acquires suppleness, texture, flexibility, and the remaining character-istics necessary for its manufacturing into leather. During the last stage, finishing, specific characteristics are imparted to the leather that the market imposes on each type of prod-uct, such as stamping, color, and touch.

The tanning of animal hide includes processes entailing high water consumption, the generation of environments with high relative humidity and, as in industrial work-places; the work environment presents low air flow and ventilation. In addition to this environment, this stage involves an important source of the bacteria and fungi that derive from the animal hide, which unite with the environment propitious for their propagation and distribution in the tanning ambit (Mohr, 2002).

At present, Mexico is found among the 10 major producers of tanned leathers at the international level, and the Mexican state of Guanajuato, specifically León City, is the greatest leather producer at the national level, generating around 65% of tanned and pro-cessed leather that is developed at >740 tanneries.[7] The tanneries present a broad range of sophistication, from small family enterprises with fewer than 10 employees and mini-mal infrastructure to modern companies with >100 employees and better infrastructure conditions.

On the other hand, the health aspects of this population of tanners comprise a theme-of-interest because, in addition to the chemical components involved, the micro-biological aspects are considered within this context. Some diseases reported in tanners include the following: tetanus; anthrax; leptospirosis; Q fever, and brucellosis, which have been contracted during the tanning process of contaminated hides that function as vectors (Gelincik et al., 2005; Seifert et al., 1997). Respiratory diseases caused by the inha-lation of fungal spores are as follows: atopic asthma; rhinitis; hypersensitivity-related pneumonitis; bronchopulmonary aspergillosis; allergic fungal sinusitis, and allergic reac-tions (Gelincik et al., 2005; Beaumont, 1988; Singh, 2005). However, the degree to which health is affected depends on individual sensitivity to the allergens, immunological ca-pacity, and exposure to the contaminants (frequency, duration, and contaminant type).

The Health Secretariat of the State of Guanajuato (SSG), through Jurisdiction VII, identified, in the municipality of León, 58 colonies with an increase in mortality caused by diarrheic and respiratory diseases in children under the age of 5 years with malnour-ishment, and an increase of cervicouterine cancer in the years from 1998 to 2001, the origin of these illnesses being viral and infectious in origin. In principle, the localization of sites with these risks is found within industrial areas, with proximity to riverbeds and brooks receiving residual waters from the industrial sector. In July 2012, in the Epidemiological Bulletin published by the SSG, reported, for León City, 4,355 cases of acute respiratory infections and 1,426 cases with acute diarrheas, these the main causes for medical ap-pointments, with reports of infectious and parasitic diseases accumulated for the Guana-juato City in week 5 of years 2015 (cases, 6,124) and 2014 (cases, 9,642).[8]

---

[7] Directorio Estadístico Nacional de Unidades Económicas DENUE, 2012.
[8] Boletín Epidemiológico de la Secretaría de Salud del Estado de Guanajuato. Julio de, 2012

## 1.2   Bacteria of Medical Importance

In non-processed animal hides, bacteria have been detected, such as Escherichia coli, Staphylococcus epidermidis, Morganella morganii, Proteus mirabilis, Proteus vulgaris, Bacillus anthracis, Bacillus subtilis, and Bacillus mycoides (Scorzoni et al., 2013). Similarly, fungi have been determined, such as the following: Penicillium commune; Penicillium glaucum; Penicillium wortmanii; Penicillium frequents; Aspergillus niger; Aspergillus flavus; Aspergillus oryzae; Aspergillus fumigatus; Alternaria; Cladosporium; Trichoderma; Fusarium; Aureobasidium, and Scopullariopsis (Orlita, 2004).

Diseases contracted by tanners from contaminated animal hides include tetanus, anthrax, leptospirosis, epizootic aphthae, Q fever, and brucellosis (Castañón, 2013). these risks derive from the management of the animal hide and the presence of microorganisms transported in the environmental air (Burge, 2002) which are related with the development of respiratory diseases (Gelincik et al., 2005).

In the interior air of the tanning industry, fungi have been reported of the genera *Scopulariopsis, Penicillium, Aspergillus, Alternaria,* and Cladosporium (Mandal & Brandl, 2011), these genera commonly cited as the cause of rhinitis and asthma (Beaumont, 1988; Arévalo-Rivas, 2005) reported for these workers, and there are added, chemical-type factors, ranging from leather tanning powders to chromium (Arévalo-Rivas, 2005; Özdilli et al., 2007; Skóra et al., 2014). The most important allergenic fungi in interior air that cause allergic asthma and tissue disease in animals as well as in humans are *Penicillium* spp. and *Aspergillus* spp (Mandal & Brandl, 2011). Additionally, yeasts of the genus *Candida* have been identified and, although these are normally found in the oral cavity, they are related with autoimmune diseases in immunosuppressed patients (Skóra et al., 2014).

The presence of 11 contamination indicator species in the tanning work environment with pathogenic potential (Arévalo-Rivas, 2005) are the following: *Bacterium pumilus; Bacterium subtilis; Bacterium cereus; Cladosporium lubricantis, Cladosporium cladosporioides; Penicillium commune; Penicillium echinulatum; Penicillium chrysogenum; Penicillium crustosum; Candida parapsilosis,* and *Candida albidus.* In this manner, the microorganisms could compromise the state of health of tanning workers due to their incidence, propagation, and concentration in the workplace. Thus, this situation does not only represent an employment health and public health problem, because these worksites could represent extramural dissemination foci. The work of Rangel (Rangel-Cordova, 2012) reports the dissemination of microorganisms toward the exterior, this of importance when the residential zone lies in its majority within the limits of the tanneries, within radii of 30–50 m, increasing when this represents an industrial zone in immediate proximity to the residential zone and the influence of the dominant wind reaches these areas. Juarez-Facio and colleagues confirm (Juárez et al., 2014) the presence of bacteria and fungi in the environment immediately proximal to tanneries adjacent to residential zones, where a total of 8 bacteria genera, 5 enterobacteria, and 11 fungi were isolated and described macro- and microscopically. Ten genera of bacteria resulted as Gram-negative and three, as Gram-positive. The bacterial genera identified were the following: *Bacillus; Agrococcus; Staphylococcus; Kocuria,* and *Exiguobacterium,* while the enterobacteria identified were *Pseudomonas, Acinetobacter,* and *Neisseria,* and finally, the fungal genera identified included

*Cladosporium, Mucor, Penicillium, Helminthosporium, Cephalosporium,* and *Aspergillus.*

At the tanneries, there are various microorganism-amplifying sources, including the following: (Odds & Bernaerts, 1994) 1) animal hide acts as a propagation medium, given its high content of nutrients; 2) the humidity of the environment (Saiki et al., 1988) which favors the period of microorganism viability; 3) the presence of fine tanning powers and solvents (Weisburg et al., 1991; Gardes et al., 1991; Maldonado-Vega et al., 2014) and 4) the workers themselves contribute, in that they are microorganism vehicles and carriers. Other important factors that exert an influence on the interior air quality comprise air renovation, air-filtration efficiency, and internal air recirculation, components found limited in the majority of tanneries.

Bacteria that are pathogenic for humans include *Escherichia coli,* the most studied prokaryote. It belongs to the Enterobacteriaceae Family and is generally found in the intestine of animals and humans. Some strains of *E. coli* (EC) give rise to different clinical conditions of diarrheic diseases. The latter are classified into six groups:

1. **EnteroToxigenic *Escherichia coli* (ETEC):** Its main mechanism of pathogenicity is the synthesis of one or both enterotoxins, denominated toxin and thermostable toxin. The sylation frequency of this pathogenic group in children with diarrhea ranges from 10–30%, it can be asymptomatic or infrequent in school-aged children and adults, it can be symptomatic and infrequent, or it can produce travelers' diarrhea. Fecal contamination of water and food is the main source of infection.

2. **EnteroHemorrhagic *Escherichia coli* (EHEC):** This has been associated with hemorrhagic colitis, which is a severe type of diarrhea, and with the hemolytic uremic syndrome, a disease capable of producing acute renal insufficiency, hemolytic anemia, microangiopathicity, and thrombocytopenia. It produces serotoxin, thus it is denominated because of its cytotoxic effect on Vero cells, a line of African green- monkey kidney cells. Among the serotypes of *E. coli* that produce serotoxin, the most common and the only one that can be identified in clinical samples, is O157:H7. Another factor of pathogenicity is the plasmid pO157 of 60 Mega Daltons (MDa), which codes for enterohemolysin. Its principal reservoir is the intestine of bovine cattle. The most common cause of this infection is the consumption of uncooked or slightly cooked meat, particularly processed chopped meat in large amounts. Its transmission can also occur due to the ingestion of contaminated water, milk, and unpasteurized juices, or because of food handlers, among others.

3. **EnteroInvasive *Escherichia coli* (EIEC):** The pathogenicity of this organism is due to its capacity for invading and destroying the epithelium of the colon, in that it is capable of evading phagolysosome lysis. This strain is associated with outbreaks of diarrhea, in which transmission can be person-to-person, because of ingesting contaminated food or water, causing dysentery on invading the epithelial cells of the intestinal mucosa; characteristic symptoms include diarrhea with blood and mucus, although in some cases, only diarrhea presents.

4. **EnteroPathogenic *Escherichia coli* (EPEC):** Its principal factor of pathogenicity is the intimate adherence between the bacteria and the intestinal epithelial membrane. The form of transmission is fecal-oral through the contaminated hands of food handlers, through contaminated water, and through meat products. It can give

rise to outbreaks or isolated cases of diarrhea and mainly affects children under the age of 2 years, although it has been isolated in healthy and sick adults, principally when there is a predisposing factor, such as diabetes. It is manifested by acute diarrhea, vomiting, fever, and poor absorption.

5. **EnteroAggregative** *Escherichia coli* **(EAEC):** This produces liquid diarrhea, with mucus, without blood, and persists for up to 20 days. These bacteria possess a mechanism of aggregative adherence characterized by auto-agglutination of the bacteria among themselves and due to its being unspecific. The target site of the damage can be the mucosa of the large and small intestine, with an incubation of at least 8 h, mainly affecting children aged less than 2 years.

6. **Diffusely Adherent** *Escherichia coli* **(DAEC):** Little is known about its mechanism of pathogenicity. It can be isolated from healthy persons as well as from individuals with diarrhea, and principally affects children aged 4–5 years. Main symptoms are diarrhea without blood and without leukocytes (Romero & Herrera, 2002; Shih et al., 1996; de Bentzmann & Plésiat, 2011).

## 1.3   Yeasts of Medical Importance

Yeasts are unicellular fungi that reproduce by means of fission, gemation, or sporulation. Heterotrophs, yeasts survive at the expense of other living beings (parasitic yeasts) or on organic material (saprophytic yeasts) (Newman et al., 2005; Li et al., 2007; Kothavade et al., 2010; Scorzoni et al., 2013). Yeasts that are of medical importance are those of the genus *Candida* (Castañón, 2013). Five *Candida* species are normally present in the oral cavity: *Candida albicans*; *Candida krusei*; *Candida parapsilosis*; *Candida tropicalis*, and *Candida* guilliermondii (González et al., 2007). These species are ubiquitous, but *Candida albicans* has been associated with oral infections, together with other species, such as *C. parapsilosis*, *C. tropicalis*, and *C. glabrata* (Li et al., 2007). Oral candidiasis is increased by facilitator factors, such as immunosuppression, endocrinopathies, nutritional deficiencies, dental prostheses, malignant neoplasms, epithelial alteration, a diet high in carbohydrates, infancy and old age, poor oral hygiene, smoking, and the use of certain drugs (Watanakunakorn & Weber, 1989; Weischer & Kolmos, 1992). It is important to underscore that the disease-related yeasts in humans are incapable of producing infection in a healthy individual; therefore, cases present when there is alteration in the host's cellular defenses, in the physiology, or in the composition of the normal flora, in order for colonization, infection or, finally, the disease to be able to be produced (Pereira-Cenci et al., 2008; Dodds et al., 2005; Dangi et al., 2010; González et al., 2007; Aguirre, 2002; Kuper et al., 2009).

The presence of *Candida* in the oral cavity ranges from 20–70%. *Candida albicans* is the species isolated with greatest frequency, and others, such as *Candida glabrata* and *Candida tropicalis*, are identified in up to 7% of persons, while yet other species, such as *Candida krusei*, *Candida guilliermondii*, or *Candida parapsilosis*, are less frequent.

Saliva constitutes the first-order antifungal fluid, because it possesses the function of mechanical scanning, which limits the adhesion of micro molecules and their antifungal power due to their protein components as follows: lysozymes; lactoferrin; lactoperoxidases, and glycoproteins (González et al., 2007). Salival pH ranges between and 5.6 and

7.8, and when this diminishes or acidifies, as occurs under removable dental prostheses, adhesion of the fungus is favored. Anti-*Candida* antibodies present in the saliva are Immunoglobin A (IgA) type, which acts by inhibiting the adherence of *Candida* to the oral mucosa. In patients with oral candidiasis, an increase in saliva has been demonstrated in the concentration of immunoglobins (Newman et al., 2005; Li et al., 2007; Kothavade et al., 2010).

## 1.4   Methods of Identification

Diverse methods facilitate the identification of bacteria and yeasts of medical importance, such as biochemical tests, selective culture media, hemolytic activity media, chromogenic media, and molecular biology methods, in addition to antibiotic and antifungal sensitivity tests.

Media such as Brilliant Green Bile Broth (BGBB) at 2% with 4-Methyl-Umbelliferyl-beta-Glucoronide (MUG) permits the investigation of the formation of gas, indole (±), and fluorescence, thus detecting the presence of coliforms such as *Escherichia coli* which possesses an enzyme, $\beta$-D-glucuronidase, that acts on the MUG substrate present in the selective culture medium, forming 4-Methylumbelliferone, which is characterized by being fluorescent on being illuminated with a 366-nm Ultraviolet (UV) lamp; additionally, the presence of *E. coli* can be confirmed with the formation of gas in Durham tubes, in that these utilize lactose as carbon source and, finally, the indole test in *E. coli* is positive. The indole is generated by reductive dissemination of the tryptophan present in the medium due to the tryptophan of the bacterium and that comes into evidence on adding Kovacs reagent to the culture, taking as positive proof the presence of indole with the formation of a red ring on the culture-medium surface (Scorzoni et al., 2013; Castañón, 2013; Cole et al., 2005; Cole et al., 2007; DeSantis et al., 2006; Gasch et al., 2000).

Another selective medium is *Escherichia coli* O157:H7 Agar, which allows the isolation and differentiation of enterohemorragic strains of *Escherichia coli* O157:H7 from diverse samples. This culture medium provides carbon, nitrogen, minerals, vitamins, oligoelements, and other essential nutrients for growth, ranging from peptone of casein, meat extract, and yeast extract (Ye et al., 2006). Sodium deoxycholate inhibits the accompanying Gram-positive flora; the pH indicator is Bromothymol Blue. Microorganisms that ferment sorbitol develop yellow colonies, and those that do not ferment it develop a greenish coloration. Sulfur thiosulfate, iron citrate, and ammonium confer a brownish-blackish color on the colonies of microorganisms that produce the precipitation of iron sulfate, mainly of the genus *Proteus*. This culture medium, similarly to that previously mentioned, also possesses the 4-MethylUmbelliferyl-$\beta$-D-Glucuronide (MUG) substrate, which reacts with the $\beta$-D-glucuronidase enzyme of *Escherichia coli*, giving rise to the formation of 4-Methylumbelliferone, which is fluorescent on irradiation with a 366-nm UV light lamp. *Escherichia coli* strains possess, as a specific characteristic, the capacity to produce the enzyme $\beta$-D-glucuronide; contrariwise, *Escherichia coli* O157:H7 cannot form this enzyme and on being illuminated with 366-nm UV light, does not produce fluorescence. *Enterobacter aerogenes* colonies have yellow growth, with a slight precipitate and without fluorescence. In this manner, the presence can be investigated of *E. coli* EHEC in samples suspected of evidencing and differentiating the presence of typical, fluorescent *E. coli* strains or the bacteria of the genera of *Proteus* or *Enterobacter* by the coloration of their colonies.

The Blood-Agar Base (BAB) medium has, as its source, carbon, nitrogen, vitamins, and growth factors, infusion of cardiac muscle and the peptone, and growth factors, cardiac muscle infusion, and the peptone; for osmotic equilibrium, they possess sodium chloride. This medium allows assessment of the presence of plasmid pO157, which is characteristic of *E. coli* EHEC on observing hemolytic activity once these are seeded in the culture medium by crossed striate and pricking above the striate. These are incubated for 24–48 h at 35°C, permitting the clear observation of hemolysis halos as a result of the bacterial action (NCCLS – Clinical and Laboratory Standards Institute, 2004).

CHROMagar *Candida* is a selective and differential chromogenic medium for direct identification of yeasts in clinical samples. It facilitates the isolation and presumptive identification of some species, such as *C. albicans*, *C. krusei*, *C. tropicalis*, and *C. glabrata* as results of the specific enzymatic reactions of the distinct species of yeasts with the chromogenic substrate present in the medium. After the corresponding enzymatic hydrolysis, the colonies can be observed. In the case of *C. albicans*, its colonies are green in color, in *C. glabrata* these are mauve, in *C. tropicalis*, blue, and in *C. krusei*, pink.

## 1.5    Sensitivity Tests

Antimicrobial sensitivity tests permit the identification of whether a microorganism (bacterium, antibiogram; fungus, antifungigram) is resistant or sensitive to a determined antibiotic/antifungal, thus allowing for the selection of the adequate treatment necessary for counteracting an infection. However, these tests do not determine the microorganism's pathogenicity.

The sensitivity of bacteria and fungi in the face of these antimicrobial or antifungal agents is based on the diminution or inhibition of growth in an antimicrobial/antimycotic culture medium at a defined concentration (Kuper et al., 2009).

The indiscriminate and uncontrolled use of drugs, antibiotics, and antifungals gives rise to resistance in bacteria and yeasts of medical importance, generating a problem of control and treatment at the worldwide level, obliging, above all, in terms of antibiotics and antifungals, an increase in the effective dose or an increase in treatment times, in that mutation-associated resistance has represented the employment of schemes involving multiple antibiotics.

## 1.6    Molecular Biology Techniques

The implementation of Molecular Biology techniques, DNA extraction, electrophoresis, PCR, purification, and sequentiation comprises part of the processes that allow for the identification and understanding, from the genetic information, the identity of bacteria- and yeasts-of interest by means of the so-called molecular sequentiation task.

One of the techniques of greatest usefulness is the Polymerase Chain Reaction) (PCR), developed in 1983 by K.B. Mullis (Saiki et al., 1988). PCR is highly specific, rapid, sensitive, and versatile in detecting minimal amounts of DNA and in amplifying these, thus facilitating their identification. PCR is an *in vitro* method of DNA synthesis in which a particular segment of DNA is specifically amplified on being delimited by a pair of feeders, initiators, or the primers that flank these. Copying is achieved exponentially through repeated cycles at different times and incubation temperatures in the presence of the thermostable DNA polymerase enzyme. Thus, in a question of hours, millions of copies of the DNA sequence desired are obtained. Each of the repetitive cycles is composed of three steps: the first consists of the breakdown of DNA hydrogen bridges denaturation, and incubation at a temperature around 95ºC for 1 min. This step exposes the nitrogenated bases of the target DNA. The second step gives rise to the hybridization of the DNA-target denatured chains with primers (single-stranded synthetic DNA) at a temperature that favors the pairing of the complementary nitrogenated bases of both types of DNA, this temperature depending on the fusion temperature (Tm) of the primers, which generally ranges from 50–60°C. The third step is effected at 72ºC, the temperature at which the polymerase extends the length of the primers, adding the different free nucleotides in the order dictated by the sequence of the chain that acts as the mold (Juárez et al., 2014; Saiki et al., 1988).

This technique is applied in Microbiology for the identification of infectious agents independently of a serological response, which represents an advantage in cases in which antibodies appear after a long infection period and sometimes unpredictably, and it also determines, by means of the presence of antibodies, whether a sign of infection derives from the past or whether is recent, as occurs with the finding of antibodies against the hepatitis C virus, or to accurately establish whether a determined virus is present or not. Molecular Biology permits rapid identification of microorganisms through the amplification of genes, as in the case of the bacteria of the gene *16SrDNA*.

Identification of bacteria from amplification of the gene *16S rDNA* is based on the utilization of universal primers (*FD1: 5´ CCG AAT TCG TCG ACA ACA GAG TTT GAT CCT GGC TCA G 3´*, and *RD1: 5´ CCC GGG ATC CAA GCT TAA GGA GGT GAT CCA GCC 3´*), (Weisburg et al., 1991) which are designed in different conserved zones in bacteria, which permits the amplification of regions with variable genus and species characteristics.

Identification of yeasts from Molecular Biology has allowed for the development of novel techniques. Various studies have demonstrated that the Internal Transcribed Spacer (ITS) region is frequently highly variable among the different species of a same genus and easily amplified from universal primers, which render this region ideal for carrying out molecular identification. The size of the ITS1 region ranges from 162–266 pb and it is localized between genes *18S* and *5.8S rDNA* (Li et al., 2007), these genes are conserved zones among species and even among different genera, families, and orders. For ITS1-region amplification, universal primers are utilized, such as *ITS1: (5´- TCC GTA GGT GAA CCT GCG G)*, which is hybridized at the end of *18S rDNA*, and *ITS2: (5´- GCT GCG TTC TTC ATC GAT GC)*, which is hybridized at the beginning of *5.8S rDNA* (Juárez et al., 2014; White et al., 1990; Makimura et al., 2000).

Sequentiation is carried out from the amplified genes of bacteria and yeasts; the genes are edited by means of different programs, such as the Ribosomal Database Project

II or the green genes project, among others, and later, identification is performed in databases such as National Center for Biotechnology Information (NCBI) by means of the Blast program,[9] thus seeking identity with the sequences of organisms already reported.

The previously described techniques, including biochemical methods, selective, differential, and chromogenic cultures, and Molecular Biology techniques are proposed as tools for characterizing and identifying isolated bacteria and yeasts from nasal and oropharyngeal mucosa samples of tanners. Studies prior to this report (Maldonado-Vega et al., 2014) evaluated the microbiological interior-air quality inside 23 tanneries and at a control site in León City, Guanajuato State, Mexico, the bacterial and fungal burden exceeded the maximal permissible values in 87 and 83% of the tanneries included in the study, respectively, taking as reference the European Regulation for Work Sites (Abel et al., 2002), due to the lack of Mexican Norms. The bacterial and fungal burden at the control site did not exceed these values. Additionally, this study revealed the presence of microorganisms in the air, inside the tanneries, related with pathogenicity in humans.

Therefore, on identifying the microorganisms present in the oropharyngeal mucosa of tanners and to compare these results with those obtained in the previous study, a correlation could be established between the work environment (its microbiological quality) and the workers' state of health, in order to identify microorganisms in the oropharyngeal mucosa of workers of a control group made up of persons working in administrative areas, at a distance from the tanning ambience. Thus, these individuals were contrasted with tannery workers.

# 2    Methods

## 2.1    Study Population

The study had a control group composed of 20 automotive-industries, administrative-area workers, localized at a distance from the work ambit of the tanneries, without proximity to animal hide and with adequate environmental control in terms of temperature and ventilation (NOM-001-STPS-1999). The study group comprised 32 tannery workers with antecedents of respiratory problems and intestinal infections, and active work activity in tanneries for >5 years. An inclusion criterion comprised presenting respiratory or intestinal conditions. The sole exclusion criterion was being a smoker.

In the first sentinel group of tanners, nasal and oropharyngeal mucosa samples were taken, which were processed separately. In a second group of tanners, as well as in the control group, a sample of oropharyngeal mucosa was taken. Each sample of nasal, as well as oropharyngeal, mucosa was processed separately.

## 2.2    Sample Taking and Processing

The samples were obtained by means of a cotton swab. A sterile swab was utilized for

---

[9] http://ncbi.nlm.nih.gov/blast

each sample type. Thus, the swab was introduced into the nasal and oropharyngeal mucosa (according to the case), and a short scrape motion was performed. Immediately thereafter, the swab was introduced into a tube containing 1 ml of Phosphate-buffered saline (PBS) solution and was duly sealed and labeled. The PBS was prepared in the following manner: for every 400 ml of distilled water, 3.2 g was added of NaCl, 0.45 g of $Na_2HPO_4$, and 0.08g of $KH_2PO_4$, adjusting the pH (7.4) and sterilizing in autoclave at 121°C for 15 min.

The samples obtained were transported to the laboratory for the performance of microbiological seeding. Each tube was gently shaken and each sample was inoculated with 200 µl in Brilliant Green Bile Agar (BGBA) and 200 µl in Sabouraud Dextrose Agar (SDA). The sample was extended over each medium using a flamed glass pipette, until it was completely absorbed. The preparation of BGBB media for bacteria and SDA for yeasts was carried out according to the manufacturer's instructions, sterilizing these in autoclave at 121°C for 15 min, and finally poured these into Petri dishes. Incubation conditions were as follows: for BGBB medium, at 37°C for 48 h, and for SDA medium, at room temperature for 72 h.

Once the incubation time had passed, the bacteria and yeasts were isolated for their description and differentiation based on their morphological characteristics.

## 2.3   Characterization and Identification of Bacterial Isolates

Different experiments were conducted, among which the bacterium *Escherichia coli* ATCC 35218 (IECSA) was included as positive control.

- **Brilliant Green Bile Broth (BGBB) at 2% with MUG (DIBICO, S.A.).** The culture broth was prepared according to the manufacturer's instructions (Hernández-Arredondo, 2010). Once prepared, it was distributed into assay tubes and a Durham tube was added to each; verification was conducted to ensure that the tube did not present air bubbles, and the tubes were sterilized in autoclave at 121°C for 15 min. Prior to seeding the different isolates, the absence was verified of air bubbles in the Durham tubes, and these were incubated in a double boiler with shaking (250 rpm) for 24 h at 37°C. At the end of this incubation time, the formation of gas was observed in the Durham tubes, and the Kovacs reagent was added to determine the presence or not of the indole.
- **Escherichia coli O157:H7 Agar (DIBICO, S.A.).** The culture medium arrived prepared in Petri dishes thus; seeding was carried out by the cross-striate technique and was incubated for 24 h at 35°C.
- **Blood-Agar Base (DIBICO, S.A.).** The culture medium was prepared according to the manufacturer's instructions; sterilized in autoclave at 121°C for 15 min, allowed to cool, and 5% of defibrinated sterile rabbit blood was added, stirring the flask gently to avoid the formation of bubbles; finally, this was poured into the Petri dishes and left to gel. The different bacterial isolates were seeded by pricking and were subsequently incubated for 48 h at 35°C.

## 2.3.1     Antibacterial Sensitivity Test by the Disk Diffusion Method

The Mueller-Hinton culture medium was prepared according to the manufacturer's instructions (DIBICO, S.A). For preparation of the McFarland turbidity standard, 0.5 ml was added of $BaCl_2$ 0.048 M ($BaCl_2$ $H_2O$ at 1,175% P/V) to 99.5 ml of $H_2SO_4$ 0.18 M (0.36 N) (1% V/V) under constant movement to maintain the suspension. The density of the standard was verified in a spectrophotometer, whose absorbance at 625 nm should be 0.08–0.10 for 0.5 of the McFarland standard. The prepared suspension will contain approximately 1–2 × $10^8$ Colony-forming units (CFU)/ml for *E. coli* American Type Culture Collection (ATCC) 25922. This was maintained in the dark at room temperature.

Two ml of PBS was divided into assay tubes according to the number of the isolates of the bacteria, plus a control (+) and (-), and 2 ml of the McFarland standard was added into an additional tube. A colony was added to each of the tubes with PBS and for visual comparison, the turbidity was adjusted to the McFarland standard. After this, each of the seeding was carried out by striate in three directions with sterile swabs in Mueller-Hinton Agar. Once the agar surface was dry, the diffusion disks were set in place (BIO-RAD) (See Tables 1 and 2). This was incubated for 18 h at 35°C.

| TIM (75/10 µg) | SAM (10/10 µg) | AMC (20/10 µg) | TZP (100/10 µg) |
|---|---|---|---|
| 21–25 mm | 13–19 mm | 17–22 mm | 24–30 mm |

**Table 1:** Antibiotics and critical diameters. Acid Control (+): Escherichia coli ATCC 35218.

| Antibiotic | Content of the Disk | Diameter in mm | | |
|---|---|---|---|---|
| | | S | I | R |
| Ticarcillin/ Clavulanic acid (TIM) | 75/10 µg | ≥20 | 15–19 | ≤14 |
| Ampicillin/ Sulbactam (SAM) | 10/10µg | ≥ 15 | 12–14 | ≤ 11 |
| Amoxycillin / Acid Clavulanic (AMC) | 20/10µg | ≥ 18 | 14–17 | ≤ 13 |
| Piperacilina / Tazobactam (TZP) | 100/10µg | ≥ 21 | 18–20 | ≤ 17 |

**Table 2:** Average diameter of the inhibition zone recommended for quality control.

## 2.3.2     Molecular Biology Techniques

The different isolates of bacteria of both study groups were seeded in 3 ml of Trypticase Soy Broth (TSB), also including a control (-), and these were incubated in a double boiler (model 4682; Lab-Line Instruments, Inc.), with shaking (250 rpm) for 12 h at 37°C.

- **DNA Extraction.** At the end of the incubation time, 3 ml of the TSB was acquired for the extraction of DNA with the *ZR Fungal/Bacterial DNA* Kit™, following the manufacturer's instructions (ENDURO™ Electrophoresis System, Lab net International, Inc.). A 1% agarose gel was prepared, placing in a flask 50 ml of TAE 1X (Tris-Acetate-

EDTA) and 0.5 g of agarose. This was gently shaken and placed in the microwave oven for 1 min; once this had cooled, 3 µl of ethidium bromide was added and gently shaken; the electrophoresis combs were set in place, and this was allowed to gel. After this, it was immediately introduced into the electrophoresis bat, the combs were removed, and it was gently shaken, and then poured over the electrophotoray, adding TAE until this was above the level of the gel. Five µl was taken of each sample of DNA and was mixed with 1 µl of charge buffer on a Parafilm paper; once mixed, 5 µl was again taken and charged in each of the gel wells. The power source was programmed at 120V and 140mA for 20 min. After this time, the agarose gels were observed in an Ultraviolet (UV) Tran's illuminator.

- **PCR.** The initial concentration of each DNA sample was measured using a Quawell Q5000 spectrophotometer, and each of the samples was 10 nanograms (ng). Prior to sequentiation, the concentration of the amplified product was measured, as well as the A260/A280 relation, which indicates the degree of purity of the DNA with respect to the presence of proteins. Amplification of gene *16S rDNA* for each of the isolates was performed in a Thermocycler (*Lab net International, Inc.*), and the primers utilized for this amplification were the following: *FD1*: 5′- CCG AAT TCG ACA GAG TTT GAT CCT GGC TCA G y *RD1*: CCC GGG ATC CAA GCT TAA GGA GGT GAT CCA GCC (Invitrogen) (Özdilli et al., 2007), which amplified a gene segment of approximately *1,500 pb*. The PCR reaction was carried out in a volume of 50 µl under the following conditions: 5 µl of 10X PCR buffer minus Mg; 1.5 µl of $MgCl_2$ (50 mM); 1 µl of dNTP solution (10 mM) (Invitrogen); 1 µl of the FD1 primer (30 mM); 1 µl of the RD1 primer (30 mM); 0.5 µl of Platinum Taq polymerase 5 U/µl (Invitrogen), and 38 µl of sterile water. In this manner, the Super Mix was prepared for the 34 isolates; each PCR tube contained 48 µl of the Super Mix plus 2 µl of each of the DNA samples, for a final volume of 50 µl. The PCR was programmed as follows: at 94°C for 5 min; 40 cycles at 94°C for 50 sec; at 55°C for 1 min; and at 72°C for 2 min, with a final extension of 10 min at 72°C.
- **Electrophoresis.** Once the PCR was finished, we proceeded to verify the products in a 1% agarose gel. This gel was prepared in the same manner as previously described, and as molecular weight marker, *1Kb plus DNA Ladder* was employed. Five ul of each sample, previously charged with 1 µl of the charge buffer, was charged, and the molecular weight marker was also charged. The power source was programmed with 120V and 140mA for 20 min; when this time had elapsed, it was observed in a UV light trans illuminator.
- **DNA Purification.** This was conducted employing the UltraClean® PCR Clean-Up kit, following the manufacturer's instructions. This was quantified in a Quawell Q5000 Nano-Spectrophotometer to determine the amount of DNA that was contained in each of the samples, and finally, the purified product was sent to the Centro de Investigación y de Estudios Avanzados (CINVESTAV)-Irapuato-México Sequentiation Laboratory. The sequences obtained were edited in Ribosomal Database Project II (Cole, et al., 2007; Cole, et al., 2005),[10] in the green genes project (DeSantis, et al.,

---

[10] https://rdp.cme.msu.edu/seqmatch/seqmatch_intro.jsp

2006),[11] and in the SILVA database project,[12] and were compared with the NCBI Data-Bank by means of the Blast program,[9] thus seeking identify with sequences of already reported organisms.

## 2.4    Characterization and Identification of Yeast Isolates

Different experiments were carried out, among which were those that included, as control (+), *Candida albicans* ATCC 90028 (DIBICO).

- **BBL™ CHROMagar™ Candida Medium (BD-Becton Dickinson & Co.).** This commercial culture medium was utilized to propagate the yeasts. Seeding was carried out by the striate technique, and this was incubated for 48 h at 37°C. BB™ CHRO-Magar™ *Candida* Medium possesses easy and efficient detection of mixed yeast cultures; thus, no other conventional identification is performed. This efficiency is due to the different colors that their colonies present thanks to the specially selected peptones supplying the nutrients in the BBL™ CHROMagar™ *Candida* Medium. The patented chromogenic mixture is made up of artificial substrates (chromogens) that release compounds of different colors on being degraded by specific enzymes. In this way, it is possible to differentiate determined species or to detect certain organisms with only a minimum of confirmation tests.

### 2.4.1    Antifungal Sensitivity Test by the Disk Diffusion Method

The antifungal sensitivity test by the disk-diffusion method[88] includes of the formation of inhibition halos, which represent the capacity of the determined antifungal to inhibit the growth of the yeast that, in this case, is under study. For the case of Fluconazole, depending on the diameter of the inhibition halo formed, the result could be interpreted as that a yeast is sensitive (≥19 mm) or resistant (≤14 mm) to Fluconazole. The diffusion disks utilized, in the antibiotic as well as in the antifungal test, were of the BIO-RAD commercial brand.

Preparation of the Mueller-Hinton culture medium was performed according to the manufacturer's instructions (DIBICO). Sterilization was conducted in autoclave at 121°C for 15 min, left to cool, and poured into Petri dishes for gelification. Immediately afterward, this was supplemented with a Methylene Blue Glucose solution. This solution was prepared in the following manner: for the *Methylene Blue stock,* 0.1 g of Methylene Blue was dissolved in 20 ml of distilled water and heated under slow heat; subsequently, the *glucose stock* solution was prepared, for which 40 g of glucose was dissolved in 100 ml of distilled water and slowly heated to dissolve it. Finally, 200 µl of the Methylene Blue stock solution was added to 100 ml of the glucose stock solution to prepare the *Methylene-Blue Glucose stock solution at a final concentration of 40% glucose and 10 µg/ml* of Methylene Blue.

These were divided into 20, 1.5-ml aliquot assay tubes (for Petri dishes 90 mm in

[11] http://greengenes.lbl.gov/cgi-bin/nph-blast_interface.cgi
[12] http://www.megx.net/gms/geographic-blast

diameter) with the *Methylene-Blue-Glucose* stock solution and sterilized in autoclave at 121°C for 15 min. After allowing these to cool, each of the aliquots was poured into the Petri dishes containing Mueller-Hinton jellified agar, spread with a glass handle on the surface of the agar in order for the supplement to be diffused in the same manner, and allowed to dry at room temperature for 4–5 h until it was completely absorbed.

Once the Mueller-Hinton medium was supplemented, inoculate were prepared in the same manner as in the antibiogram. A 2-ml assay tube of the McFarland standard was added. Twenty assay tubes were used of 2 ml of PBS each, to which was added a colony of each isolate and a control (+) colony. Turbidity was adjusted for visual comparison with the McFarland standard. Sterile swabs were utilized: these were submerged separately into each of the tubes; then, the excess of liquid was eliminated by pressing the swab against the sides of the tube, and subsequently, seeding was performed in three different directions on the surface of the agar. Once the agar's surface was dry, the Fluconazole diffusion disk (BIO-RAD) was set in place (See Tables 3 and 4), and finally, this was incubated for 18 h at 35°C.

| Antifungal agent | Content of the Disk | Zone of the Diameter of Inhibition in mm | | |
|---|---|---|---|---|
| | | R | S-DD | S |
| Fluconazole | 25 µg | ≤14 | 15–18 | ≥19 |

**Table 3:** Interpretative standard of the zone of inhibition for Fluconazole.

| Antifungal agent | Content of the Disk | *Candida albicans* ATCC 90028 |
|---|---|---|
| Fluconazole | 25 µg | 28–39 mm |

**Table 4:** Range of diameter of the zone of inhibition recommended for quality control.

The controls utilized in this test were the following: 1). Quality control, which consists of the seeding of the yeast *Candida albicans* ATCC 90028 in the presence of the diffusion disk containing Fluconazole; this quality control should give rise to an inhibition halo with a diameter of between 28 and 39 mm and 2). Sterile control, consists of the solid medium without yeast and without a diffusion disk, to ensure the effectiveness of the medium, discarding possible contamination.

## 2.4.2    Molecular Biology Techniques

The different yeasts isolated from both of the study groups were seeded in 3 ml of Sabouraud Dextrose Broth (SDB), in addition including a control (-), and these were incubated in a double boiler (model 4682; Lab-Line Instrument, Inc.) with shaking (250 rpm) for 72 h at 37°C.

- **DNA extraction:** At the end of the incubation time, 3 ml of the SDB was taken to carry out DNA extraction by means of the *ZR Fungal/Bacterial DNA* Kit™ following the manufacturer's instructions.

- **Electrophoresis:** A 1% agarose gel was prepared in the same manner as in the previously mentioned electrophoreses. Three µl of each DNA sample was taken and mixed with 3 µl of charge buffer. Then, these were charged in the different agarose-gel wells. The power source was programmed with 120V and 140mA for 20 min, and after this time, it was observed in a UV light trans illuminator.

- **PCR:** The initial concentration of each DNA sample was measured using a Quawell Q5000 spectrophotometer; the concentration in each of the sample was 10 nanograms (ng). For amplification of region ITS1, *ITS1: (5´- TCC GTA GGT GAA CCT GCG G9)* was used, which is hybridized at the end of *18S rDNA*, and *ITS2: (5´- GCT GCG TTC TTC ATC GAT GC)*, which is hybridized at the beginning of *5.8S rDNA* (de Bentzmann & Plésiat, 2011; Kothavade et al., 2010), and these amplify the 62–266-pb segment, which is localized between genes *18S rDNA* and *5.8S rDNA* (Li et al., 2007). The PCR reaction was carried out in a total volume of 50 µl under the following conditions: 5 µl of 10X PCR Buffer minus M, 1.5 µl of $MgCl_2$ (50 mM), 1 µl of dNTP solution (10 mM) (Invitrogen), 1 µl of each primer (30 mM), and 0.25 µl of Platinum Taq DNA polymerase 5 U/µl. The amplification program was performed in a thermocycler (Lab net International, Inc.) under the following conditions: at 96°C for 5 min; 40 cycles at 94°C for 30 sec; at 58°C for 30 sec, and at 72°C for 30 sec, with a final 5-min extension at 72°C.

- **Electrophoresis:** Again, a 1% agarose gel is prepared under the same conditions as previously described. *1Kb plus DNA Ladder* is employed as molecular weight marker; 3 µl of each DNA sample was taken and each was mixed with 3 µl of the charge buffer on Parafilm paper. Immediately thereafter, 3 µl of this mixture was poured into the different agarose-gel wells, as well as 3 µl of the molecular weight marker. The power source was programmed with 120V and 140mA for 20 min, after which time this was observed in a UV light trans illuminator.

- **DNA Purification:** This was conducted employing the Ultraclean® PCR Clean-Up kit, following the manufacturer's instructions, and was quantified in a nanospectrophotometer to determine the amount of DNA contained in each of the samples. Finally, some of the purified products were randomly selected for delivery to the CINVESTAV-Irapuato-México Sequentiation Laboratory.

Presumptive identification was performed of all of the yeast isolates through CHROMagar *Candida*. Later, in order to carry out molecular identification from the extraction of the DNA, three yeasts were selected at random from the group of tanners and two yeasts were chosen from the control group. Once the sequentiation was performed, these were edited by means of the following programs: Ribosomal Database Project II (Cole, et al., 2007; Cole, et al., 2005);[10] green genes project (DeSantis, et al., 2006),[11] and the SILVA database project,[12] and were subsequently compared with the NCBI Database through the Blast program,[9] thus seeking identity with the sequences of organisms already reported.

# 3   Results

## 3.1   Sample Taking and Processing

With regard to the taking of the nasal and oropharyngeal sample from tanners, this took two sites into consideration. The first group of tanners was evaluated in their work environment (the sentinel group), within the tanneries offices. For the second group of tanners, as well as the control group workers, sample-taking was conducted at a clinical laboratory distant from the tanners' environment.

The samples of nasal and oropharyngeal mucosa taken from the tanners (the sentinel group) demonstrated a high burden of bacteria and yeasts, with values up to $76 \times 10^7$ CFU/ml for bacteria and $80 \times 10^7$ CFU/ml for yeasts (Table 5), observing bacterial and fungal growth in all of the participants (Table 6).

The nasal-mucosa results of the second group of tanners and of the control group, in which the sample was taken at the clinical laboratory, confirmed the presence of bacteria and fungi previously observed in the first tanners' group; however, the concentration was less with respect to the sentinel group of tanners, with values of $1.5 \times 10^3$ CFU/ml and $1.9 \times 10^3$ CFU/ml for bacteria and yeasts, respectively (Table 7).

In this second group of tanners, 63% presented growth from bacteria as well as for the oropharyngeal-mucosa yeasts (See Table 8), in contrast with the oropharyngeal samples of the control group, in which maximal values were $4 \times 10^1$ CFU/ml and $1.1 \times 10^3$ CFU/ml for bacteria and yeasts, respectively (Table 9), resulting in bacterial growth in 15% of the workers and with fungal growth in 45% of workers (Table 10).

For the tannery worker's group, observation and macroscopic description corresponded to 31 colonies of bacteria and 14 of yeasts; in contrast, for the control group, this comprised only three different bacterial colonies of bacteria and four different yeast colonies. Comparison between both groups evidences greater contamination and microbiological concentration in the tanners.

## 3.2   Characterization and Identification of Bacterial Isolates

### 3.2.1   BGBB at 2% with MUG

In this selective culture broth for detection of the coliform group, the production was evaluated of gas and indole. In the tanners' group isolates, it was observed that 48% did not present the production of gas nor of indole. In this case, the culture broth did not present turbidity or the broth was scarce; 31% presented only the production of gas, 14% the production of gas and indole, and 7% were positive only for the indole test. In all cases in which the production of gas and/or indole was observed, turbidity was observed in the culture broth; in contrast, in the culture broth in control-group isolates, none presented turbidity, nor gas production, and were negative for the indole test. BGBB at 2% with MUG is selective for the detection of the coliform group, the presence of gas after incubation (24–48 h at 35°C) is a positive test for the presence of a *Coli–Enterobacter* group, and the indole test confirms the presence of *E. coli*; thus, in both groups (control and tanners),

| Oropharyngeal sample | Bacteria CFU/ml | Yeasts CFU/ml |
|---|---|---|
| E1 | 400 | 3,400 |
| E3 | 100 | 160,000 |
| E5 | 650 | 3,700 |
| E6 | 950 | 3,000 |
| E7 | 1,200 | 750 |
| E9 | 760,000,000 | 800,000,000 |
| E10 | 170 | 17,000 |
| E11 | 12,000 | 12,000 |
| E12 | 40,000,000 | 15,000,000 |
| E13 | ND | ND |
| E14 | 20,000 | 62,000 |
| E15 | ND | 12,000 |
| E16 | 70,000,000 | 200,000 |

ND: Not Determined.; Culture media: BGBB and SDA; Temperature and Incubation Time: 37°C for 48 h (bacteria); room temperature (25°C) for 72 h (yeasts).

**Table 5:** Concentration of bacteria and yeasts found in samples of nasal and oropharyngeal mucosa of Tannery workers (E) and whose samples were taken at the tannery offices, i.e. their work environment. The high number can be observed of bacteria and yeasts can be observed in the workers

| | Total | 13 |
|---|---|---|
| **Bacterias** | Positives | 13 (100%) |
| | Negatives | 0 |
| | Total | 13 |
| **Levaduras** | Positives | 13 (100%) |
| | Negatives | 0 |

**Table 6:** It can be observed that in oropharyngeal and nasal mucosa samples taken from the first group of tanning workers presented 100% of growth of bacteria as well as yeasts.

| Oropharyngeal sample | Bacteria CFU/ml | Yeasts CFU/ml |
|---|---|---|
| E17 | 10 | 310 |
| E18 | 50 | 0 |
| E19 | 1,535 | 1,870 |
| E20 | 15 | 5 |
| E21 | 1,000 | 105 |
| E22 | 0 | 5 |
| E23 | 0 | 0 |
| E24 | 0 | 0 |
| E25 | 55 | 0 |
| E26 | 25 | 25 |
| E27 | 40 | 95 |
| E28 | 85 | 410 |
| E29 | 0 | 0 |
| E30 | 85 | 10 |
| E31 | 5 | 15 |
| E32 | 0 | 400 |
| E33 | 0 | 0 |
| E34 | 15 | 25 |
| E35 | 0 | 0 |

Culture media: BGBB and SDA; temperature and incubation time: 37°C for 48 h (bacteria); room temperature (25°C) for 72 h (yeast).

**Table 7:** Concentration (Colony-forming units [CFU]/ml) of bacteria and yeasts found in samples of the oropharyngeal mucosa of Tannery workers (E) and whose samples were taken at a clinical laboratory, i.e. a place distant from their work environment. The concentration (CFU/ml) is observed of bacteria and yeasts as diminished.

| | | |
|---|---|---|
| **Bacteria** | Total | 19 |
| | Positive | 12 (63%) |
| | Negative | 7 |
| **Yeasts** | Total | 19 |
| | Positive | 12 (63%) |
| | Negative | 7 |

**Table 8:** It is observed that the oropharyngeal mucosa samples taken from the second group of tanners presented 63% of bacterial growth, as well as of yeasts

| Oropharyngeal sample | Bacteria CFU/ml | Yeasts CFU/ml |
|---|---|---|
| C1 | 0 | 65 |
| C2 | 0 | 0 |
| C3 | 0 | 0 |
| C4 | 0 | 35 |
| C5 | 0 | 1,105 |
| C6 | 0 | 0 |
| C7 | 25 | 605 |
| C8 | 0 | 150 |
| C9 | 0 | 0 |
| C10 | 0 | 0 |
| C11 | 0 | 25 |
| C12 | 15 | 0 |
| C13 | 0 | 0 |
| C14 | 0 | 320 |
| C15 | 0 | 0 |
| C16 | 40 | 20 |
| C17 | 0 | 45 |
| C18 | 0 | 0 |
| C19 | 0 | 0 |
| C20 | 0 | 0 |

Culture media: BGBB and SDA; temperature and incubation time: 37°C for 48 h (bacteria); room temperature (25°C) for 72 h (yeast).

**Table 9:** Concentration (Colony-forming units [CFU]/ml) of bacteria and yeasts present in the oropharyngeal mucosa samples of the control group, that is, of workers located at a distance from the Tanning environment (T). These samples were taken at a clinical laboratory. A concentration is importantly observed (CFU/ml) of bacteria and yeasts much fewer in number than in the previously mentioned groups

| Bacteria | Total | 20 |
|---|---|---|
| | Positive | 3 (15%) |
| | Negative | 17 |
| Yeasts | Total | 20 |
| | Positive | 9 (45%) |
| | Negative | 11 |

**Table 10:** It is observed that the oropharyngeal mucosa samples taken of the control group presented 15% of bacterial growth and 45% presented yeast growth

there is a great difference in the type of bacteria present; according to these results in the group of tanners, the presumptive presence of coliforms was identified.

### 3.2.2     Escherichia coli O157:H7 Agar

Bearing the previous results in mind, the presence was demonstrated of coliforms, and possibly among these, *Escherichia coli*. Seeding was undertaken of the different isolates in a selective culture medium for the isolation and differentiation of enterohemorrhagic strains of *Escherichia coli* O157: H7, whose colonies should present as greenish in color and without fluorescence on illumination with the 366-nm UV light. Which is characteristic of whether or not these were typical colonies of *Escherichia coli* After incubation at 35°C for 24 h, it was observed that 65% presented colonies that were yellow in color, 6% cream, 3%, dark orange, 3%, blackish, and 26% did not present bacterial growth. This was illuminated with 360-nm UV light, and one of the isolates that had grown yellow in color, said to be sorbitol-positive, presented fluorescence. The positive control utilized was *Escherichia coli* ATCC 35218, whose colonies grew yellow in color and, on being illuminated with 366-nm UV light, presented fluorescence. Due to this, the presence was noted of enterohemorrhagic strains of *Escherichia coli* O157:H7 and, at the same time, the presence of *Escherichia coli* in the nasal and oropharyngeal mucosa samples of workers exposed to tanning environments.

In control-group colonies, a cream color was observed and without fluorescence on being illuminated with 366-nm UV light. Thus, the presence of *Escherichia coli* was discarded.

### 3.2.3     Blood-Agar Base

To assess the absence of enterohemorrhagic strains of *Escherichia coli* O157:H7, all of the isolates were seeded in Blood-Agar Base (BAB), investigating hemolytic activity in this manner. *Escherichia coli* O157: H7 possesses pO157 as a characteristic plasmid, which gives rise to hemolysis halos around the colonies developed on plates of this nutritive culture medium. None of those isolated from the tanners' group presented hemolysis halos, completely discarding the presence of this highly pathogenic strain in the samples evaluated.

### 3.2.4     Antimicrobial Sensitivity Tests for the Disk Diffusion Method

Antimicrobial sensitivity tests were carried out through the disk diffusion method from the different isolated of the nasal and oropharyngeal mucosa samples of workers exposed to tannery environments, in which different percentages of resistance were observed, among which are the following:
- Piperacillin/TaZobactam (TZP): 10%
- Ticarcillin/Clavulanic Acid (TIM): 13%
- Ampicillin/Sulbactam (SAM): 26%
- Amoxicillin/Clavulanic Acid (AMC): 42%

Taking the results of the sequentiation into account with respect to these bacteria, we are able to state the following: *Kluyvera ascorbata* strain ATCC 33433, *Rahnella aquatilis* HX2 strain HX2, *Citrobacter murliniae* strain CDC 2970-59, *Klebsiella Pneumoniae* sub spp. *Pneumoniae* strain MGH 78578 ATCC 700721, *Stenotrophomonas maltophilia* strain IAM 12423, *Proteus vulgaris* strain DSM 30118, *Alcaligenes faecalis* sub spp. *Parafaecalis* sub spp. *Parafaecalis* sub spp. *G, Acinetobacter johnsonii* strain ATCC 17909, *Neisseria bacilliformis* ATCC BAA-1200 strain MDA2833, *Neisseria subflava* strain U37, *Pseudomonas psychrotolerans* strain C36, *Achromobacter xylosoxidans* strain A8A8, and *Escherichia coli* strain U 5/41 were sensitive to the four antibiotics employed: TIM; SAM; AMC, and TZP. The remainder of the bacteria exhibited behavior with variable sensitivity, among which are the following: *Enterobacter asburiae* strain JCM6051, sensitive to TIM, SAM, and TZP and resistant to AMC; *Enterobacter cloacae* subspp. *Dissolvens* strain LMG 2683, sensitive to TIM and TZP, resistant to AMC, and with an intermediate range for SAM; *Pseudomonas brenneri* strain CFML 97-391, resistant to TIM, SAM, and AMC, but sensitive to TZP; *Enterobacter aerogenes* strain JCM1235, sensitive to TIM and TZP, resistant to AMC, and with an intermediate range for SAM; *Pseudomonas aeruginosa* strain PAO1 PAO1, sensitive to TIM and TZP and resistant to SAM and AMC; *Neisseria bacilliformis* ATCC BAA-1200 strain MDA2833, sensitive to TIM and TZP and resistant to SAM and AMC; *Klebsiella pneumoniae* subspp. *Pneumoniae* strain MGH 78578 ATCC 700721, sensitive to TIM, SAM, and TZP, but resistant to AMC, and finally, *Serratia marcescens* subspp. *Sakuensis* strain KRED, with sensitivity to TIM and TZP, resistance to AMC, and with an intermediate range for SAM (Table 11).

Therefore, TZP presented greatest antimicrobial response, with an effectiveness of 90%, followed by TIM, SAM, and finally, AMC.

Within the control group, only two of three oropharyngeal samples isolated were submitted to the antimicrobial sensitivity test, and with one sample, the extraction of DNA was achieved, in addition to its later sequentiation for its identification, which corresponded to *Neisseria polysaccharea* strain NCTC11858; with respect to the isolates of the two remaining samples, these presented resistances to the four antibiotics (Table 11).

### 3.2.5    Sequentiation

The amplification products of the gene *16S rDNA* of bacteria and ITS1 of yeasts were sequenced, and the information indicates that 53% of bacteria found in the nasal and oropharyngeal mucosa of workers exposed to tanning environments belong to the Enterobacteriaceae Family (Table 12). Within this group, the following are found: *Kluyvera ascorbate; Citrobacter murliniae; Enterobacter asburiae; Klebsiella pneumoniae* subspp. *Pneumoniae; Enterobacter cloacae* subspp. *Escherichia coli; Serratia marcescens* subspp. *Sakuensis; Proteus vulgaris; Enterobacter* aerogenes, and *Rahnella aquatilis HX2*, while the other families of bacteria were found at a lesser percentage: 16% belonging to the Pseudomonadaceae Family, 10% to the Neisseriaceae Family, 10% to the Alcaligenaceae Family, 5% to the Moraxellaceae Family, and the remaining 5%, to the Xanthomonadaceae Family. A high percentage of the bacteria found are pathogens to humans or opportunistic pathogens; this listing represents information on environmental as well as personnel contamination for the tanneries considered as a sample of these sites, representing an element for establishing procedures that reduce the effects on the health of the personnel. It is evident that

| Isolate | TIM | | SAM | | AMC | | TZP | |
|---|---|---|---|---|---|---|---|---|
| E1* | 27 | S | 21 | S | 25 | S | 25 | S |
| E2* | 29 | S | 23 | S | 26 | S | 30 | S |
| *Kluyvera ascorbata* strain *ATCC 33433* | 28 | S | 25 | S | 30 | S | 28 | S |
| *Citrobacter murliniae* strain *CDC 2970-59* | 35 | S | 32 | S | 30 | S | 35 | S |
| *Enterobacter asburiae* strain *JCM6051* | 29 | S | 16 | S | (--) | R | 24 | S |
| *Klebsiella pneumoniae* subspp. *Pneumoniae* strain *MGH 78578 ATCC 700721* | (-) | S | (-) | S | (-) | S | (-) | S |
| *Enterobacter cloacae* subspp. *Dissolvens cepa LMG 2683* | 29 | S | 13 | I | (--) | R | 31 | S |
| *Pseudomonas brenneri* strain *CFML 97-391* | (--) | R | (--) | R | (--) | R | 37 | S |
| *Rahnella aquatilis* HX2 strain *HX2* | (-) | S | (-) | S | (-) | S | (-) | S |
| *Stenotrophomonas maltophilia* strain *IAM 12423* | (-) | S | (-) | S | (-) | S | (-) | S |
| *Proteus vulgaris* strain *DSM 30118* | 33 | S | 23 | S | 25 | S | 37 | S |
| E12* | 26 | S | (--) | R | 18 | S | 36 | S |
| *Enterobacter aerogenes* strain *JCM1235* | 28 | S | 14 | I | 10 | R | 27 | S |
| E14* | (-) | S | (-) | S | (-) | S | (-) | S |
| *Alcaligenes faecalis* subspp. *Parafaecalis* strain *G* | 44 | S | 37 | S | 37 | S | 42 | S |
| *Acinetobacter johnsonii* strain *ATCC 17909* | 25 | S | 32 | S | 25 | S | 25 | S |
| *Neisseria bacilliformis* ATCC BAA-1200 strain *MDA2833* | (-) | S | (-) | S | (-) | S | (-) | S |
| *Pseudomonas aeruginosa* strain *PAO1 PAO1* | 21 | S | (--) | R | (--) | R | 29 | S |
| *Neisseria bacilliformis* ATCC BAA-1200 strain *MDA2833* | 21 | S | (--) | R | (--) | R | 29 | S |
| *Neisseria subflava* strain *U37* | (-) | S | (-) | S | (-) | S | (-) | S |
| *Pseudomonas psychrotolerans* strain *C36* | (-) | S | (-) | S | (-) | S | (-) | S |
| *Achromobacter xylosoxidans* strain *A8 A8* | (-) | S | (-) | S | (-) | S | (-) | S |
| *Escherichia coli* strain *U 5/41* | 32 | S | 26 | S | 27 | S | 30 | S |
| E20F* | (--) | R | (--) | R | (--) | R | (--) | R |
| *Enterobacter asburiae* strain *JCM6051* | 28 | S | 18 | S | (--) | R | 26 | S |
| *Klebsiella pneumoniae* subspp. *Pneumoniae* strain *MGH 78578 ATCC 700721* | 29 | S | 15 | S | 8 | R | 27 | S |
| *Serratia marcescens* subspp. *Sakuensis* strain *KRED* | 28 | S | 14 | I | 10 | R | 27 | S |
| E26* | (--) | R | (--) | R | (--) | R | (--) | R |
| E27* | (--) | R | (--) | R | (--) | R | (--) | R |
| E30* | (-) | S | (-) | S | (-) | S | (-) | S |
| *Enterobacter asburiae* strain *JCM6051* | 27 | S | 11 | R | 7 | R | 27 | S |
| E1* | (--) | R | (--) | R | (--) | R | (--) | R |
| *Acinetobacter* [*calcoaceticus*] strain NCCB 22016 | (--) | R | (--) | R | (--) | R | (--) | R |
| Quality Control: *Escherichia coli* ATCC 35218 | 21 | | 13 | | 17 | | 26 | |

(Rows above grouped under the left-margin labels: **Tanners' Group** (E1* through E30* / *Enterobacter asburiae* strain JCM6051) and **Control** (E1* / Acinetobacter [calcoaceticus] strain NCCB 22016 / Quality Control).)

(-): Without Growth; (--): Without Inhibition Halo with Growth; R: Resistant; I: Intermediate; S: Sensitive. The diameters of the zone of inhibition are expressed in mm. *: No significant similarities are found in NCBI.

**Table 11:** Antimicrobial sensitivity test of tannery workers and a control group.

| Bacteria | Family |
|---|---|
| *Kluyvera ascorbata strain ATCC 33433* | Enterobacteriaceae |
| *Citrobacter murliniae strain CDC 2970-59* | Enterobacteriaceae |
| *Enterobacter asburiae strain JCM6051* | Enterobacteriaceae |
| *Klebsiella pneumoniae subspp. Pneumoniae strain MGH 78578 ATCC 700721* | Enterobacteriaceae |
| *Enterobacter cloacae subspp. Dissolvens strain LMG 2683* | Enterobacteriaceae |
| *Escherichia coli strain U 5/41* | Enterobacteriaceae |
| *Rahnella aquatilis HX2 strain HX2* | Enterobacteriaceae |
| *Serratia marcescens subspp. Sakuensis strain KRED* | Enterobacteriaceae |
| *Proteus vulgaris strain DSM 30118* | Enterobacteriaceae |
| *Enterobacter aerogenes strain JCM1235* | Enterobacteriaceae |
| *Pseudomonas brenneri strain CFML 97-391* | Pseudomonadaceae |
| *Pseudomonas psychrotolerans strain: C36* | Pseudomonadaceae |
| *Pseudomonas aeruginosa strain PAO1 PAO1* | Pseudomonadaceae |
| *Neisseria bacilliformis ATCC BAA-1200 strain MDA2833* | Neisseriaceae |
| *Neisseria subflava strain U37* | Neisseriaceae |
| *Achromobacter xylosoxidans A8 A8* | Alcaligenaceae |
| *Alcaligenes faecalis subspp. Parafaecalis strain G* | Alcaligenaceae |
| *Acinetobacter johnsonii strain ATCC 17909* | Moraxellaceae |
| *Stenotrophomonas maltophilia strain IAM 12423s* | Xanthomonadaceae |

**Table 12:** Bacteria found in the samples of nasal and oropharyngeal samples of tannery workers.

| Bacteria | Family |
|---|---|
| *Neisseria polysaccharea strain NCTC 11858* | Neisseriaceae |
| *Acinetobacter calcoaceticus strain NCCB 22016* | Moraxellaceae |

**Table 13:** Bacteria found in samples of oropharyngeal mucosa of the control group (workers distant from the tanning environment).

interaction presents of microorganisms at the interior of the environment of the tanneries in terms of the personnel involved, which is in contrast with the control group with minimal microbiological exposure, and (See Table 13) only 15% of the control group's oropharyngeal samples exhibited bacterial growth, identified among this, the bacterium of the Neisseriaceae Family: *Neisseria polysaccharea* strain *NCTC11858* and *Acinetobacter calcoaceticus* strain NCCB 22016, which belongs to the Moraxellaceae Family. These live as commensals in the oropharynx of healthy persons.

## 3.3    Characterization and Identification of the Yeast Isolates

### 3.3.1    BBL™ CHROMagar™ Candida Medium

The different colors that yeast colonies present are thanks to the specially selected peptones that supply the nutrients in BBL™ CHROMagar™ *Candida* medium. The patented
chromogenic mixture is made up of artificial substrates (chromogenes), which release
compounds of different colors on being degraded by specific enzymes. These colonies,
which are pink or mauve in color, ranging from light to dark, in this medium indicate
*Candida glabrata*, and large colonies, flat, light-pink-to-pink in color, and edges acquiring
a whitish color indicate *Candida krusei*. Colonies that are light green in color indicate *Candida albicans*, while colonies that are blueish-grey in color with or without a violet-colored
halo indicate *Candida tropicalis*.

Seeding in CHROMagar *Candida* is carried out from yeasts already isolated in solid
Sabouraud Dextrose Agar (SDA) medium. As mentioned in the methodology, each sample was seeded in solid SDA medium; once the incubation time had ended, morphologically different yeasts were isolated in solid SDA medium and, once this incubation time
was finished, each isolated yeast was seeded in solid CHROMagar *Candida* medium

This chromogenic culture medium permits the presumptive identification of some
species of medical importance. Isolates of the nasal and oropharyngeal mucosa samples
of workers exposed to tannery environments presented the following percentages: in 57%
of the isolates a mauve color was observed, indicating the presence of *Candida glabrata*;
21% were green in color, indicating the presence of *Candida albicans*; 7% were blue in color,
indicating the presence of *Candida tropicalis*, 7% were pink, which indicates the presence
of *Candida krusei*, and 7% of the isolates exhibited no growth.

In contrast, in the control group, 75% of the isolates grew with a mauve color, indicating the presence of *Candida glabrata*, and 25% of isolates were green in color, which
corresponds to *Candida albicans*. The positive control, *Candida albicans* ATCC 90028, grew
green in color in CHROMagar *Candida* medium

Antibiotics were not employed in the culture media for inhibition of bacteria; however, the low pH of the SDA medium resulted favorable for the growth of fungi and
slightly inhibitory for bacteria. On its part, the CHROMagar *Candida* medium contains,
among its components, Chloramphenicol, which inhibits the majority of the bacterial contaminants.

In the nasal and oropharyngeal mucosa samples of the groups of tanners, by means
of CHROMagar, the yeasts *C. glabrata*, *C. albicans*, *C. tropicales*, and *C. krusei* were identified, while in control-group samples, only *C. glabrata* and *C. albicans* were identified. Thus,
the yeasts *C. tropicalis* and *C. krusei* were found only in workers exposed to the tanning
environment. On the other hand, in the interior air of the tannery environment, the yeasts
*C. krusei* and *C. glabrata* were identified. The latter allows supposing that the yeast *C.
krusei*, present in the nasal and oropharyngeal mucosa of the tanners and not in the control group, derives from the work environment, able to be acquired by inhalation or ingestion in the workers.

These yeasts can be found living naturally in humans; however, in recent years, they are considered as opportunistic and nosocomial pathogens. Although >17 pathogens have been reported, 90% of infections are attributed to *C. albicans*, *C. krusei*, *C. glabrata*, *C. parasilopsis*, and *C. tropicalis*. The species identified in the tannery environment, *C. krusei* and *C. glabrata*, are customarily resistant to azolytic compounds, and the finding of these as infectious agents involved in intrahospitalary systemic diseases has increased over recent years (Castañón, 2013).

### 3.3.2    Antifungal Sensitivity Tests by the Disk Diffusion Method

In the growth of yeasts from workers exposed to the tannery environment, it was observed that 81% of nasal and oropharyngeal samples presented yeast growth in SDA medium (Tables 5 and 7), from which, by macroscopic comparison, the isolation of 14 different colonies was achieved.

In antifungal sensitivity tests by the disk diffusion disk method, Fluconazole (25-μg) disks were utilized and, as positive control, *Candida albicans* ATCC 90028 (Table 4). In isolates of the group of tanners, 21% presented resistance to Fluconazole and 79% were sensitive to this antifungal (Table 14).

Therefore, yeasts from the tanners' group exhibited a low degree of resistance to Fluconazole; thus, the majority can be treated with this antifungal. In contrast, in the control group, it was observed that only 45% of samples presented yeast growth in SDA medium (Tables 9 and 10) and, by macroscopic comparison, four isolates were carried out, of which four were resistant to Fluconazole, while the remaining 50% were Fluconazole-sensitive (Table 14). Therefore, in both environments (tanning and control), there are yeasts that are resistant to, as well as yeasts that are sensitive to, Fluconazole.

### 3.3.3    Sequentiation

With regard to yeasts, some of the isolates were selected at random in that they had been presumptively identified by means of CHROMagar *Candida* (three yeast isolates from the tanners' group and two from the control group), and their later identification was carried out by means of the extraction of the DNA. Two of the isolates studied from the group of tanners coincided in the identification of sequentiation, such as *C. albicans*, with a 100% percentage of identity, confirming the result obtained from CHROMagar *Candida*, and one isolate from the tanners' group by means of the molecular test was identified as *C. albicans*, with 98% identity, which had been presumptively identified by means of CHRO-Magar *Candida* as *C. glabrata*. Regarding the yeast isolates of the control group, this was performed randomly from two isolates that had been identified as *C. albicans* with 100% identify in the molecular test for each of these, thus confirming the result obtained through presumptive identification of the CHROMagar *Candida* medium.

Summing up the five yeast isolates, only four coincided in both identification tests for the presumptive test with CHROMagar *Candida*, and molecular identification from DNA extraction identified these isolates as *C. albicans* with 100% identity in the molecular test, and one of the isolates from the DNA extraction was identified as *C. albicans*, with 98% identity in the molecular test.

| | ISOLATE | Fluconazole 25 µg | |
| --- | --- | --- | --- |
| | | Diameter of the Zone of Inhibition (mm) | Sensitivity |
| Tanners' Group | Candida glabrata • | (--) | R |
| | Candida krusei • | 30 | S |
| | Candida glabrata • | (-) | S |
| | Candida glabrata • | (-) | S |
| | Candida glabrata • | (-) | S |
| | Candida tropicalis • | (-) | S |
| | L7 * | 40 | S |
| | Candida glabrata • | (-) | S |
| | Candida glabrata • | (--) | R |
| | Candida albicans strain Hb37 | 45 | S |
| | Candida albicans strain Hb37 | 35 | S |
| | Candida albicans strain YN50-151205 | 33 | S |
| | Candida glabrata • | (-) | S |
| | Candida albicans strain L8278 | (--) | R |
| Control | Candida albicans strain Hb20 | 30 | S |
| | Candida glabrata • | (--) | R |
| | Candida glabrata • | (--) | R |
| | Candida albicans strain L3805 | 35 | S |
| | Quality Control: Candida albicans ATCC 90028 | 32 | |

(-): Without Growth; (--): Without Inhibition Halo with Growth; R: Resistant; S: Sensitive. •: Presumptive Identification through CHROMag *Candida*. *: Without Growth in CHROMagar.

**Table 14:** Antifungigram of the yeast present in tannery workers and in the control group.

The GenBank Database isolates that allowed the establishment of the sequence of isolates corresponding to *Candida albicans* are the following:

| | Description | Identified (%) |
| --- | --- | --- |
| Tanners' Group | C. albicans strain Hb37 | 100% (168/168) |
| | C. albicans strain YN50-151205 | 100% (164/164) |
| | C. albicans strain L8278 | 98% (165/169) |
| Control | C. albicans strain Hb20 | 100% (146/146) |
| | C. albicans strain L3805 | 100% (168/168) |

The GenBank Database isolates that permitted the establishment of the sequence of isolates corresponding to bacteria are as follows:

| | Description | Identity (%) |
|---|---|---|
| | *Kluyvera ascorbata* strain ATCC 33433 | 99% (848/852) |
| | *Citrobacter murliniae* strain *CDC 2970-59* | 99% (863/867) |
| | *Enterobacter asburiae* strain *JCM6051* | 99% (902/910) |
| | *Klebsiella pneumoniae* subspp. *Pneumoniae* strain *MGH 78578 ATCC 700721* | 96% (885/919) |
| | *Enterobacter cloacae* subspp. *Dissolvens* strain *LMG 2683* | 98% (890/911) |
| | *Escherichia coli* strain *U 5/41* | 99% (826/836) |
| | *Rahnella aquatilis* HX2 strain HX2 | 100% (967/967) |
| | *Serratia marcescens* subspp. *Sakuensis* strain *KRED* | 99% (935/940) |
| **Tanners'** | *Proteus vulgaris* strain *DSM 30118* | 99% (967/979) |
| **Group** | *Enterobacter aerogenes* strain *JCM1235* | 99% (832/844) |
| | *Pseudomonas brenneri* strain *CFML 97-391* | 99% (851/858) |
| | *Pseudomonas psychrotolerans* strain *C36* | 100% (819/819) |
| | *Pseudomonas* aeruginosa strain *PAO1 PAO1* | 100% (903/903) |
| | *Neisseria bacilliformis* ATCC BAA-1200 strain *MDA2833* | 99% (916/917) |
| | *Neisseria subflava* strain *U37* | 99% (879/890) |
| | *Achromobacter xylosoxidans* A8 A8 | 98% (647/660) |
| | *Alcaligenes faecalis* subspp. *Parafaecalis* strain *G* | 99% (884/888) |
| | *Acinetobacter johnsonii* strain *ATCC 17909* | 99% (888/895) |
| | *Stenotrophomonas maltophilia* strain *IAM 12423* | 99% (904/911) |
| **Control** | *Neisseria polysaccharea* strain *NCTC11858* | 99% (760/771) |
| | *Acinetobacter [calcoaceticus]* strain *NCCB 22016* | 99% (614/619) |

In bacteria, both *16S rDNA* amplicon chains were sequenced, and the sequences obtained were edited in the following databases: Ribosomal Database Project II (Cole et al., 2005; Cole et al., 2007),[10] green genes project, [11] and the SILVA database project.[12] For genus and species identification of the isolates, the sequences were aligned and compared with *16S RNAr*/ITS1 sequences already registered in the National Center for Biotechnology Information (NCBI) data bank through the BLAST program (Gasch et al., 2000).

# 4   Data Analysis

Among the bacterial isolated obtained from the nasal and oropharyngeal mucosa samples from the group of workers exposed to tannery environments, different characterization and identification methods were applied, such as molecular biology techniques, which permitted the identification of the presence of pathogenic bacteria present in workers of different tanneries. The propagation of some bacteria and yeasts was not possible in the laboratory, possibly due to the specific and different requirements of those tested here, considering non-cultivable microorganisms as having nutritional requirements and physicochemical conditions that are not known and factors necessary for their cultivation. In addition, information on the symbiotic, commensal, or parasitic relationship that the members of a microbial community maintain is limited; thus, some members will require, or not, these relationships for their normal development in the laboratory (Weisburg et al., 1991; Gasch et al., 2000; Keller & Zengler, 2004). In second place, some DNA samples did not possess sufficient purity, giving rise to poorly secure sequences; therefore, similarities were not found in the NCBI databases.

The human body naturally has microorganisms in the skin, hair, and digestive system; in fact, various microorganisms have been reported as natural inhabitants of the oropharyngeal mucosa (Mohr, 2002; Abel et al., 2002; Shih et al., 1996). This supports the results of this study, in that in the microbiological burden in both study groups, some coincide for the tanners and for the automotive company administrators (control group); however, the differences lie in the microbiological burden in tanners, which reached concentrations of up to $10^8$ CFU/ml (first group of tanners) and of $10^3$ CFU/ml (second group of tanners), while the bacterial burden of the control group was scarcely $10^1$ CFU/ml, and that of yeasts, $10^3$ CFU/ml. Although there are normally microorganisms in the oropharyngeal mucosa, the difference in concentration present in tanners with respect to the controls is quite significant, up to 7 orders-of-magnitude. While the concentration of yeasts of the second group of tanners and of the control group was of the same order-of-magnitude, the difference can be noted in the percentage of tanners who had yeast growth: 63% with respect to the percentage of administrators (control), which was 45%.

This difference between the tanners' oropharyngeal- mucosa microbiological burden and that of the automotive-industry control-group participants that is demonstrated is due in part to the work environment to which the tanners are exposed during 8–12-h workdays. The work environments of the tanneries and the automotive industry are significantly different because of various reasons, some of these comprising the raw material (animal skin) utilized in the tanning industry, which serves as a mechanism of transport and as a source of microorganisms (Scorzoni et al., 2013). The environmental conditions at the interior of each work site, such as a temperature >30°C, relative humidity >80%, low ventilation, and even the eating habits inside the workplaces, among others, leading to high microbiological burdens in interior environments. The tanneries that had been previously evaluated (Maldonado-Vega et al., 2014) reported relative-humidity values of up to 80% inside the tanneries, different from that reported at the control group's work site, which was 32%. This is explained due to the high consumption of water required in the tanning process, generating a humid environment. Additionally, wind velocity in the interior of the tanneries was measured; generally, this parameter was 0.0 m/sec at both work sites; however, the highest value found inside the tanneries was 0.8 m/sec and at the control site, this was 2.2 m/sec. Therefore, both work sites present different environmental conditions, which exert an influence on the interior, thus the microbiological burden and its dispersion present in the oropharyngeal mucosa of the workers, which can be acquired through inhalation.

The microbiological burden in the environmental air at the work sites (tannery and administration area in the automotive industry) (Maldonado-Vega et al., 2014) reported a concentration of up to $10^4$ CFU/m$^3$ of fungi and $10^3$ CFU/m$^3$ of bacteria, while at the control group's workplace, the reported concentration was $10^2$ CFU/m$^3$ of bacteria and

fungi. The presence of microorganisms in the environment is normal; the difference between the microbiological burdens at the interior of the tanneries was significant, even
up to two orders-of-magnitude for the case of the fungi and one order-of-magnitude for
the case of the bacteria. For the control site, this appears to represent a normal microbiological burden, while for the tanneries, this appears to represent microbiological contamination.

In Mexico, there are no norms or guidelines that establish maximal concentrations
of microorganisms in interior environmental air, nor of work sites; thus, the concentrations reported in this work were previously compared with value limits established in
Swedish guidelines,[95] which establish, for bacteria, a value limit of 500 CFU/m$^3$ and for
fungi, an allowed value limit of 300 CFU/m$^3$ in inside air. In this manner, it can be confirmed that the microbiological burden present in interior environmental air was exces-
sively elevated, exceeding the permitted limits established in European requirements, in
contrast with the microbiological burden present at the control group's work site, which
did not surpass these values.

In that prior work, the identification was carried out of bacteria, fungi, and yeasts.
The bacterial families identified were Bacillaceae, Corynebacteriaceae, Enterobacteriaceae, Moraxellaceae, Nocardiopsaceae, Pseudomonadaceae, and Staphylococcaceae.
The genera of fungi identified were mainly *Aspergillus* and *Penicillium*, which are considered the most significant allergenic fungi in air, and these have been associated with adverse effects on human and animal health (Keller & Zengler, 2004). Finally, the yeasts
identified were *Candida krusei* and *Candida glabrata,* which have been associated with adverse effects on the health of immunosuppressed individuals (Siarabrigaditte, 2014;
Castañón, 2013; Cole et al., 2005; Cole et al., 2007; DeSantis et al., 2006; Gasch et al., 2000;
Keller & Zengler, 2004).

Some of the microorganisms identified in the oropharyngeal mucosa of the workers effectively form part of the biological flora or natural microbiota of the human body;
however, many of these microorganisms have been associated with affectations of the
health state. Some pathogens and opportunists affect the workers' health, depending on
their immunological system and nutritional status. In some cases, the microorganisms are
acquired in the work environment, because bacterial families have been identified in common with the interior air of tanneries and in the oropharyngeal mucosa of tanners, these
families including Enterobacteriaceae, Moraxellaceae, and Pseudomonadaceae, while the
yeasts present in common in tannery environments and in the oropharyngeal mucosa of
tanners were *Candida krusei* and *Candida glabrata.*

In this study, bacteria identified in oropharyngeal mucosa revealed the presence of
pathogenic bacteria in tanners, while the bacteria identified in the control group corresponded to normal flora. The family identified with greatest frequency was Enterobacteriaceae, which was also present in the interior air of the tanneries (Maldonado-Vega et al.,
2014). the pathogenicity of Enterobacteriaceae has already been reported (Baylis et al.,
2011). Enterobacteriaceae comprises a family that is important in medical terms, serving
as a biological indicator of risk to health.

The species identified within this family were the following: *Klebsiella pneumoniae,*
which can live in the respiratory and digestive tracts and that, has been correlated with

infections of the urinary tract, diarrhea, and pulmonary abscesses. This bacterium has been considered opportunistic, able to cause pneumonia and bacteremia, and strongly correlated with nosocomial infections (Zarzoso et al., 1999). *Enterobacter aerogenes* has been related with Urinary tract infections (UTI), pneumonia, and wound infections, and also acts as a catalyzer for other infections (Ye et al., 2006). *Enterobacter cloacae* had been associated with opportunistic infections that affect the urinary and respiratory tracts, and it also has the capacity to cause septicemia and meningitis (Romero & Herrera, 2002; Harrell et al., 1989; Christiaens et al., 1987). *Proteus vulgaris*, also considered an opportunistic pathogen, has been isolated from infections in immunosuppressed patients (Stewart & Quirk, 2001; Paton, 1996), *Rahnella aquatilis* has been isolated from respiratory samples in which it causes infections. It has also been correlated with urinary infections and in the wounds of immunosuppressed patients and with endocarditis in patients (Shih et al., 1996). *Citrobacter* spp. has been found in water, soil, and in the intestinal tract, being correlated with respiratory and intestinal infections (Shedlak, 1973; Shih et al., 1996; de Bentzmann & Plésiat, 2011). *Kluyvera ascorbata* has been described as an opportunistic pathogen (Zarzoso et al., 1999). *Enterobacter asburiae* has been found in human biological samples, such as blood, urine, and feces; this pathogen has been reported as the cause of interhospitalary pneumonia (Stewart & Quirk, 2001). *Escherichia coli* resides in the human intestinal tract; however, there are pathogenic strains that cause respiratory-tract infections, sepsis, meningitis, and diarrhea (Romero-Cabello, 2007). Additionally, non-pathogenic strains of this species have already been correlated with opportunistic infections, such as pneumonia in hospitalized patients with an immunosuppressed system. *Serratia marcescens* was reported as an opportunistic pathogen, frequently associated with pneumonia and sepsis in patients receiving chemotherapy.

Other identified species belonging to the Families Pseudomonadaceae, Neisseriaceae, Alcaligenaceae, Moraxellaceae, and Xanthomonadaceae have been reported as opportunistic pathogens, such as the following: *Pseudomonas aeruginosa*;[40,] *Neisseria bacilliformis* (Han et al., 2006); *Neisseria subflava* (Shih et al., 1996); *Achromobacter xylosoxidans*; *Alcaligenes faecalis* (Dangi et al., 2010); *Acinetobacter johnsonii*, and *Stenotrophomonas maltophilia*.

In contrast, bacteria identified in the control group corresponded to normal flora, among which was found *Neisseria polysaccharea*, reported in the upper respiratory tract of 0.5% of individuals and which has not been described as part of pathogenic processes (Castañón, 2013). *Acinetobacter calcoaceticus* of the Moraxellaceae Family is a natural inhabitant of human skin and can be a commensal in oropharyngeal mucosa (Pfaller et al., 2002).

With respect to yeasts, in the tanners' as well as in the control group, the yeasts *Candida glabrata* and *Candida albicans* were identified, and additionally, in the tanners' group, the yeasts *Candida tropicalis* and *Candida krusei* were identified. *Candida* species are considered opportunistic in humans, although *C. albicans* form as part of normal flora colonizing mucocutaneous surfaces (oral cavity, gastrointestinal tract, and vagina) of healthy humans, although it has been the pathogen most prevalently correlated with systemic infections and infections in mucosa (Weisburg et al., 1991; Pfaller et al., 2002). While *Candida* is not normally the cause of diseases, some species of this genus, on arriving in immunosuppressed commensals or altered microflora, can be transformed into oppor-tunistic pathogens, as is the case of *C. albicans* (Newman et al., 2005), which has been associated in pharynx with pneumonitis (Li et al., 2007). *C. glabrata* has been considered a non-pathogenic saprophytic microorganism, found in the normal flora of healthy indi-viduals; however, *C. glabrata* has emerged as an important opportunistic pathogen pre-sent in the oral musoca (Kothavade et al., 2010) and, in recent years, its prevalence has increased in systemic infections. *C. tropicalis* has been identified as a pathogenic species of yeasts of the most-prevalent *Candida* group. *C. tropicales*-associated candidiasis infec-tions have increased drastically on a global scale; thus, this is emerging as a pathogenic yeast. *C. krusei* is an opportunistic pathogen that presents intrinsic resistance to Flucona-zole, and it has been described as a causal agent of infections disseminated in susceptible patients (Scorzoni et al., 2013).

The present work does not include an evaluation of the state of health of the work-ers. However, the application of a questionnaire directed to knowing, in a general man-ner, their health state indicated that the workers in their majority are asymptomatic. The lack of symptoms in the workers can be due to more than one reason; notwithstanding this, based on the results of this work, it could be supposed that this is due to that the microorganisms identified are mainly opportunistic. Thus, adverse effects on the worker's health will depend on the nutritional and immunological status of these indi-viduals.

# 5   Conclusions

In tanneries, workers have an important burden of pathogenic bacteria and opportunistic yeasts, which appear to exert effect on the health state of personnel with problems of malnutrition of immunodeficiency. Tannery workers present pathogenic bacteria in nasal and oropharyngeal mucosa, with the recognition of important species, such as *Enterobac-teria*, *Pseudomonas*, and opportunistic yeasts such as *Candida albicans*.

Eighty one percent of the nasal and oropharyngeal mucosa samples of tannery workers exhibit yeast growth in Sabouraud Dextrose Agar (SDA) medium, while in the control group, this was only 50%. Seventy eight percent of nasal and oropharyngeal mu-cosa samples of workers exposed to tannery environments presented BGBB bacterial growth, in contrast to 15% of the control group. This indicated that tannery work envi-ronments and those of the automobile industry are distinct, and the microbiological bur-den can be influenced by diverse factors, such as ventilation, the presence of biological matter, the presence of pets and plants, and the form of the construction. The tanneries that participated in this study were characterized by having poorly ventilated environ-ments, high humidity, high temperatures, and limited means of hygiene and prevention, creating an optimal environment for the viability and propagation of microorganisms in the environment that can be acquired by their workers through inhalation, ingestion, or contact, because some of the enterobacteria identified in tanneries are also identified in the air inside the tanneries.

Fifty three percent of the bacteria found in the isolates of workers exposed to tannery environments belong t0 the Enterobactericeae Family as an indicator of contamination, while in the control group, these were not identified. As has been described, the majority of, the microorganisms identified are related with diarrheic and respiratory diseases, thus converting these into a problem of work health, in addition to possible effects on the familial health of the workers. Forty two percent of bacteria associated with respiratory diseases have 5% of bacteria that are also related with diarrheic diseases. This allows correlating with the incidence of cases reported in the Epidemiological Bulletin of the Ministry of Health of the State of Guanajuato, Mexico.

Microbial sensitivity tests applied battery of bacteria isolated from nasal and oropharyngeal mucosa demonstrated the presence of microorganisms resistant to each of the four antibiotics employed; therefore, in Amoxycillin/Clavulanic Acid (AMC), 42% of resistance was observed, in Ampicillin/Sulbactam (SAM) 26%, in Ticarcillin/Clavulanic Acid (TIM) 13%, and finally, for Piperacillin/Tazobactam (TZP), 10% of resistance. In sum, TZP presented 90% efficiency on the bacterial isolates, while with respect to the yeasts obtained, 79% presented sensitivity to Fluconazole (25 µg) and 21%, resistance to Fluconazole.

This work demonstrates that tanners represent a population at risk of contamination by bacteria, fungi, and yeasts, which can integrate into mucosa, above all respiratory and digestive mucosa, and although the registry of workers appears to denote asymptomatology, respiratory and diarrheic diseases were found at a greater frequency, all of this added to the manipulation of animal hides in which, due to their origin, the transference is highly probable of microorganisms that, under ideal conditions, are propagated, achieving greater dispersion.

# Acknowledgement

This project was funded by the council on science and technology Guanajuato *CON-CYTEG GTO-2011-C04-16449. 2012-2013.*

# References

Abel E, Ande RJV, Dawido WN, et al. (2002). *The Swedish key action "the healthy building" – research results achieved during the first three years period 1998–2000. In: Indoor Air 2002. Proceedings of the 9th International Conference on Indoor Air Quality and Climate, Monterey, California (Ed Levin H), Santa Cruz, California, 996–1001.*

Aguirre UJM. (2002). *Candidiasis Orales. Rev Iberoam Micol, 19:17–21.*

Ajello L, Georg LK, Kaplan W, and Kaufman L. (1963). *CDC laboratory manual for medical mycology. PHS Publication No. 994, U.S. Government Printing Office, Washington, D.C.*

Arévalo-Rivas BI. (2005). *Evaluación de riesgos en la salud en una población de trabajadores de tenería. Universidad de Guanajuato. Tesis de Maestría.*

Barry A, Bille J, Brown S, Ellis D, et al. (2003). Quality control limits for fluconazole disk susceptibility tests on Mueller-Hinton agar with glucose and methylene blue. J. Clin. Microbiol, 41:3410–3412.

Baylis C, Uyttendaele M, Joosten H, Davies A. (2011). The Enterobacteriaceae and their Significance to the Food Industry. ILSI Europe Report Series, 17–28.

Beaumont F. (1988). Clinical manifestations of pulmonary Aspergillus infections. Mycoses, 3: 5–20.

Bouquete MT. Marcos C. Saez-Nieto JA. (1986). Characterization of Neisseria polysaccharea sp. nov. (Riou 1983) in previously identified noncapsulated strains of Neisseria meningitides. J Clin Microbiol, 23:973–975.

Burge HA. (2002). An update on pollen and fungal spore aerobiology. J Allergy Clin Immunol, 1110: 544–52.

Cann KJ and Rogers TR. (1989). The phenotypic relationship of Neisseria polysaccharea to commensal and pathogenic Neisseria sp. J Mol Microbiol, 39:351–354.

Castañón Olivares RL. (2013). Candidiasis. Departamento de Microbiología y Parasitología, Facultad de Medicina, UNAM. 2013. (acceso en febrero de 2013). http://www.facmed.unam.mx/deptos/microbiologia/micologia/candidosis.html

Christiaens E, Hansen W. and Moinet J. (1987). Isolament des expectorations d´un patient attaint de leucemie lymphoide chronique et de broncho-emphyeme d´une Enterobacteriaceae nouvellement decrite: Rahnella aquatilis. Med Maladies Infect, 17:732–734.

Cole JR, Chai B, Farris RJ et al. (2007). The ribosomal database project (RDP-II): introducing myRDP space and quality controlled public data. Nucleic. Acids. Res, 35, D169-72.

Cole JR, Chai B, Farris RJ, et al. (2005). The Ribosomal Database Project (RDP-II): sequences and tools for high-throughput rRNA analysis. Nucleic. Acids. Res, 33, D294-6

Dangi YS, Soni ML, Namdeo KP. (2010). Oral candidiasis: a review. Int J Pharm Pharm Sci, 2(4):3641.

de Bentzmann S and Plésiat P. (2011). The Pseudomonas aeruginosa opportunistic pathogen and human infections. Environ Microbiol, 13 (7):1655–1665.

Demmler GJ, Couch RS, Taber LH. (1985). Neisseria subflava bacteremia and meningitis in a child: report of a case and review of the literature. Pediatric Infectious Disease. 4(3):286–288.

DeSantis TZ, Hugenholtz P, Larsen N, et al. (2006). Greengenes, a chimera-checked 16S rRNA gene database and workbench compatible with ARB. Appl. Environ. Microbiol. 72, 5069–72

Dodds MWJ, Johnson DA, Yeh CK. (2005). Health benefits of saliva: a review. Journal of Dentistry, 33, 223–233

Gales AC, Jones RN, Turnidge J et al. (2001). Characterization of Pseudomonas aeruginosa isolates: Occurrence rates, antimicrobial susceptibility patterns and molecular typing in the Global SENTRY Antimicrobial Surveillance Program, 1997–1999. Clin Inf. Dis, 32: S146–55.

Gardes et al. (1991). Identification of indigenous and introduced symbiotic fungi in ectomycorrhizal by amplification of nuclear and mitochondrial ribosomal AND. Canadian Journal of Botany. 69: 180–190.

Gardes M, and Bruns TD (1993). ITS primers with enhanced specificity for basidiomycetes application to the identification of mycorrhizae and rusts. Mol. Ecol. 2:113–118.

Gasch AP, Spellman PT, Kao CM, Carmel-Harel O, et al. (2000). Genomic expression programs in the response of yeast cells to environmental changes. Mol. Biol. Cell. 11, 4241–57.

Gelincik AA, Büyüköztürk S, Gül H, Güngör G, İşsever H, Çağatay A. (2005). The effect of indoor fungi on *the symptoms of patients with allergic rhinitis in Istanbul. Indoor Built Environ, 14 (5):427–32.*

*González Gravina H, González de Morán E, Zambrano O, et al. (2007). Oral Candidiasis in children and adolescents with cancer. Identification of Candida.spp Med Oral Patol Oral Cir Bucal, 12: E419–23.*

*Han XY, Hong T and Falsen E. (2006). Neisseria baciliformis sp. nov. Isolated from human infections. J. Clin. Microbiol, 44:474–479.*

*Harrell Li, Cameron ML, O´Hara CM (1989). Rahnella aquatilis an unusual gramnegative rod isolated from the bronchial washing of a patient whit acquired immunodeficiency syndrome. J Clin Microbiol, 27:1671–1672.*

*Hernández-Arredondo VR. (2010). Emisión De Disolventes Derivados De Hidrocarburos En Ambientes Laborales De Industrias Procesadoras De Calzado. División de Ciencias Exactas, Campus Guanajuato. Tesis de Licenciatura*

*Juárez Facio AT, Maldonado-Vega M, Castellanos-Arévalo A, Rangel-Cordova AA. (2014). Efecto De Las Tenerías Sobre La Calidad Del Aire Circunvecino En Zona Urbana. Verano de la Ciencia CONCYTEG.*

*Kavuncuoglu A, Unal N, Oguzhan B, Tokgoz O, Oymak C, Utas. (2010). First Reported Case of Alcaligenes faecalis Peritonitis. Perit Dial Int, 30(1):118–9*

*Keller M and Zengler K. (2004). Tapping into microbial diversity. Nature Reviews 2: 141–150.*

*Kothavade RJ, Kura MM, Valand AG, Panthaki MH. (2010). Candida tropicalis: its prevalence, pathogenicity and increasing resistance to fluconazole. J Med Microbiol, 59(8):873–80*

*Kuper KM, Boles DM, Mohr JF, Wanger A. (2009). Antimicrobial Susceptibility Testing: A Primer for Clinicians. Pharmacotherapy, 29 (11):1326–1343.*

*Li L, Redding S, Dongari-Bagtzoglou A. (2007). Candida glabrata, an Emerging Oral Opportunistic Pathogen J Dent Res, 86:204*

*Makimura K, et al. (2000). Species identification and strain typing of Malassezia species stock strains and clinical isolates based on the DNA sequences of nuclear ribosomal internal transcribed spacer 1 regions. J.Med. Microbiol, vol. 49: 29–35.*

*Maldonado-Vega M, Peña-Cabriales JJ, Guzmán de Peña, DL, Arévalo-Rivas BI, Calderón-Salinas JV, et al. (2014). Detección de factores biológicos involucrados en el desarrollo de enfermedades diarreicas y respiratorias en el manejo de pieles bovinas en curtidurías. Editorial Trillas, ISBN: 978-607-17-1850-1, 92–9*

*Mandal J, Brandl H. (2011). Bioaerosols in indoor environment — a review with special reference to residential and occupational locations. Open Environ Biol Monit J, 4: 83–96.*

*Manual de Procedimientos para el Manejo Adecuado de los Residuos de la Curtiduría. (1999). Instituto Nacional de Ecología SEMARNAP, Primera Edición.*

*Miles D and Kevin GK. (1998). Microbiological and Clinical Aspects of Infection Associated whit Stenotrophomonas maltophilia. Clin. Microbiol, 11(1):57–80.*

*Mohr AJ. (2002). Fate and transport of microorganisms in air. In: Hurst CJ (Ed) Manual of Environmental Microbiology. 2nd ed. Washington: ASM Press, 827–838.*

*Muder RR, Harris AP, Muller S, et al. (1996). Bacteremia Due to Stenotrophomonas (Xanthomonas) maltophilia: A Prospective, Multicenter Study of 91 Episodes. Clin. Infect. Dis, 22(3):508–512.*

*NCCLS – Clinical and Laboratory Standards Institute. (2004). Method for Antifungal Disk Diffusion Susceptibility Testing of Yeasts. Approved Guideline. NCCLS document M44-A (ISBN 1-56238-532-*

*1). Vol. 24, No 15. USA.*

Newman SL, Bhugra B, Holly A, Morris RE. (2005). *Enhanced Killing of Candida albicans by Human Macrophages Adherent to Type 1 Collagen Matrices via Induction of Phagolysosomal Fusion Infect Immun, 73(2):770–777.*

Odds F, Bernaerts R. (1994). *CHROMagar Candida, a new differential isolation medium for the presumptive identification of clinically important Candida species. J Clin Microbiol, 32 (8):1923–1929.*

Orlita A. (2004). *Microbial biodeterioration of leather and its control: A review. Int Biodeterior Biodegrad, 53(3):157–63.*

Özdilli K, Issever H, Özyildirim BA, et al. (2007). *Biological Hazards in Tannery Workers. Indoor Built Environ, 16(4):349–357.*

Paton AW. Paton JC. (1996). *Enterobacter cloacae producing a shiga-like toxin II-related cytotoxin associated whit a case of hemolytic-uremic syndrome. J. Clin Microbiol, 34:463–465.*

Pereira-Cenci T, Del Bel Cury AA, Crielaard W, Ten Cate JM. (2008). *Development of candida-associated denture stomatitis: new insights. J Appl Oral Sci, 16(2):86–94.*

Pfaller MA, Diekema DJ, Jones RN, Messer SA, Hollis RJ (2002). *Trends in antifungal susceptibility of Candida spp. isolated from pediatric and adult patients with bloodstream infections: SENTRY Antimicrobial Surveillance Program, 1997 to 2000. J Clin Microbiol, 40:852–856*

Rangel-Cordova AA. (2012). *Evaluación de bioaerosoles en ambiente exterior de zonas industriales de curtiduría en León, Gto. Tesis Técnico Universitario. Universidad Tecnológica de León.*

Romero C and Herrera B. (2002). *Síndrome Diarreico Infeccioso. México: Editorial Médica Panamericana, 93–110.*

Romero-Cabello R. (2007). *Microbiología y Parasitología Humana: Bases etiológicas de las enfermedades infecciosas y parasitarias. 3rd ed. México: Editorial Médica Panamericana, 746, 747, 748, 805.*

Saiki RK, Gelfand DH, Stoffel S, Scharf SJ, Higuchi R, Horn GT, Mullis KB, et al. (1988). *Primer-directed enzymatic amplification of DNA with a thermostable DNA polymerase. Science 239: 87–491.*

Sakurad A. (2012). *Achromobacter xylosoxidans. Revista chilena de infectología, 29(4):453–4.*

Scorzoni L, de Lucas MP, Mesa-Arango AC, Fusco-Almeida AN, Lozano E, Cuenca-Estrella M, Mendes-Giannini MJ, Zaragoza O. (2013). *Antifungal Efficacy during Candida krusei Infection in Non-Conventional Models Correlates with the Yeast In Vitro Susceptibility Profile. PLoS ONE, 8(3):1–13.*

Seifert H, Dijkshoom, L. Gerner-Smidt P, et al. (1997). *Distribution of Acinetobacter species on human skin: comparison of phenotypic identification method. J. Clin Microbiol, 35:2819–2825.*

Seifert H, Strate A, Schulze A, Pulverer G. (1993). *Vascular Catheter – Related Bloodstream Infection Due to Acinetobacter johnsonii (Formerly Acinetobacter calcoaceticus var. lwoffii): Report of 13 cases.*

Shedlak J. (1973). *Present knowledge and aspects of Citrobacter. Curr. Top. Microbiol. Inmunol. 62:41–59.*

Shih CC, Chen YC, Chang SC, et al. (1996). *Bacteremia Due to Citrobacter Species: Significance of Primary Intraabdominal Infection. Clinical Infectious Diseases, 23:543–9*

Siarabrigaditte de Jesús. (2014). *Evaluación clínica de trabajadores de la curtiduría relacionándola carga de agentes biológicos en ambiente laboral. Ciencias Médicas. Departamento de Ciencias Médicas, División de Ciencias de la Salud, Campus León, Universidad de Gto. Tesis de Especialidad.*

Singh J. (2005). *Toxic molds and indoor air quality. Indoor Built Environ, 14: 229–34.*

Skóra J, Gutarowska B, Stępień Ł, et al. (2014). The evaluation of microbial contamination in the working environment of tanneries. Medycyna Pracy, 65(1):15–32.

Stern FB. (1998). Health Effects and Disease Patterns. In Stellman JM (ed.) Encyclopedia of Occupational Health and Safety. 4th ed. ILO, Geneva, 88.8

Stewart JM, Quirk JR. (2001). Community-acquired pneumonia caused by Enterobacter asburiae. Am J. Med, 111:82:83.

Tiedje JM and Stein JL (1999). Microbial diversity: strategies for its recovery. In: Manual of Industrial Microbiology and Biotechnology. Demain A. L. and J. E. Davies (Eds). ASM Press. Washington, D.C. USA. 682–692.

Visca P, Seifert H and Towner KJ. (2011). Acinetobacter Infection – an Emerging Threat to Human Health. IUBMB Life, 63 (12):1048–1054.

Watanakunakorn C and Weber J. (1989). Enterobacter bacteremia: A review of 58 episodes. Scand J. Infect. Dis, 21:1–8.

Weisburg WG. Barns SM, Pelletier DA, Lane DJ. (1991). 16s ribosomal DNA amplification for phylogenetic study. Journal of Bacteriology. 173: 697–703.

Weischer M and Kolmos HJ. (1992). Retrospective 6-years study of Enterobacter bacteremia in a Danish university horpital. J. Hosp. Infect, 20:15–24.

White T, Bruns T, Lee S. and Taylor, J. (1990). Amplification and direct sequencing of fungal RNA genes for phylogenetics. PCR Protocols: a Guide to Methods and Applications. San Diego, 315–322, CA: Academic Press.

White T, Bruns T, Lee S. and Taylor, J. (1990). Amplification and direct sequencing of fungal RNA genes for phylogenetics. PCR Protocols: a Guide to Methods and Applications. San Diego, 315–322, CA: Academic Press.

Ye Y, Li JB, Ye DQ, Jiang ZJ. (2006). Enterobacter bacteremia: Clinical features, risk factors for multiresistance and mortality in a Chinese University Hospital. Infection, 34 (5):252–7.

Yogev R. and Kozlowski S. (1990). Peritonitis due to Kluyvera ascorbata: Case report and review. Rev. Infect. Dis. 12:399–402.

Zarzoso E, Belloch M, Uruburu F and Querol A. (1999). Identification of yeasts by RFLP analysis of the 5.8S rRNA gene and the two ribosomal internal transcribed spacers, International Journal of Systematic Bacteriology 49, 329–337.

# Chapter 8

# Can Glucocorticoids Against Severe Sepsis Act As Causal Drugs?

Thomas Scior[1], Itzel Gutierrez-Aztatzi[2] and Jorge Lozano-Aponte[2]

## 1 Introduction

In day-to-day clinical practice in medicine complications may arise in three mayor fields: for the patients themselves, their sufferings due to detrimental effects of the disease evolution as well as the applied treatments in response to symptoms and clinical parameters, and for the care-taking and decision-taking Medical personal or the family members. Not to speak about the economic impact and need of adequate infrastructure in hospitals and at home.

In the present work we focus on complications which arise from the fact that there is no causal therapy in hospitalized cases of what specialists call "generalized septicemia" and septic shock syndrome, all of which frequently associated with a fatal outcome for the patients.

Clinically speaking, the term "sepsis" refers to the starting stage of a three-stage syndrome caused by endotoxins from Gram-negative bacteria. Stage 1 sepsis is then followed by "severe sepsis" and "septic shock". Fortunately, developing the three-stage sepsis is a rare clinical complication for infected patients. But, once passing from stage 1 to 2, it shows an extremely unfavorable prognostic aspect with variably high mortality rates (30–50 %) because no causal treatment has been invented so far (Dellinger et al., 2013). In

[1] Department of Pharmacy, Faculty of Chemical Sciences, Benemérita Universidad Autónoma de Puebla, Mexico.
[2] Faculty of Chemical Sciences, Laboratory of Computational Molecular Simulations, Benemérita Universidad Autónoma de Puebla, Mexico.

a worst case scenario, a generalized infection causes a life-threatening drop in blood pressure – called septic shock – leading to the failure of vital organs in the patient's body. In addition, "septicemia" refers to the infectious process in the blood stream.

There is an urgent need to develop new drugs for the causal treatment of septic shock patients suffering from Gram-negative septic infections also known as endotoxicity reaction (Scior, Alexander et al., 2013).

The situation is complicated not only for the patient her- or himself but also for the Medical personal and the patient's family. The complications can be described with the following words of Clinical experts in sepsis disease management and care-taking in intensive care units (ICU) as follows: "…the majority of ICU patients receive full support with aggressive, life-sustaining treatments. Many patients with multiple organ system failure or severe neurologic injuries will not survive or will have a poor quality of life… Decisions to provide less-aggressive life-sustaining treatments or to withdraw life-sustaining treatments in these patients may be in the patients' best interest and may be what patients and their families' desire… Physicians have different end-of-life practices based on their region of practice, culture, and religion…"(Dellinger et al., 2013).

In sight of this health problem and patient suffering, six years ago we started a multi-disciplinary and bi-centric molecular modeling project (at Research Center Borstel, Hamburg, Germany, and at Pharmacy Department, BUAP University in Puebla, Mexico). Here the purpose of our ongoing research studies is to contribute to the understanding of the molecular events through computational simulations. Precisely, the (molecular) structure – (endotoxic) activity relationships of known septic agents – lipopolysaccharides (LPS) – and their derivatives by means of ligand – receptor docking and molecular dynamics methods allow us analyzing their interactions with their biomolecular targets: the human cell surface receptors, called TLR4/MD-2 complex. They function as mini-antennae or nanosensors to capture traces of LPS moieties stemming from the bacterial membranes, and thusly alerting the living body of an imminent bacterial invasion.

The Toll-like receptor 4 (TLR-4) / myeloid differentiation 2 (MD-2) receptor complexes are thought to confer endotoxicity by activating the innate immune system. Endotoxicity is triggered by bacterial lipopolysaccharides (LPS) which act as agonistic ligands to the TLR4 / MD-2 receptor complex on the cell surface of Mammalian species reaction (Scior, Alexander et al., 2013).

Prior to the present study we reviewed and identified specific amino acids of these biomolecular structures (TLR4 / MD-2 complexes) which could confer the endotoxicity differences which are reported for Mammals like humans, mice, dogs and horses etc. reaction (Scior et al., 2014).

In the first place (data not shown) the amino acid sequences of the biomolecules from the aforementioned four Mammalian species (human, murine, canine and equine) are aligned in such a way that the corresponding (identical or similar) amino acids are located in the same position. This procedure is known as Multiple Sequence Alignments. It can be carried out in bioinformatics tools on academic Web servers in the internet. The positions with nonidentical and not similar amino acids are marked as different amino acids by a certain color. They are called "differential amino acids" in our published work

reaction (Scior, Alexander et al., 2013; Scior, Lozano et al., 2013). Comparing the four protein sequences (of four species) the species-dependency becomes manifest on an atomic
scale, i.e. the possible concert of mechanistically relevant side chains varies to a certain
degree switching from one animal model to another. The computed three-dimensional
(3D-) models of the proteins form a triangle: inside this "wedge" molecular interactions
between TLR4, MD-2 and ligands take place (Figure 1). Our earlier molecular modeling
studies (Scior, Alexander et al., 2013; Scior, Lozano et al., 2013) identified two regions
where agonists and antagonists like lipid IVA can possess a species-dependent dual activity. Lipid IVA is a derivative, i.e. a simpler compound than LPS because it has less fatty
acids than LPS. It is therefore labeled as "under-acylated" in view of its binding into the
MD-2 protein pocket. It constitutes a weak antagonist in the TLR4/MD-2 receptor complex of the human innate immune system. The reason for this strange behavior is a reduced phosphate attraction force in the "wedge" caused by nonhomologous (nonidentical or not similar) amino acids. Precisely these are the aforementioned "differential amino
acids" when compared to known crystal structures (x-ray crystallographic images) and
computed models (when x-ray data do not exist) of the corresponding murine and equine
TLR4/MD-2 system (Scior, Lozano et al., 2013).

Clinically the intravenous administration of hydrocortisone in adult septic shock
patients is recommended at a dose of 200 mg per day (Dellinger et al., 2013). Substantial
improvements of the drug are observed as significant effects on shock reversal with steroid therapy in cases of relative adrenal insufficiency (defined as post-adrenocorticotropic
hormone, ACTH (Dellinger et al., 2013). The improvements seem plausible because of the
direct and causal endocrinologic link between ACTH and corticoid hormones. The report
of Dellinger and colleagues of the expert groups concluded, however, that the published
reports give a contradicting picture. On the one side publications showed missing benefits to lower the mortality rate while on the other side published clinical research work
showed effective mortality reduction under low-dose hydrocortisone therapy in septic
shock by means of statistical meta-analyses of original clinical trial studies (statistical significance). The expert group emitted recommendation for the clinical personal and we,
experts in molecular simulations, strongly recommend to read their original article to un-
derstand the differential diagnostics and therapeutic conclusions thereof, for instance, the
fact that "not using intravenous hydrocortisone to treat adult septic shock patients if adequate fluid resuscitation and vasopressor therapy are able to restore hemodynamic stability...", or the particularities of pediatric patients where they endorsed "...the timely
hydrocortisone therapy in children with fluid-refractory, catecholamine-resistant shock
and suspected or proven absolute (classic) adrenal insufficiency..." (Dellinger et al.,
2013).

We focus on the molecular events to shed new light on the possible causal relationship and mechanism of action for hydrocortisone hormone therapy and the cell surface
receptors which are thought of being the first step in triggering endotoxic molecular signaling into the body cells of the patients. Molecular modeling – at least – may contribute
to settle the question whether or not glucocorticoids possess a causal interference with
the endotoxicity signaling at its very beginning, that is the binding of invading LPS to the
cell membrane-bound TLR4/MD-2 complex receptor system.

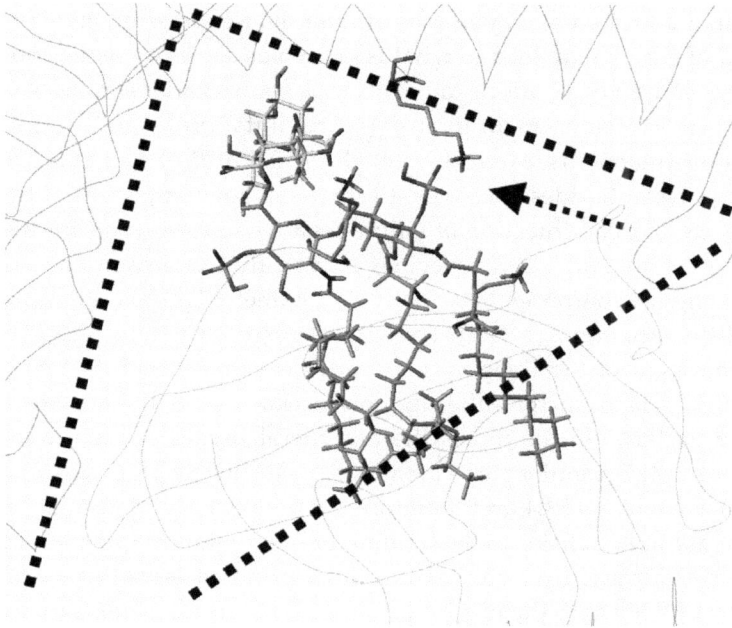

**Figure 1:** A lipopolysaccharides (LPS) from a Gram-negative bacterium entered the binding cavity of the Mammalian cell surface receptor system (TLR4 / MD-2) which is the initial step of the innate immune system recognition of a potentially life-threatening invasion through bacterial infection. The binding cavity is surrounded by three biomolecules forming a whole (cavity or empty pocket) of a triangular shape (see dashed lines of triangle). This central part we called "the wedge" (Scior, Alexander et al., 2013; Scior, Lozano et al., 2013). The lower dashed line is the MD-2 protein the upper two lines are 2 TLR4 proteins. As an illustration a particular lysine amino acid is in display (uppermost atoms on the TLR4 backbone line). The cationic lysine is in atom-to-atom interaction (see arrow) with one of two anionic phosphate groups sitting on the LPS molecule (nearest atoms to the lysine head group). This type of interaction is called ion-ion attraction (or salt bridge) which is induced by electrostatic forces (Coulomb's law). The nonpolar fatty acids of LPS are deeply buried into a large cavity (nonpolar or hydrophobic pocket) of the MD-2 receptor (see lowermost atoms in the middle). The sugar rest of LPS is located on top (apex of the wedge).

## 2    The Biochemical Aspects of LPS, TLR4 and Sepsis

The innate immune system response is the first step of defense against exogenic pathogens. The activation of innate immune system leads to the release of proinflammatory cytokines such as IL-1β y TNF-α, which help to prevent the infection. Besides they are enhancers of the adaptive immunity. The principles of the latter refers to antigen-specific immune responses by adaptive antibody production (Aderem & Ulevitch, 2000). Such cytokines act in a detrimental way in case of their over-expression and henceforth over-production, all of which may lead to what is known as sepsis or septic shock syndrome. The septic shock caused by Gram-negative bacteria shows variable rates of mortality with approximately 20 % incidences in intensive care units, prolonged hospitalization and high costs of after-treatments (Meng, Lien et al., 2010; Carillo-Esper et al., 2010).

The lipopolysaccharides (LPS) constitute the major component of the outer membrane of the bacteria in an infection of Gram-negative bacteria, and for historic reasons denominated as "endotoxin". LPS molecules activate the innate immune system by binding through a complex composed of two proteins, namely: Toll-like 4 receptor (TLR4) and the Myeloid differentiation 2 (MD-2). The active substructure which can be isolated as a molecular component of the lipopolysaccharides is called Lipid A (LA), a partly conserved glycolipid which anchors the lipopolysaccharides at the surface membrane of Gram-negative bacteria. In Mammals the peripheral tissues – like monocytes, macrophages and neutrophil granulocytes – greatly express the receptors cluster of differentiation 14 (CD14) as well as TRL4 and therefore are the primary molecular targets on host cells for the invading LPS. Prior to the binding of LPS to the complex of TLR4 and MD-2 on the human cell surface, two other extracellular proteins assist the specific LPS recognition: bacterial LPS binds to the human protein CD14 but the latter is in need of another human protein, called lipopolysaccharide-binding protein (LBP).

The mononuclear human cells constitute a highly sensitive cell type to endotoxic LPS exposition (agonists). The threshold for the activation of human monocytes through LPS from enterobacteria in whole blood *in vitro* samples or in living cell cultures with blood serum amounts to approximately 10 pg / ml (picomolarity, $10^{-12}$ molar). The hypersensitization of these cyto-sensors to incoming LPS provokes the production of interferon-$\gamma$ (IFN-$\gamma$), which augments the sensitivity, the extent and the maintenance of the answer of monocytes to LPS *in vitro* (Meng, Lien et al., 2010; Alexander & Rietschel, 2001). The activation of mononuclear cells through endotoxic forms of LPS or LA, lead – *in vitro* – to the secretion of a multitude of endogenous mediators such as colony stimulating factor (CSFs), platelet activating factor, Prostaglandin E2 (PGE2), thromboxane A2, leukotrienes, reduced oxygen species, hydroxyl radicals, nitric oxide (NO, nitrogen monoxide), cytokines like TNF-$\alpha$, IL-1$\beta$, IL-6, IL-8, IL-12, IL-15 or IL-18. Particularly, the pro-inflammatory cytokines TNF-$\alpha$, IL-1$\beta$ and IL-6 show the faculty to trigger a complex pathway of secondary reactions, e.g. the acute phase stimulation of the protein secretion by hepatocytes in the liver, the activation of lymphocytes, thrombocytes, basophils and eosinophils, in addition to an increased haematopoietic activity in the bone marrow and a generalized pro-coagulatory state in augmentation (Aderem & Ulevitch, 2000; Alexander & Rietschel, 2001; Takeuchi & Akira, 2010; Saavedra et al., 2011).

# 3    The Molecular Aspects of LPS, TLR4 and Sepsis

At the molecular level, the pivotal activation step is the most forward one – namely the sensing of the invading LPS by TLR4/MD-2 receptors on the extracellular side of cell membranes expressed in certain cell types and tissues (Figure 2).

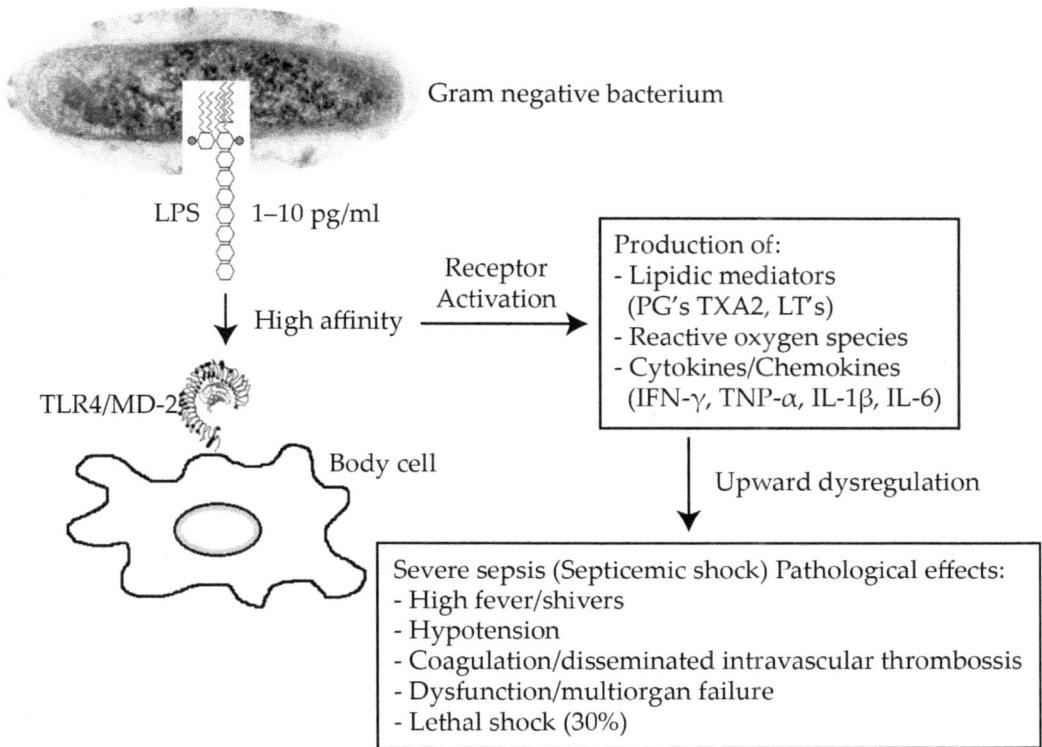

**Figure 2:** Schematic synoptic view of the molecular and biochemical processes which lead to the final stage of fatal septic shock syndrome in infected patients. The starting point is the presence of a Gram-negative bacteria (see first arrow, topmost to the left) is followed by the atom to atom contact between a lipopolysaccharide of the bacteria and the human receptor molecules on the cell surfaces of specialized immune-competent cells (arrow to the right). In the biochemical pathway a plethora of interwoven steps are concerned but only a few are shown for illustration (downwards arrow).

The TLR receptor family has been identified as the initial step of the signaling cascade for LPS endotoxic reactions in tissues of Mammals. Even though the TLR4 is commonly referred to as "t h e" receptor of invading bacterial LPS, LPS does not directly bind to it, rather to an associated protein in the complex, namely the MD-2 protein with its hydrophobic central huge pocket, surrounded by the secondary structure of beta sheets of its amino acids (Aderem & Ulevitch, 2000; Meng, Lien et al., 2010; Alexander & Rietschel, 2001; Takeuchi & Akira, 2010; Ohto et al., 2012; Scior, Alexander et al., 2013).

LPS is one of the most potent immune system-stimulating agents since its presence in picomolar concentration is all what is needed to trigger the body response to the invading bacteria. It is generally assumed that the LA substructure is the core part of the complex LPS to infer that immune response on a molecular level (Meng, Lien et al., 2010a;

Alexander & Rietschel, 2001; Takeuchi & Akira, 2010; Scior, Alexander et al., 2013). The principal chemical components of the scaffold (structural basis) of LA from *Escherichia coli* is a so-called di-glucosamino-di-phosphate backbone. A variable number of up to six fatty acids are attached to the backbone (acyl or amide groups, with noncyclic aliphatic carbon chains). The fatty acids are inserted in the lipid layer of the bacterial membrane and they can also deeply bind into the MD-2 lipophilic pocket. Whereas a LPS embraces more components like a variable sugar or sugar-like chains ("glycol" units, oligosaccharide O-chain) (Alexander & Rietschel, 2001; Scior, Alexander et al., 2013; Ittig et al., 2012).

The presence of both phosphate groups (P1: $1\alpha$-GlcN I y P2: 4'-GlcN II) contribute to the dimerization of the TL4 / MD-2 / LPS complex. The structural variability of the LPS molecules also confer a range of endotoxic activities, .e.g. the LPS form *Capnocytophaga canimorsus* is 100-fold less potent as the LPS of *E. coli*. A structure - activity relationship study reveals that this is due to the penta-acylated di-glucosamino-mono-phosphate (ester groups of five fatty acids) and without the phosphate group in position 4' of glucosamine Nr. 2 (four prime of GlcN II) which is present in the more potent LA from *E. coli* (Scior, Lozano et al., 2013).

And to complicate matters a well-identified precursor of LA, denominated in allusion to its four acyl attachments (4 fatty acid chains) – Lipid IVa (L4a) – acts as an antagonist in human cells, but in rat tissue L4a acts as an agonist (Meng, Lien et al., 2010; Akashi et al., 2001; Meng, Drolet et al., 2010). Not knowing why the very same ligand / binder to the TLR4 / MD-2 receptor complex either enhances or gladly reduced endotoxic reactions, constitutes a severe setback to the pharmaceutical endeavor to develop an antidote of the septic fatal reactions, not even to think about the application as new drug candidate to the national and international health authorities. If an animal model like rats or mice, hamster, dogs and others show different test outcome, the biological effect becomes species-dependent, a fact that is extremely unusual in experimental pharmacology and in urgent need of explanations to dominate the situation (Alexander et al., 2013; Meng, Lien et al., 2010; Akashi et al., 2001).

## 3.1    TLR4 / MD-2 Complex Activation by LPS and its Congeners

In the first step LPS compounds are peeled off the outer membrane of Gram-negative bacteria and followed by the binding to CD14 assisted by LBP (see above). In the next step it is not the TLR4 but the associated MD-2 to which LPS can anchor (Dziarski et al., 2001). MD2 can be regarded as a co-receptor – a protein of 25 kDa consisting of 160 amino acids – because it is permanently associated to TLR4 on the cell surface (Figure 3) (Ittig et al., 2012). Furthermore it was reported, that the CD14 proteins and the LPS-binding protein (LBP) augment the response to LPS because the can act as transporter proteins.

The effect-bearing substructure of LPS is the LA lipoprotein. Its lipid part (the fatty acids) becomes deeply buried into the hydrophobic empty pocket of MD-2. The di-glucosamine backbone is flanked by a phosphate anionic group on either side. They reach out in the space to specific side chains of amino acids of the TLR4 and to the second TLR4 (counter TLR4*) by ionic interactions, sometimes called salt bridges (cationic amino acids to phosphate anions). Formally, when the TLR4 / MD-2 / LPS complex comes together twice, a dimerization occurs forming a larger complex of [TLR4 / MD-2 / LPS]₂ which is also written as [TLR4 / MD-2 / LPS / TLR4* / MD-2* / LPS]. The [TLR4 / MD-2] complex is considered in biochemistry as a functional "monomeric unit", even though it is chemically speaking a hetero-dimer (two different proteins, namely TLR4 and MD-2). The dimeric complex has an "m" shape due to the two large units "banana-shaped" proteins: TLR4 and its completely identical counterpart, the TLR4* (Figure 3) (Park et al., 2009).

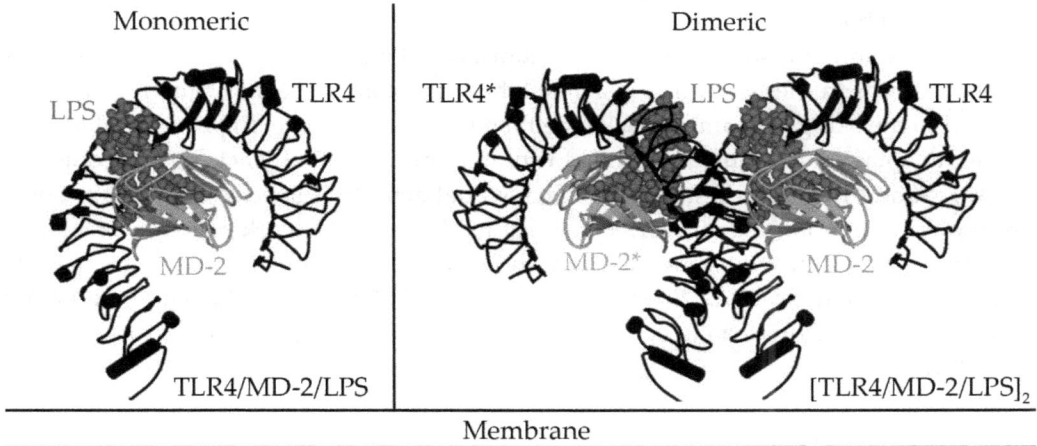

**Figure 3:** Representation of the "monomeric" complex (left) and the homodimeric complex (right). The latter is a duplication of the former which is composed of one "banana"-shaped TLR4 associated to one "empty basket-like" MD-2 protein where the LPS-related agonists or antagonists can bind as a ligand. (Modified and adapted from: Takeuchi & Akira, 2010; Kang & Lee, 2011).

# 4    Computational Molecular Simulations for LPS and TLR4

In the following we present three mayor concepts of Computer-aided drug design all of which have been applied in our ongoing computational molecular simulations concerning the aforementioned initial step of the endotoxicity process which may then develop a full-scale fatal severe sepsis at the clinical level in the living patient.

## 4.1    Structure – Activity Relationships Studies

It is assumed that the dimerization of the extracellular LPS - recognition complex is the initial step toward the intracellular signaling pathway which ends up in endotoxicity (Park et al., 2009, Scior , Alexander et al., 2013). This conclusion was drawn from the three-dimensional structural data made available by x-ray crystallography: the "m"-shaped [TLR4 / MD-2 / LPS]₂, representing the situation of a natural agonist, LPS. In stark contrast, antagonists like Eritoran or L4a were also co-crystalized albeit they only appear in monomeric complexes: [TLR4/MD-2/Eritoran] or [MD-2/L4a], respectively. Seemingly, while agonists induce dimerization, antagonistic binders can only lead to a liganded (ligand-bound) monomer protein complex (Park et al., 2009; Meng, Lien et al., 2010; Meng, Drolet et al., 2010; Scior, Alexander et al., 2013; Scior, Lozano et al., 2013).

There seems to be a link between the faculty of agonistic ligands to form dimeric complexes to the fact that in case of agonists, the sugar unit glucosamine-I-phosphate (1$\alpha$) is oriented in its MD-2 bound form toward the dimerization interface between TLR4 / TLR4*. In contrast to all hitherto known antagonist crystal structures where the di-glucosamine backbone turns around by flipping around 180º. In addition they are even more deeply buried into the MD-2 pocket than agonists do (Park et al., 2009). Structure – activity relationships studies show that in general the antagonists have not so many fatty acids attached to their di-glucosamine backbone than the agonists have. In particular L4a constitutes an antagonist in humans, while Eritoran more consistently acts as antagonists in human, rat and horse cell test systems. L4a 's dual activity is species-dependent, but it can be also seen more as an imperfect agonist tending to "not work properly as an agonist", the behavior of which then becomes notable as "antagonism" (Meng, Lien et al., 2010; Scior, Alexander et al., 2013; Meng, Drolet et al., 2010; Scior, Lozano et al., 2013; Scior et al., 2014; Scior, Lozano et al., 2009; Scior, Medina et al., 2009; Lozano-Aponte & Scior, 2012).

## 4.2    Ligand – Receptor Docking Studies

Docking is a common tool in molecular modeling to simulate how well does a smaller (often organic) compound (often drugs) can bind to a larger biomolecule (often a protein, enzyme), called receptor. To this end, a large number of ligand positions in the receptor cavity are predicted and afterwards become evaluated by another computed process, called scoring functions. They assess the likelihood of how "natural" and probable are the proposed ligand orientations and positions in space (the docking poses). There are also numerical measurements by estimating binding enthalpies, entropies and the overall free energy of binding (Gibbs), regrouping of positions into clusters (groups) of similar geometries etc. (Halperin et al., 2002). In principle, two different kinds of atom to atom interactions exist: (1) steric hindrance and repulsions due to the specific ion or atom radii; or (2) Electronic attraction and repulsion due to atomic partial charges or cations and anions. For instance, double bonds localize electron densities (negative partial charges) on the double bonds, leading to п-п stacking, edge to face attractions and so forth. Software can be either commercial – therefore must be licensed – or can be downloaded from the internet without fees: Chimera (Meng, Pettersen et al., 2006), Swiss PDB Viewer (Johansson et al., 2012), as well as Vega ZZ (Pedretti et al., 2004).

## 4.3    Molecular Dynamics Studies

We also applied another *in silico* (computational) method called molecular dynamics (MD). It is in need of huge computational resources, large scaled super computers with many hundreds and thousands of processors and Terabytes of RAM memory or equivalents. In our case this was provided by the LNS - BUAP, Mexico, an acronym standing for "National Super-computation laboratory" at the *Benemerita Universidad Autonoma de Puebla*, City of Puebla, Mexico.

A MD simulation follows the physic-chemical (sometimes over-) simplification of the so-called "molecular mechanics concept" (Lozano-Aponte & Scior, 2014). All atoms are modelled as small point in space. They have to obey the classical rules of physics / mechanics of the macroscopic world. This refers fundamentally to the popular school text book knowledge about normal-sized bodies according to Newton's Second Law of Motion (F = m a). Used in a more scientific way, and down-scaled to the world of atoms and molecules, the force of a ball-shaped (spherical) atom is equal to the mass of that atom times its acceleration. All atoms exercise forces upon their neighbor atoms and all force contributions are summed up to estimate the acceleration. Mechanical forces at an atomic scale is the key and is reflected in the word "dynamics". The concept of speed and acceleration are related by a simple equation of classical physics. This allows the numerical and precise description of the change in locations (movement) during a given period of time. The force contributions are now calculated by predefined quantities (force field parameters like atom distances, angles, torsions, bending, vibrations, electrostatic attraction and repulsion of point charges on each atom). The sheer amount of date to calculate can be imagined thinking that in order to assess the location and velocities of each atom during the time of simulation is required. And the number of atoms is very huge. The ligand is normally small, say 50 to 200 atoms, no more, but a protein receptor may contain ten thousands of atoms, while when simulating the natural liquid water bath and dissolved ions, or cellular membrane fragments, millions of atoms are added to the simulation model. In order to cope with all those atoms, electronic effects between the bonded or nonbonded atoms are not considered. They can however be calculated otherwise, by so-called ab initio quantum mechanical approaches, which is not part of this study here because they are only applicable to a very limited number of atoms, say one or two hundreds. Electric charges have to be calculated too, and bond types assigned between atoms. This is done by the force field atom types. Since these atom attributes remain permanently the calculations may run astray because the natural behavior of atoms is different: new bonds may be formatted leading to different atom types, like a 4-bonded carbon (4 simple bonds) could become a 3-bonded one (showing one double bond and 2 single bonds), etc. Another inconsistency are the natural occurrence of electronic fluctuations (polarizations) or even changes in total charge (ionizations). So the models must have limited interpretation when assumptions of such chemical events cannot be ruled out. The atoms in MD must be predefined and averaged to keep the error small. In supercomputers such calculations are carried out by computer practitioners with a background formation of biophysics, theoretical chemists and pharmacists with a specialization in Medicinal chemistry or bioinformatics (Scior, Lozano et al., 2009). Another way to save CPU time would be to jump from a given moment in time to another one leaving a discrete time interval in-between without calculating the atom movements in that time step. This way MD can advance faster and cover larger time windows for observations like atom vibrations, conformational changes of amino acid side chains and protein backbones or domain rotations etc. (discretization error). But due to the time interval not calculated imprecisions and wrong behavior may occur. So, all told the MD method, like all computational molecular simulations is by far, not fool-proof.

# 5   Computed Results of the Glucocorticoid Study

Our docking study was carried out between glucocorticoids (GCs) as ligands and the TLR4 / MD-2 receptor complex in order to unravel possible – but hitherto unknown molecular processes – between steroids and the first step of endotoxicity signaling, when the aforementioned cell surface antennae (receptors) receive the invading LPS molecules as ligands (Figure 4, left). Other mechanisms of actions of GCs do not lie in the scope of our simulation study.

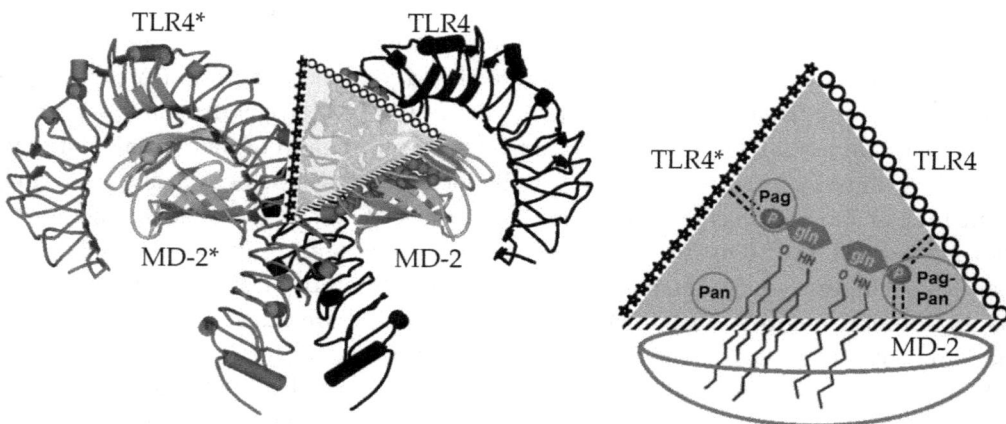

**Figure 4:** Three dimensional model of the complex containing the wedge (right) and schematic view of the wedge with more details (left) (Scior, Lozano et al., 2013). In this triangular cavity between TLR4, counter TLR4* (of the dimerization complex) and MD-2 (basket at the bottom, left) we devised three discrete sites where the phosphate groups of the LPS-like ligands may bind to: the Pag-Pan site (Oval cycle, leftmost corner of the wedge) is a location where the phosphate group (P) of the diglucosamine backbone will always bind to – regardless whether the ligand acts as an agonist (ag) or an antagonist (an). The Pag site is only "visited" by agonists, here shown with LPS (right, sugar part and backbone located in the wedge; and fatty acids partly below the bottom of the wedge; atoms with volumes in opaque triangle) or LA (left; no sugar rests; schematic drawing). As can be seen the agonists protrude (stay off), while an antagonists will occupy with one phosphate group the Pag-Pan site and the Pan site with its second phosphate group, leading to a position with the fatty acids more deeply buried into the MD-2 cavity (basket), filling it up with fewer fatty acids ("under-acylation"). The wedge and the Pag, Pan, PagPan sites were postu Scior, Lozano et al., 2009ted by our group prior to this work to explain the observed activities and crystal structures (Scior, Lozano et al., 2009).

Our structure – activity relationships study compared the chemical models of the ligands to recognize atomic differences and correlated them with the clinically known biological activity of the substances (Figures 4 and 5). The conclusion drawn is that the complicated LPS structure alone is not necessary to induce endotoxicity. A much simpler derivative – called Lipid A (LA) – acts in the same way while cutting off one of both phosphate groups from the LA causes the complete loss of endotoxic activity (Figure 5).

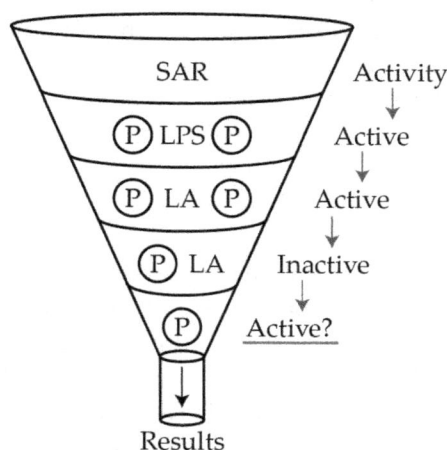

**Figure 5:** The funnel-shaped scheme displays the four complexity levels coming down from a complete LPS ligand toward a mere phosphate anion. Of note, a monophosphate derivative is not active any more, while LPS or its substructure LA show endotoxicity (Alexander & Rietschel, 2001; Scior, Alexander et al., 2013; Scior, Lozano et al., 2013; Ittig et al., 2012; Amano et al., 1982; Mata-Haro et al., 2007; Park, 2009; Berezow et al., 2009; Galanos et al., 1984)

The docking simulation taking the TLR4/MD-2 complex as a receptor and the glucocorticoid (hydrocortisone drug) as a potential binder to this cell surface receptor were successfully carried out on a normal PC and compared to the docking results of a similar situation which was studied and resolved by x-ray crystallography: the binding of a phytosteroid hormone in the plant tissue in order to stimulate apical plant growth (Santiago et al., 2013; Bojar et al., 2014; Jiang et al., 2013; He et al., 2013).

All proteins of the TLR protein family contain substructures which are known as leucine-rich repeats (LRR). The LRR segments are also present in protein complexes which do not belong to the TLR family. For instance, the membrane receptor kinase brassinosteroid insensitive 1 (BRI1) of plants. Intriguingly, these extracellular BRI1 receptors a capable of binding phytosteroids at the vegetal cell surface and therein can activate the cytoplasmic kinase domain of the receptor (within the plant cells). Plant physiology research discovered that the phytosteroids like Brassinosteroids control plant growth and development (Santiago et al., 2013).

We took a phytosteroid hormone out of its natural known binding site of a protein segment [LRR / LRR*] dimeric receptor protein and successfully docked it back into that cavity with a nanomolar affinity ($10^{-9}$ molar concentration) which is a quite normal concentration range for typical hormones to act in living organisms (Figure 6). The docking of the steroid drug against sepsis, hydrocortisone, yielded a roughly one million-fold drop (into a micro-molarity range) for the affinity towards the dimeric [TLR4 / TLR4*] complex (Figure 7).

It is save to utter that our computed results simulating the steroid drug attachment to the TLR4 receptors are correct. The reason is that the binding affinity differences are so overwhelmingly huge that our future more precise calculations will not shepardize this numerical tendency in its overall proportions.

# 6   Conclusions

The motivation of this study was about the medical complication that a causal drug therapy against severe sepsis or septic shock is still missing. Our *in silico* (computational) study was carried out in our Computational Molecular Simulations Laboratory at the University of Puebla (BUAP), Mexico. We simulated the association of the hydrocortisone drug with the cell surface receptor complex TLR4 / MD-2 of the innate immune system which recognizes invading Gram-negative bacteria on a molecular level. The numerical calculations estimated the complex binding affinities and we compared them to a known steroid phytohormone which can bind to structurally related LRR which practically shares the same shape and secondary structure, namely a beta helix made of parallel beta strands. After interpretation of the obtained results we concluded that – while steroid – LRR binding is highly effective in a nanomolar range – steroid binding to TLR4 is far weaker (one million-fold drop). Hence, a hydrocortisone drug interference with the TLR4 biochemical signaling pathways of endotoxicity can be ruled out and with a great confidence. As yet the present preliminary research results have to be completed (as of February 2016). There is literature evidence that, for instance, in renal tissues LPS infections reflect association and signaling cooperativity between TLR4 and TLR2 (Good et al., 2012). In 2012 another article confirmed aforementioned *in vivo* findings, in that certain TLR4 activities are assisted by a TLR2 component (Castoldi et al., 2012). The absence of TLR4 in healthy mice lowers the risk of endotoxicity which was observed in TLR4 knock-out mice. They become endotoxin hyporesponsive mice (abnormality) (Silverstein & Johnson, 2003). R. Silverstein and D. Johnson also mentioned that the therapeutic value of GC administration to sepsis patients "remains controversial" (Silverstein & Johnson, 2003). In sight of the known picomolar LPS sensitivity of the innate immune response to microbial exposition, the normal biochemical situation could inversely be qualified as "entoxin hyper-responsiveness". The present study focused on the TLR4-dependent signaling pathway because it is triggered by LPS. Further downstream in the intracellular signaling pathway this leads to the biosynthesis of pro-inflammatory cytokines, all of which could induce sepsis in the final stage of LPS-induced signaling (Supajatura et al., 2002). The same article also experimentally confirmed that not LPS and its congeners but

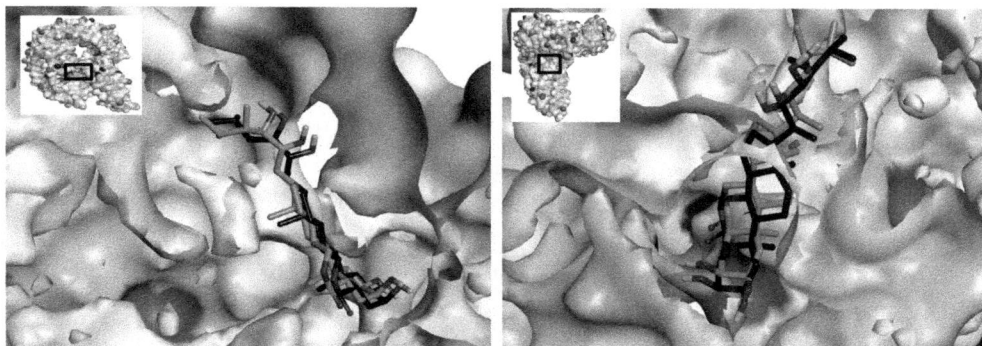

**Figure 6:** The final three-dimensional models between the [LRR / LRR*] receptor complex and the computed pose of its natural ligand (light gray sticks) and its crystallographically observed pose (darker sticks, PDB code: 4LSX) (Santiago et al., 2013). By eye-sight it can be judged that the software (here Autodock: 4.2 (Morris et al., 2009) is capable of predicting the natural binding behavior of the steroid phyto-hormone to its receptor in plant tissues. Such simulations are called back-docking to proof that the chosen software can also handle similar cases with un-known ("blind docking") solutions of binding complexes. The two sides represent the 3D model in orthogonal view (90 degrees rotation). The two inlay panels display the entire complex on white backgrounds and mark the ligand site by a box.

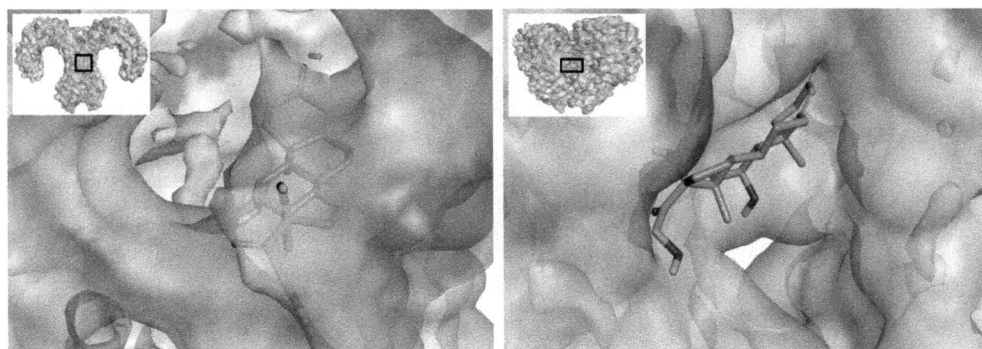

**Figure 7:** Display of the computed blind docking simulation between the TLR4 receptor and the hydrocortisone drug molecule to test whether or not the corticosteroid could be a potential binder to the TLR4 receptor. The human [TL4 / TLR4*] complex (PDB code: 3FXi (Park et al., 2009) is displayed by its surface which is built up by the atom volumes. This viewing methods allows to see the cavity and crevices, clefts and other empty wholes in the protein. The hydrocortisone drug molecule lies between the two TLR4 proteins in a cleft which forms the natural interface between both. Our theoretical results suggest that the steroid drugs are poor binders to the TLR4 receptor protein. Hence it can be ruled out that corticoid therapy could have a direct, causal influence on the initial step of the pathway triggering endotoxic cell reactions.

peptidoglycan derivatives can trigger inflammation through a signaling cascade which starts at the cell surface with TLR2 receptors. Thus, whether TLR2 would also interact with GC drug treatment is a question that deserves further scrutiny.

Hopefully, in the near future we can contribute with the complete molecular study to discard the hydrocortisone interaction on other biomolecules (TLR2 etc) and the final results could become available on the web (NCBI, Pub Med Entrez, SciFinder, Science Direct, Scopus, Web of Science). This way we may shed valuable light upon the biochemical underpinnings for a better understanding of the molecular processes leading to the clinical manifestation of sepsis in patients.

In good keeping to our work where computer simulations is related to *in vivo* observations the contemporary literature also includes publications where *in silico* work is validated by *in vivo* findings (Leach et al., 2010; Shi et al., 2015; Unzue et al., 2014; Wang & Li, 2014; Sohn et al., 2005; Yadav et al., 2014).

In an even more general view, molecular computational simulations assist the researchers in the field of Medicinal sciences to visualize molecular disease-related events or find physic-chemical properties as well as biochemical behaviors to describe the physiopathologic processes in addition to the administered drug effects and – why not? – devise new drugs for future treatments.

## Acknowledgement

We are much beholden to Prof. Dr. Ulrich Schaible, Prof. Dr. Ulrich Zaehringer and Dr. Christian Alexander at Leibniz Research Center Borstel (Hamburg, Germany) for discussions and three visits of TS. We wish to thank Pharmacy exchange student Sarah Guethlein from University Erlangen, Germany, and graduate student Viridiana Vargas Castro for trial reading and manuscript revisions. For financial support we feel grateful to CONACyT for the scholarships of doctoral student Jorge Lozano Aponte (CONACyT id: 244868, 2013–2017) and Masters student Itzel Gutiérrez Aztatzi (CONACyT id: 304615, 2014–2015), and to Faculty of Chemical Sciencies as well as Vicerrectoría de Investigación y Estudios de Posgrado, Dr. Ygnacio Martínez Laguna, Vicerrector VIEP-BUAP.

## References

Aderem, A., Ulevitch, R. J. (2000). Toll-like receptors in the induction of the innate immune response. Nature, 406, 782–787.

Akashi, S., Nagai, Y., Ogata, H., Oikawa, M., Fukase, K., Kusumoto, S., Kawasaki, K., Nishijima, M., Hayashi, S., Kimoto, M., Miyake, K. (2001). Human MD-2 confers on mouse Toll-like receptor 4 species-specific lipopolysaccharide recognition. International Immunology, 13, 1595–1599.

Alexander, C., Rietschel E T. (2001). Bacterial lipopolysaccharides and innate immunity. Journal of Endotoxin Research, 7, 301–308.

Bojar, D., Martinez, J., Santiago, J., Rybin, V., Bayliss, R., Hothorn, M. (2014). Crystal structures of the phosphorylated BRI1 kinase domain and implications for brassinosteroid signal initiation. Plant J, 78,

31–43.

Castoldi, A., Braga, T. T., Correa-Costa, M., Aguiar, C. F., Bassi, Ê. J., Correa-Silva, R., Elias, R. M., Salvador, F., Moraes-Vieira, P. M., Cenedeze, M. A., Reis, M.A., Hiyane, M. I., Pacheco-Silva, Á., Gonçalves, G. M., Saraiva, C. N. O. (2012). TLR2, TLR4 and the MYD88 signaling pathway are crucial for neutrophil migration in acute kidney injury induced by sepsis. PLoS One. 7, e37584.

Carrillo-Esper, R., Carrillo-Córdova, J. R., Carrillo-Córdova, L. D. (2010). Estudio epidemiológico de la sepsis en unidades de terapia intensiva mexicanas. Cirugía y Cirujanos, 77, 301–308.

Dellinger, R. P., Levy, M. M., Rhodes, A., Annane, D., Gerlach, H., Opal, S. M., Sevransky, J. E., Sprung, C. L., Douglas, I. S., Jaeschke, R., Osborn, T. M., Nunnally, M. E., Townsend, S. R., Reinhart, K., Kleinpell, R.M., Angus, D. C., Deutschman, C. S., Machado, F. R., Rubenfeld, G. D., Webb, S., Beale, R. J., Vincent, J. L., Moreno, R. and the Surviving Sepsis Campaign Guidelines Committee including the Paediatric Subgroup (2013). Surviving Sepsis Campaign: International Guidelines for Management of Severe Sepsis and Septic Shock: 2012. Intensive Care Med, 39, 165–228.

Dziarski, R., Wang, Q., Miyake, K., Kirschning, C. J., Gupta, D. (2001). MD-2 Enables Toll-Like Receptor 2 (TLR2)-Mediated Responses to Lipopolysaccharide and Enhances TLR2-Mediated Responses to Gram-Positive and Gram-Negative Bacteria and Their Cell Wall Components. The Journal of Immunology, 166, 1938–1944.

Good, D. W., George, T., Watts, B. A. 3rd. (2012). Toll-like receptor 2 is required for LPS-induced Toll-like receptor 4 signaling and inhibition of ion transport in renal thick ascending limb. J Biol Chem. 8, 287, 20208–20220.

Halperin, I., Ma, B., Wolfson, H., Nussinov, R. (2002). Principles of Docking: An Overview of Search Algorithms and a Guide to Scoring Functions. Proteins: Structure, Function and Genetics, 47, 409–443.

He, K., Xu, S., Li, J. (2013). BAK1 directly regulates brassinosteroid perception and BRI1 activation. J Integr Plant Biol, 55, 1264–1270.

Ittig, S., Lindner, B., Stenta, M., Manfredi, P., Zdorovenko, E., Knirel, Y. A., dal Peraro, M., Cornelis, G. R., Zähringer, U. (2012). The Lipopolysaccharide from Capnocytophaga canimorsus Reveals an Unexpected Role of the Core-Oligosaccharide in MD-2 Binding. Plos, 8, 1–18.

Jiang, J., Zhang, C., Wang, X. (2013). Ligand perception, activation, and early signaling of plant steroid receptor brassinosteroid insensitive 1. J Integr Plant Biol, 55, 1198–1211.

Johansson, M. U., Zoete, V., Michielin, O., Guex, N. (2012). Defining and searching for structural motifs using DeepView/Swiss-PdbViewer. BMC Bioinformatics, 13, 173.

Kang, Y., Lee, J. (2011). Structural Biology of the Toll-Like Receptor Family. Annual Review of Biochemistry, 80, 917–941.

Leach, K., Loiacono, R. E., Felder, C. C., McKinzie, D. L., Mogg, A., Shaw, D. B., Sexton, P. M., Christopoulos, A. (2010). Molecular mechanisms of action and in vivo validation of an M4 muscarinic acetylcholine receptor allosteric modulator with potential antipsychotic properties. Neuropsychopharmacology. 35, 855–869.

Lozano-Aponte, J., Scior, T. (2012). Que sabe usted de QSAR? Revista Mexicana de Ciencias Farmacéuticas, 43, 82–84.

Lozano-Aponte, J., Scior, T. (2014). ¿Qué sabe Ud. Acerca de... Dinámica Molecular? Revista Mexicana de Ciencias Farmacéuticas, 45, 86–88.

Meng, E. C., Pettersen, E. F., Couch, G. S., Huang, C. C., Ferrin, T. E. (2006). Tools for integrated sequence *structure analysis with UCSF Chimera. BMC Bioinformatics, 12, 339.*

Meng, J., Drolet, J. R., Monks, B. G., Golenbock, D. T. (2010). *MD-2 Residues Tyrosine 42, Arginine 69, Aspartic Acid 122, and Leucine 125 Provide Species Specificity for Lipid IVA. The Journal of Biological Chemistry, 285, 27935–27943.*

Meng, J., Lien, E., Golenbock, D. T. (2010). *MD-2-mediated ionic interactions between lipid A and TLR4 are essential for receptor activation. The Journal of Biological Chemistry, 285, 8695–8702.*

Morris, G. M., Huey, R., Lindstrom, W., Sanner, M. F., Belew, R. K., Goodsell, D. S., Olson, A. J. (2009). *AutoDock4 and AutoDockTools4: Automated docking with selective receptor flexibility. Journal of Computational Chemistry, 30, 2785–2791.*

Ohto, U., Fukase, K., Miyake, K., Shimizu, T. (2012). *Structural basis of species-specific endotoxin sensing by innate immune receptor TLR4/MD-2. PNAS, 109, 7421–7426.*

Park, B. S., Song, D. H., Kim, H. M., Choi, B., Lee, H., Lee, J. (2009). *The structural basis of lipopolysaccharide recognition by the TLR4–MD-2 complex. Nature, 458, 1191–1195.*

Pedretti, A., Villa, L., Vistoli, G. (2004). *VEGA—an open platform to develop chemo-bioinformatics applications, using plug-in architecture and script programming. J Comput Aided Mol Des, 18, 167–73.*

Saavedra, P. G., Vásquez, G. M., González, L. A. (2011). *Interleucina-6: amiga o enemiga? Bases para comprender su utilidad como objetivo terapéutico. Iatreia, 24, 157–166.*

Santiago, J., Henzler, C., Hothorn, M. (2013). *Molecular mechanism for plant steroid receptor activation by somatic embryogenesis co-receptor kinases. Science, 341, 889–892.*

Scior, T., Alexander, C., Zaehringer, U. (2013). *Reviewing and identifying amino acids of human, murine, canine and equine TLR4 / MD-2 receptor complexes conferring endotoxic innate immunity activation by LPS/lipid A, or antagonistic effects by Eritoran, in contrast to species-dependent modulation by lipid Iva. Computational and Structural Biotechnology Journal, 5, 1–13.*

Scior, T., Lozano-Aponte, J., Echeverria, D. (2009). *CAMD Y CADD. Simulaciones moleculares computacionales de fármacos. Parte 1. Informacéutico, 16 (5), 46–50.*

Scior, T., Lozano-Aponte, J., Echeverria, D. (2009). *CAMD Y CADD. Simulaciones moleculares computacionales de fármacos. Parte 2. Informacéutico, 16 (6), 32–35.*

Scior, T., Lozano-Aponte, J., Figueroa-Vazquez, V., Yunes-Rojas, J. A., Zähringer, U., Alexander, C. (2013). *Three-dimensional mapping of differential amino acids of human, murine, canine and equine TLR4/MD-2 receptor complexes conferring endotoxic activation by lipid A, antagonism by Eritoran and species dependent activities of Lipid IVA in the mammalian LPS sensor system. Computational and Structural Biotechnology Journal, 7, 1–11.*

Scior, T., Medina, F. J. L., Do, Q-T., Martínez-Mayorga, K., Yunes-Rojas, J. A., Bernard, P. (2009). *How to Recognize and Workaround Pitfalls in QSAR Studies: A Critical Review. Current Medicinal Chemistry, 16, 4297–4313.*

Scior, T., Paiz-Candia, B., Islas, Á. A., Sánchez-Solano, A., Millan-Perez, Peña, L., Mancilla-Simbro, C., Salinas-Stefanon, E. M. (2015). *Predicting a double mutant in the twilight zone of low homology modeling for the skeletal muscle voltage-gated sodium channel subunit beta-1 (Nav1.4 β1). Comput Struct Biotechnol J. 13, 229–240.*

Scior, T,. Verhoff, M., Gutierrez-Aztatzi, I., Ammon, HP., Laufer, S., Werz, O. (2014). *Interference of boswellic acids with the ligand binding domain of the glucocorticoid receptor. J Chem Inf Model, 54, 978–986.*

Shi, X. N., Li, H., Yao, H., Liu, X., Li, L., Leung, K. S., Kung, H. F., Lu, D., Wong, M. H., Lin, M. C.(2015). In Silico Identification and In Vitro and In Vivo Validation of Anti-Psychotic Drug Fluspirilene as a Potential CDK2 Inhibitor and a Candidate Anti-Cancer Drug. PLoS One. 10, e0132072.

Silverstein, R., Johnson, D. C. (2003). Endogenous versus exogenous glucocorticoid responses to experimental bacterial sepsis. Journal of Leukocyte Biology , 73, 417–427.

Sohn, J., Parks, J. M., Buhrman, G., Brown, P., Kristjánsdóttir, K., Safi, A., Edelsbrunner, H., Yang, W., Rudolph, J. (2005). Experimental validation of the docking orientation of Cdc25 with its Cdk2-CycA protein substrate. Biochemistry. 44, 16563–16573.

Supajatura, V., Ushio, H., Nakao, A., Akira, S., Okumura, K., Ra, C., Ogawa, H. (2002). Differential responses of mast cell Toll-like receptors 2 and 4 in allergy and innate immunity. J Clin Invest. 109, 1351–1359.

Takeuchi, O., Akira, S. (2010). Pattern Recognition Receptors and Inflammation. Cell, 140, 805–820.

Unzue, A., Dong, J., Lafleur, K., Zhao, H., Frugier, E., Caflisch, A., Nevado, C. (2014). Pyrrolo[3,2-b]quinoxaline derivatives as types I1/2 and II Eph tyrosine kinase inhibitors: structure-based design, synthesis, and in vivo validation. J Med Chem. 57, 6834–6844.

Wang, J., Li, W. (2014). Discovery of novel second mitochondria-derived activator of caspase mimetics as selective inhibitor of apoptosis protein inhibitors. J Pharmacol Exp Ther. 349, 319–329.

Yadav, D. K., Dhawan, S., Chauhan, A., Qidwai, T., Sharma, P., Bhakuni, R. S., Dhawan, O. P., Khan, F. (2014). QSAR and docking based semi-synthesis and in vivo evaluation of artemisinin derivatives for antimalarial activity. Curr Drug Targets. 15, 753–761.

# Chapter 9

# Diabetes Mellitus And Hearing Loss

Prasanna Venkatesan Eswaradass[1], Swapna Anandan[2],
Hari Krishnan Nair[3] and Mohammed Ismail[4]

## 1 Introduction

Diabetes mellitus is a chronic disease characterized by hyperglycemia and is associated with microvascular and macrovascular complications. The microvascular complications affect the retina, peripheral nerves, and kidneys, while the macrovascular complications include coronary artery disease, peripheral artery disease and stroke. Sensorineural hearing loss (SNHL) may also be an under-recognized complication of diabetes, and as diabetes becomes more common worldwide, the diabetes-associated sensorineural hearing loss may become a significant contributor to hearing impairment in the general population (Bainbridge et al., 2008).

Diabetes mellitus is associated with a gradually progressive, bilateral sensorineural hearing loss affecting predominantly higher frequencies[1]. The hearing loss is about twice as common in adults with diabetes compared to non-diabetics and is a major public health concern. The risk for hearing impairment is associated with male sex, lower education, industrial or military occupation, smoking, and leisure time noise exposure. Prevalence varies substantially with age, sex, and race, and it is estimated that the proportion of hearing loss in diabetics exceeds 30% among those aged 65 years or more (Plies & Lethbridge-Cejku, 2006; Muhr et al., 2006).

The pathologic changes that accompany diabetes involves injury to the vasculature or the neural system of the inner ear, resulting in sensorineural hearing impairment. Two

---

[1] Calgary Stroke Program, University of Calgary, Calgary, AB, Canada
[2] Griffin Hospital, Derby, CT, United States
[3] St. Elizabeth's Medical Center, Tufts University School of Medicine, Boston, MA, United States
[4] Kasturba Medical College Mangalore, Manipal University, Karnataka, India

studies described evidence of such pathologic changes on autopsy in diabetics, which showed sclerosis of the internal auditory artery, thickened capillaries of the stria vascularis, atrophy of the spiral ganglion, and demyelination of the eighth cranial nerve (Makishima & Tanaka, 1971; Jorgensen, 1961).

In this study, pure-tone audiometry was used to compare the hearing impairment in diabetics with non-diabetics.

## 1.1   Aim and Objectives

1.   Study of hearing impairment in diabetic patients and to assess whether diabetes is an independent risk factor for sensorineural hearing loss.

2.   To assess the relation between glycemic status of diabetic patients and the severity of sensorineural hearing loss.

# 2   Materials And Methods

We recruited 50 known diabetics (cases) and 50 non-diabetics (controls) from the outpatient clinic in the Department of Medicine at Government Wenlock Hospital in Mangalore, Karnataka, India. The study was done from August 2008 to August 2009. We analyzed all 100 patients with pure-tone audiometry (PTA). The results of the PTA were classified as mild to moderate (25-40 dB) hearing loss, moderate to severe (40-60 dB) hearing loss, and severe to profound (>60 dB) hearing loss. People aged 70 years and above were excluded due to the high incidence of presbycusis that might be a confounding factor. The study was adjusted for age, sex, and other risk factors.

## 2.1   Inclusion Criteria for Cases

1.   Age between 20 and 69 years

2.   Known diabetic patients as diagnosed by American Diabetes Association (ADA) criteria

## 2.2   Inclusion Criteria for Controls

1.   Non-diabetic patients aged between 20 and 69 years

2.   Fasting blood sugar <100 mg/dL

## 2.3   Exclusion Criteria

1.   History of occupational noise exposure (loud noise at work that requires speaking in a loud voice)

2.  History of intake of ototoxic drugs

    a.  NSAIDS

    b.  Aminoglycosides

    c.  Loop diuretics

    d.  Chemotherapeutic drugs

3.  History of head trauma

4.  Family history of hearing loss

5.  History of ear discharge

6.  History of smoking

# 3   Pure Tone Audiometry

Pure Tone Audiometry (PTA) is also known as an audiogram. The patient is made to sit in a sound-proof room and the ability to hear pure tones of frequencies 250 Hz, 500 Hz, 1000 Hz, 2000 Hz, 4000 Hz and 8000 Hz are assessed by the audiologist. Pure-tone thresholds (PTTs) indicate the softest sound audible to an individual at least 50% of the time. Hearing sensitivity is plotted on an audiogram, which is a graph displaying intensity as a function of frequency. The equipment required depends on the testing method used and may include the following:

1.  Headphones

2.  Insert earphones

3.  Speakers

4.  Bone-conduction oscillator

The hearing is tested with both bone and air conduction. Air conduction tests the ability to listen with earphones via the external auditory canal, tympanic membrane and middle ear. Bone conduction is tested with a bone oscillator placed on either side of the mastoid. The stimulating noise bypasses the middle ear and sets the cochlea in motion by bone vibration. The gap between air and bone conduction is an air-bone gap consistent with conductive hearing loss (DeBonis & Donohue, 2003).

## 3.1   Types of Hearing Loss

### 3.1.1   Conductive Hearing Loss

It is secondary to an external ear or middle ear abnormality. The abnormality reduces the air-conducted signal reaching the cochlea, but it does not affect the bone-conducted signal that does not pass through the outer or middle ear. Causes of conductive hearing loss are chronic suppurative otitis media, wax impaction in the external ear, and otosclerosis.

### 3.1.2    Sensorineural Hearing Loss

It is secondary to cochlear abnormalities and/or an abnormality of the eighth cranial nerve or the central auditory pathways. Here, the outer ear and middle ear do not reduce the signal intensity of the air-conducted signal, both air- and bone-conducted signals are effective in stimulating the cochlea. Pure-tone air- and bone-conduction thresholds are within 10 dB. Causes of sensorineural hearing loss are ototoxic drugs affecting the eighth cranial nerve, acoustic schwannoma affecting central auditory pathway and presbycusis.

### 3.1.3    Mixed Hearing Loss

Includes both conductive and sensorineural components.

## 3.2    Degree of Hearing Loss

1.   Normal hearing (0-25 dB): No symptoms.

2.   Mild hearing loss (26-40 dB): Difficulty in hearing soft speech due to difficulty in suppressing background noise.

3.   Moderate hearing loss (41-55 dB): Can affect normal language development and patients may have difficulty in hearing normal conversations.

4.   Moderate-to-severe hearing loss (56-70 dB): Patients have difficulty in engaging with any conversation.

5.   Severe hearing loss (71-90 dB): May affect voice quality.

6.   Profound hearing loss (>90 dB): With profound hearing loss (deafness), speech and language deteriorate (Ferraro et al., 1994).

## 3.3    Glycated Hemoglobin (HbA1c)

HbA1c is a test used to find the three-month average plasma glucose concentration in an individual. High-pressure liquid chromatography (HPLC) separates HbA1c from other Hemoglobin A components by passing the blood sample through special liquids under pressure and finally separates the mixture into different components. HbA1c level more than 6.5 is noted in diabetic patients.

## 4    Results and Analysis

Table 1 shows the characteristics of patients at baseline. Figure 1 to Figure 6 respectively show the distribution of hearing impairment among: (1) cases and controls, (2) cases with HbA1c < 7 and HbA1c > 7, (3) age, (4) diabetes, (5) males and females, and (6) cases and controls in terms of age.

| Characteristic | Case | Control |
|---|---|---|
| Mean age (years) | 63.5 | 64.5 |
| Sex | Men: 36 | Men: 34 |
| Hypertension | 27/50 | 28/50 |
| Mean BMI | 27.7 | 28.9 |
| Coronary artery disease | 15/50 | 16/50 |

**Table 1:** Characteristics of patients at baseline.

### Distribution of Hearing Impairment

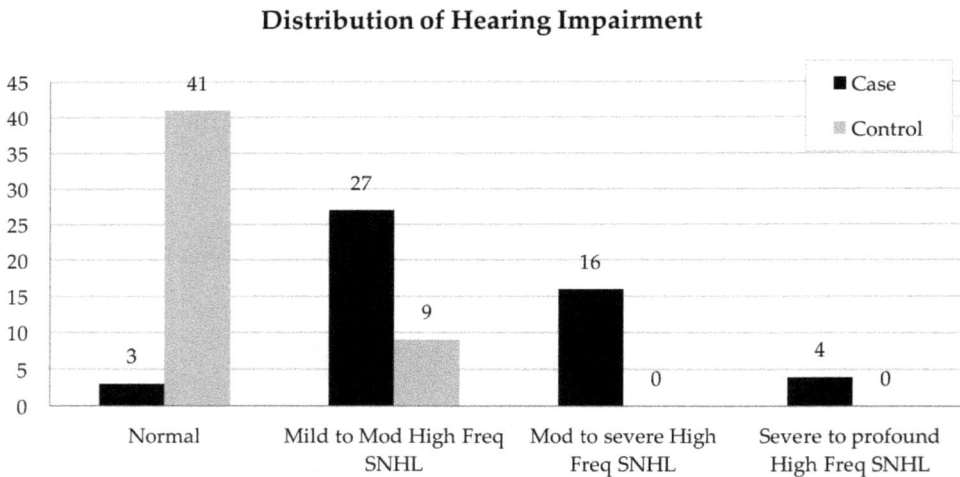

**Figure 1:** Distribution of hearing impairment among cases and controls. Among cases, only 3 were normal, 27 patients had mild to moderate high-frequency SNHL, 16 had moderate to severe high-frequency SNHL, and the rest had profound hearing impairment. In controls, 41 were normal, and the rest had mild to moderate SNHL.

## HbA1C and Hearing Impairment

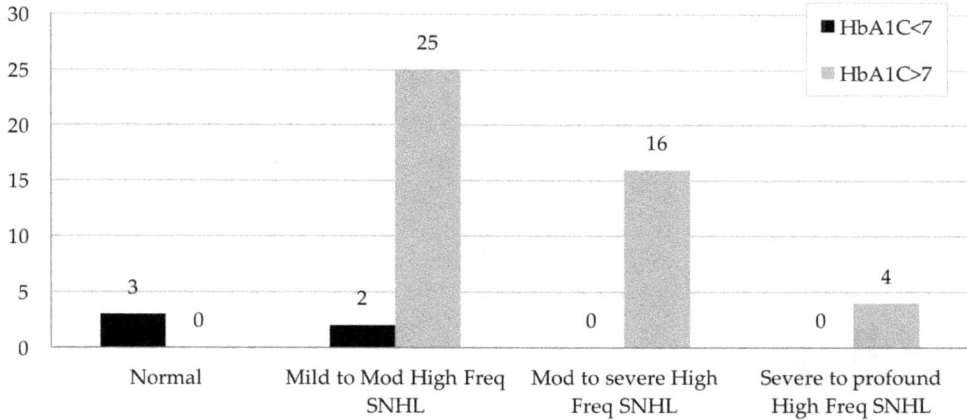

**Figure 2:** Distribution of hearing impairment among cases with HbA1c < 7 and HbA1c > 7. Among the cases, 5 patients had HbA1c < 7 and 45 had HbA1c > 7. In the first group, 3 had normal hearing, and 2 had mild to moderate high-frequency SNHL. In the group with HbA1c > 7, all patients had SNHL of varying severity, 25 patients had mild to moderate high-frequency SNHL, 16 had moderate to severe high-frequency SNHL, and 4 had profound high-frequency SNHL respectively.

## Age and Hearing Impairment

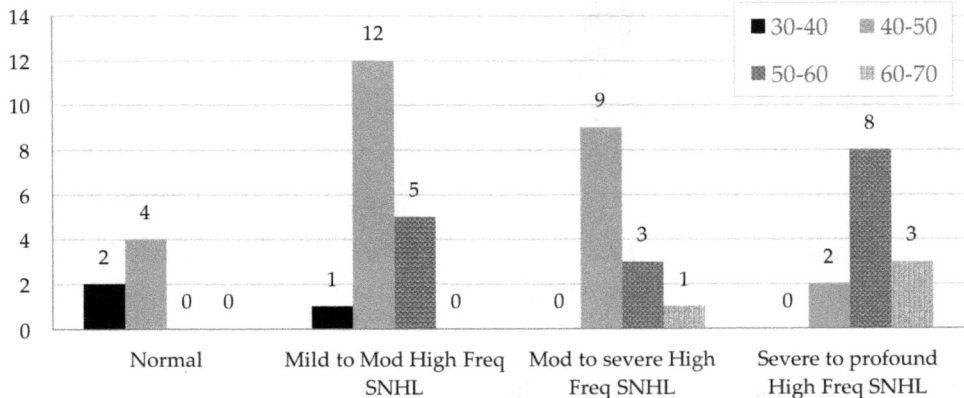

**Figure 3:** Distribution of age and hearing impairment. Among cases aged <50 years, 24 had SNHL, but cases aged >50 years had SNHL of greater severity. In the age group > 50 years, 4 patients had profound high-frequency SNHL, while none had profound SNHL in the age group <50 years.

## Duration of Diabetes and Hearing Impairment

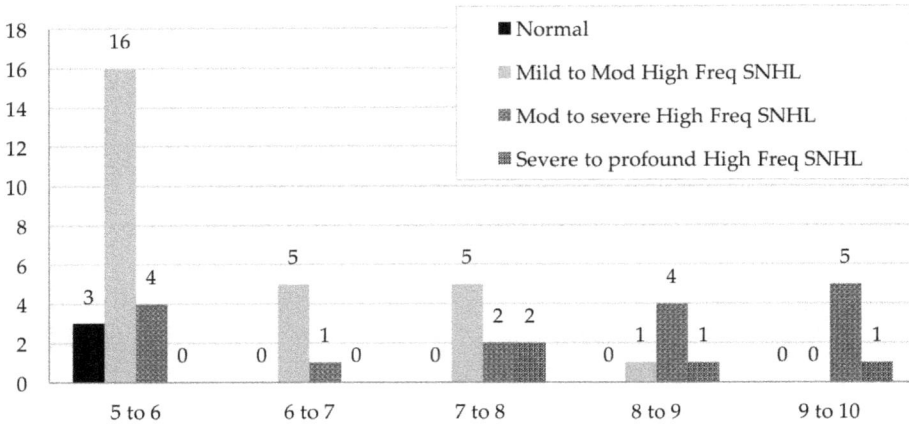

**Figure 4:** Distribution of duration of diabetes and hearing impairment. Among cases of duration < 7 years, 26 had hearing impairment, whereas cases of duration >7 years had hearing impairment of greater severity.

## Gender and Hearing Impairment

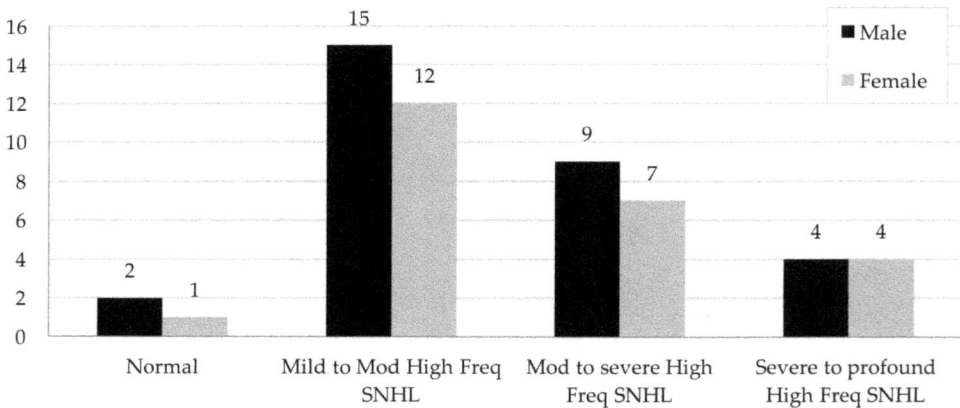

**Figure 5:** Distribution of hearing impairment among males and females. Among cases, 28 males and 19 females had SNHL, while 2 males and a female had no hearing loss. It had no statistical significance.

**Cases and Controls**

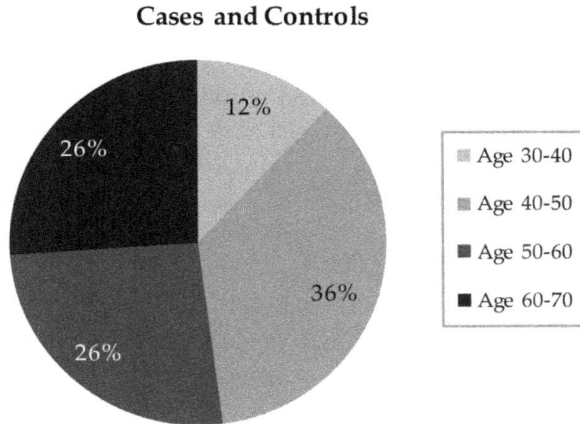

**Figure 6:** Age distribution of cases and controls.

# 5   Discussion

There has been a dramatic rise in the worldwide prevalence of diabetes mellitus over the past two decades. In this study, we evaluated the association between diabetes and audiometrically assessed hearing impairment in Government Wenlock Hospital, Mangalore, Karnataka, India. We also tried to find the correlation between duration of diabetes and sensorineural hearing loss (SNHL) and also between glycemic status of diabetes patients and severity of SNHL. The strength of the association of diabetes and SNHL that we observed was similar to that in previous population-based studies. We found that SNHL was significantly higher in cases (94%) as compared to controls (18%) ($p$=0.01).

Bainbridge and colleagues reported an increased risk of hearing loss in persons with self-reported diabetes. It was a cross-sectional study, where they used the National Health and Nutrition Examination Survey to determine the relative risk of sensorineural hearing loss in a community-based random sample of patients who reported a history of diabetes. They found that persons with diabetes were at increased risk for hearing loss (adjusted odds ratio, 2.2 to 2.4). They estimated a prevalence of low- to mid-frequency hearing impairment in 28%. Bainbridge et al. (2008) reported SNHL in 67% of cases as compared to 30% in controls. This high prevalence was not just limited to old age, smokers or those exposed to loud noise and ototoxic drugs. Diabetics of both sexes, all ethnicities, race, and all age groups were affected.

In another study, Cullen and Cinnamond used a large population-based data set and reported an odds ratio for hearing loss of 1.41 in non-insulin-dependent diabetics (Cullen & Cinnamond, 1993). A possible explanation for the divergent results between this study and that of Bainbridge and colleagues is that Cullen and Cinnamon excluded patients younger than 48 years and patients with non-insulin-dependent diabetes. The possible hypothesis for SNHL in diabetes was attributed to microvascular disease affecting the cochlea. Microvascular disease of stria-vascularis affects the endolymph production and machine transduction of hair cells resulting in SNHL in diabetes.

In another comparative study, the association of diabetes and SNHL among non-elderly population was studied. The study included 160 subjects with no history of occupational noise exposure. Among the 160 patients, 80 had diabetes while 80 were age- and sex-matched controls. It was found that 45% of diabetics and 20% of controls had SNHL. They concluded that diabetes is a risk factor for SNHL regardless of age and smoking (Mozaffari et al., 2010).

In a study by Kakarlapudi et al. (2003), electronic medical records from 12,575 diabetic patients and age-matched 53461 non-diabetic controls were reviewed. They looked into serum creatinine, serum triglyceride, serum cholesterol, speech discrimination and pure-tone hearing (dB). They found that SNHL was more prevalent in the diabetic group than in the non-diabetic group. The severity of the hearing loss correlated with an increase in the serum creatinine levels rather than with HbA1c. This may have been due to microangiopathic disease in the inner ear. However, these results should be interpreted with caution as it is a retrospective study.

Konrad-Martin et al. (2015) studied the cross sectional data from a baseline visit of a longitudinal study of veterans with and without diabetes. They assessed the possible differences in age-related peripheral and central auditory function among the two groups. The outcomes measured were pure-tone thresholds, word recognition, and an inventory assessing the self-perceived impact of hearing loss on Quality of Life (QOL) subscales. They concluded that significant hearing dysfunction was present among subjects with poorly-controlled diabetes, and that hearing dysfunction in type 2 diabetes may be prevented or delayed through tight metabolic control. However, these findings need to be corroborated using longitudinal assessments.

Sakuta et al. (2007) evaluated the association of diabetes with hearing loss in middle-aged people from self-defense forces. They found that hearing loss was more prevalent among diabetics than subjects with normal glucose tolerance. The odds ratio (OR) was 1.87 (95% confidence interval 1.20-2.91, $p$=0.006) derived from a logistic regression analysis adjusted for age, rank, cigarette smoking and ethanol consumption. In conclusion, Type 2 diabetes is associated with hearing loss independent of lifestyle factors, in middle-aged men.

de León-Morales et al. (2005) compared diabetic patients with age- and sex-matched healthy subjects. Patients with type 2 diabetes mellitus were found to have a subclinical hearing loss and impaired auditory brainstem evoked response independent of peripheral neuropathy, retinopathy or nephropathy, compared to non-diabetic subjects. There was also a correlation between duration of diabetes and the age of patients with hearing impairment. Gupta et al. (2013) studied the brain stem evoked potentials in 126 diabetic patients and 106 healthy subjects. He found that diabetic patients had an early involvement of central auditory pathway, which could be detected with fair accuracy with auditory evoked potential studies.

A meta-analysis by Horikawa et al. (2012) of 13 eligible studies was done in Japan, and the hearing loss between diabetic and non-diabetic patients was compared. They concluded that there was a higher prevalence of hearing impairment in diabetic patients compared to non-diabetic patients regardless of age.

In our study, we also found an association between glycemic status of the patient and severity of hearing loss. In patients with HbA1c greater than 7, 100% had SNHL whereas in patients with HbA1c less than 7, only 40% had SNHL, which was statistically significant (p=0.01). Similarly, in patients with duration of diabetes more than 8 years, 8.33% had mild-to-moderate hearing loss, 75% had moderate-to-severe hearing loss, and 16.67% had severe-to-profound hearing loss. The corresponding figures for those with duration less than 8 years were 68.4%, 18.4%, and 5.2%. However, 87.5% of cases aged less than 50 years had SNHL, in contrast to 100% in those more than 50 years of age.

The main limitation of this study is that it is a small pilot study and hence requires validation after another study in a larger population. Another limitation is that age might be a confounding factor.

In conclusion, high-frequency SNHL is a very common but underdiagnosed complication of diabetes. This becomes all the more significant with the increasing lifespan of diabetics, and consequently the increasing number of elderly people with diabetes. SNHL increases in severity with a longer duration of diabetes mellitus and poorer glycemic status.

# References

Bainbridge KE, Hoffman HJ, Cowie CC (2008). Diabetes and hearing impairment in the United States: audiometric evidence from the National Health and Nutrition Examination Survey, 1999 to 2004. Annals of Internal Medicine, 149 (1), 1-10.

Plies JR. Lethbridge-Cejku (2006). Summary health statistics for US adults: National Health Interview Survey.

Muhr P, Månsson B, Hellström PA (2006). A study of hearing changes among military conscripts in the Swedish Army: Estudio de Los cambios auditivos en conscriptos de la Armada Sueca. International Journal of Audiology, 45 (4), 247-251.

Makishima K, Tanaka K. Pathological changes of the inner ear and central auditory pathway in diabetics (1971). The Annals of Otology, Rhinology, and Laryngology, 80 (2), 218.

Jorgensen MB (1961). The inner ear in diabetes mellitus: histological studies. Archives of Otolaryngology, 74 (4), 373-381.

DeBonis DA, Donohue CL (2003). Survey of Audiology: Fundamentals for audiologists and health professionals. Allyn & Bacon.

Ferraro JA, Durrant JD, Katz J (1994). Handbook of Clinical Audiology.

Cullen JR, Cinnamond M (1993). Hearing loss in diabetics. Journal of Laryngology and Otology, 107 (3), 179-182.

Fowler MJ. Microvascular and macrovascular complications of diabetes. Clinical Diabetes, 26 (2), 77-82.

Mozaffari M, Tajik A, Ariaei N, Ali Ehyaii F, Behnam H (2010). Diabetes mellitus and sensorineural hearing loss among non-elderly people. Eastern Mediterranean Health Journal, 16 (9), 947–952.

*Kakarlapudi V, Sawyer R, Staecker H (2003). The effect of diabetes on sensorineural hearing loss. Otology and Neurotology, 24 (3), 382-386.*

*Konrad-Martin D, Reavis KM, Austin D, Reed N, Gordon J, McDermott D, Dille MF (2015). Hearing impairment in relation to severity of diabetes in a veteran cohort. Ear and Hearing, 36 (4), 381.*

*Sakuta H, Suzuki T, Yasuda H, Ito T (2007). Type 2 diabetes and hearing loss in personnel of the Self-Defense Forces. Diabetes research and Clinical Practice, 75 (2), 229-234.*

*de León-Morales LV, Jáuregui-Renaud K, Garay-Sevilla ME, Hernández-Prado J, Malacara-Hernández JM (2005). Auditory impairment in patients with type 2 diabetes mellitus. Archives of Medical Research, 36 (5): 507-510.*

*Gupta S, Baweja P, Mittal S, Kumar A, Singh KD, Sharma R (2013). Brainstem auditory evoked potential abnormalities in type 2 diabetes mellitus. North American Journal of Medical Sciences, 5 (1): 60.*

*Horikawa C, Kodama S, Tanaka S, Fujihara K, Hirasawa R, Yachi Y, Shimano H, Yamada N, Saito K, Sone H. Diabetes and risk of hearing impairment in adults: a meta-analysis (2012). The Journal of Clinical Endocrinology and Metabolism, 98 (1): 51-58.*

# Chapter 10

# Unscarred Gravid Uterine Rupture: A Rare Obstetrical Emergency

Nabil Abdalla[1], Monika Pazura[1], Robert Piorkowski[1], Krzysztof Cendrowski[1], Wlodzimierz Sawicki[1]

## 1. Introduction

Unscarred uterine rupture is a very rare, life-threatening obstetrical emergency. Uterine rupture may occur during pregnancy or, more frequently, during labor (Gueye et al., 2012). Spontaneous rupture of a non-gravid uterus has also been reported (Gowda et al., 2010). Clinical diagnosis may be delayed due to nonspecific symptoms and signs (Abdalla et al., 2015). A retrospective study by Gibbins et al. with 20 cases revealed that the most common signs are non-reassuring fetal heart rate patterns (50%), vaginal bleeding (45%), and abdominal pain (30%) (Gibbins et al., 2015). Early surgical intervention is the primary management of unscarred uterine rupture. Uterine rupture should be considered in the differential diagnosis of abdominal pain, abnormal cardiotocography (CTG), vaginal bleeding, and/or hemodynamic instability, even in the absence of a major risk factor, i.e., a previous caesarean section (Bank et al., 2011; Haakman et al., 2015). Due to the rarity of this disease, data on unscarred gravid uterine rupture have mainly been analyzed in case reports or retrospective studies.

## 2. Epidemiology

Rupture of an unscarred uterus is rare. The incidence rate ranges from 1:12,500 to

[1] Chair and Clinic of Obstetrics, Gynecology and Oncology, Second Faculty of Medicine, Medical University of Warsaw, Poland.

1:16,849 deliveries (Bank et al., 2011). The incidence rate of unscarred uterine rupture is higher in developing countries than developed countries. In a study by Ahmadi et al. based on 72,283 deliveries, the incidence rate was one rupture in 2,581 deliveries. The higher incidence rate can be attributed to multiparity, lack of antenatal care, neglected labor dystocia, and low socio-economic status of the patients (Ahmadi et al., 2003). The actual incidence of unscarred uterine rupture and its complications is underreported in developing countries, which can be attributed to the difficulty in accessing medical centers in these countries or a lack of autopsies in sudden-death cases (Punguyire et al., 2011). In developed countries, the estimated incidence of rupture of an unscarred gravid uterus is 0.6–0.8 per 10,000 deliveries. Most cases are associated with the use of oxytocic agents during labor induction (Cash et al., 2011). In studies by Eze et al. in Nigeria and Chen et al. in Singapore, the ratio of scarred to unscarred uterine ruptures was 1:1.7 and 1:0.3, respectively, indicating that scarring of the uterus is the dominant cause of uterine rupture in developed countries (Chen et al., 2007, Eze et al., 2010). Most cases of unscarred uterine rupture occur in women between 30 and 34 years old (Eze et al., 2010).

# 3. Risk factors

The main risk factor for uterine rupture is a prior history of caesarean section (Mizutamari et al., 2014). In cases of unscarred uteri, many non-specific risk factors have been mentioned in the literature, including excessive fundal pressure in the second stage of labor, a history of uterine instrumentation, endometriosis, fibroids, and a twin pregnancy (Cash et al., 2011). Many of these risk factors can coexist with each other, and the exact cause of uterine rupture cannot be established in some cases (Palmer et al., 2008). Langton et al. reported a spontaneous rupture of an unscarred uterus at 32 weeks of gestation without any known risk factors (Langton et al., 1997). The following risk factors have been reported to be associated with unscarred uterine rupture.

## 3.1. Multiparity

Unscarred uterine rupture occurs more often in multiparous than in nulliparous patients (Ekpo, 2000). The highest incidence of uterine rupture was reported in a study by Ekpo et al. among grandmultipara patients (Ekpo 2000). Multiparity is the leading cause of uterine rupture in developing countries, and it is related to social factors, including the desire to have a male child (Gurudut et al., 2011).

## 3.2. Previous gynecological procedures

Therapeutic curettage of the uterus may be a risk factor for uterine rupture. Unscarred uterine rupture has been reported by Abdalla et al. in a patient in her third pregnancy, where the only possible risk factor was uterine curettage after a miscarriage in the first pregnancy. An unrecognized rupture may weaken the wall of the uterus. Although the second pregnancy in this case was uneventful, the role of this surgical procedure should be considered. A second pregnancy and labor may further weaken the uterine wall, rendering it more susceptible to rupture (Abdalla et al., 2015). Manual removal of the placenta has been reported to be a possible cause of unscarred uterine rupture in a subsequent pregnancy (Esmans et al., 2004). Jo et al. suggested amniocentesis as a possible cause of a large amniocele and subsequent uterine rupture (Jo et al., 2012). Ozdemir et al. reported unscarred uterine rupture in the second trimester in a patient with two previous suction curettages due to molar pregnancies (Ozdemir et al., 2014).

## 3.3.  Prolonged labor

Prolonged labor has been reported as a risk factor for unscarred uterine rupture (Khan, 1993). Prolonged labor is associated with a larger fetal weight, feto-pelvic disproportion, and the use of oxytocin in the management of labor (Bank et al., 2011). A study by Chuni based on 101 cases of unscarred uterine rupture showed that obstructed labor was the most common cause of ruptures, accounting for 46.5% of cases (Chuni, 2006). A study by Ekpo based on 48 patients with unscarred uterine rupture showed that 46% of these cases were related to cephalo-pelvic disproportion and 21% were due to malpresentation (Ekpo, 2000).

## 3.4.  Trauma

Motor vehicle accidents, domestic violence, and falls are the most common causes of blunt trauma during pregnancy. Over 83% of hospitalizations following motor vehicle accidents during pregnancy involved a motorcycle (Sisay Woldeyes et al., 2015). Pan et al. reported a case of unscarred uterine rupture at 40 weeks of gestation after application of fundal pressure due to maternal exhaustion (Pan et al., 2002). Kurdoglu et al. reported fundal pressure as a cause of uterine rupture that was diagnosed 32 hours after vaginal delivery (Kurdoglu et al., 2009). Repeated vomiting for three days was reported by Sun et al. as a clinical presentation of uterine rupture in the second trimester. The authors suggested the possible, although difficult to prove, effect of increased intraabdominal pressure during vomiting on the uterine musculature (Sun et al., 2012).

## 3.5.  Uterotonic agents

Induction and augmentation of labor with oxytocin is a risk factor for uterine rupture (Bank et al., 2011). Misoprostol is a synthetic prostaglandin E1 analogue, and its use has been reported to be a cause of unscarred uterine rupture (Al-Hussaini, 2001). Misoprostol should be used with extreme caution, especially in multiparous patients, even if used in the context of intrauterine death or pregnancy termination (Khabbaz et al., 2001; Syed et al., 2011). Oxytocin may augment the uterotonic effect of the prostaglandin E1 analogue (Al-Hussaini, 2001; Fatfouta et al., 2008). Intracervical application of dinoprostone without the use of oxytocin has been reported to be associated with unscarred uterine rupture (Heckel et al., 1993). Ekpo suggested the possibility of an oxytocin-like effect of herbal preparations used by traditional birth attendants (TBAs) as a risk factor for unscarred uterine rupture (Ekpo, 2000).

## 3.6.  Instrumental delivery

Faria et al. reported a case of unscarred uterine rupture that was diagnosed after in-strumental delivery using vacuum extraction (VE) (Faria et al., 2012). Forceps-assisted deliveries were also reported as a risk factor for unscarred uterine rupture in 5 of 20 cases in the study by Gibbins et al. (Gibbins et al., 2015). Interpretation of these findings should be made with caution. VE and forceps are used in the second stage of labor in cases with abnormal CTG findings, which may indeed be a sign of uterine rupture. It is a matter of debate whether instrumental delivery is a risk factor for unscarred uterine rupture (Gibbins et al., 2015).

## 3.7.  Placental pathologies

Placenta accreta occurs when all or part of the placenta attaches abnormally to the my-ometrium. The most mild form is placenta accreta. Placenta increta is characterized by partial invasion of the chorionic villi into the myometrium, whereas placenta percreta is characterized by complete penetration. Placental pathologies have been reported to be a risk factor for unscarred uterine rupture (Gherman et al., 2004; Esmans et al., 2004; Pierzynski et al., 2012).

## 3.8.  Cocaine abuse

A history of cocaine abuse has been reported as a cause of unscarred uterine rupture (Agarwal et al. 2011; Gonsoulin et al., 1990). Enhanced uterine contractions caused by cocaine may be the cause of uterine rupture, and the vasoconstrictive role of cocaine may also be a factor. The situation may be further worsened by weakening of the uter-ine wall by a morbidly adherent placenta. Cocaine is also reported to cause abnormal placentation (Agarwal et al., 2011).

## 3.9.  Chronic steroid use

Chronic steroid use for systemic lupus erythematosus (SLE) has been suggested by Noh et al. as a possible cause of unscarred uterine rupture. The exact mechanism by which uterine rupture occurs in these cases is not completely understood. It has been suggest-ed that this type of rupture is caused by low estrogen levels and antibodies blocking the estrogen receptors that are capable of inducing cell-cycle progression and preventing the apoptotic cascade. Chronic steroid use may lead to insufficient growth of the uterus to accommodate rapid fetal growth and associated stretching of the uterine muscula-ture, resulting in uterine rupture (Noh et al., 2013).

## 3.10.  Other risk factors

A retained second twin, breech presentation, labor outside of the hospital, and lack of antenatal care have been reported to be associated with unscarred uterine rupture. The placement and removal of a Shirodkar cerclage during pregnancy have also been reported to be associated with unscarred uterine rupture (Fox et al., 2009). Second trimester termination of pregnancy by extra-amniotic instillation of ethacridine lactate was reported by Malhotra et al. as a cause of unscarred uterine rupture (Malhotra et al., 2007). Adenomyosis, characterized by the presence of endometrial tissues in the uterus, has been suggested as a cause of spontaneous uterine rupture in primigravid women during the early third trimester (Nikolaou et al., 2013). A procured abortion should be investigated when in doubt (Musson et al., 1977). A multiple pregnancy is a risk factor for uterine rupture due to overstretching of the uterus (Tarney et al., 2013). Samuels et al. suggested that uterine congenital anomalies may be possible causes of unscarred uterine rupture (Samuels et al., 2005). Uterine anomalies are risk factors for uterine rupture due to abnormal uterine anatomy that will rupture due to further stretching by the growing fetus. Mullerian duct anomalies may be associated with focal myometrial defects (Mizutamari et al., 2014). Tola reported first trimester spontaneous rupture in a young primigravida with a bicornuate uterus (Tola, 2014). Porcu et al. suggested exposure to diethylstilbestrol in utero as a cause of unscarred uterine rupture in the first trimester (Porcu et al., 2003).

# 4.  Classification

Uterine defects can be partial or complete (Langton et al., 1997; Nkwabong et al., 2007). In the partial type, i.e., uterine dehiscence, only the muscular layer is ruptured while the uterine serosa is intact. In the complete type, the uterine muscular layer and serosa are interrupted and the abdominal and uterine cavities communicate with each other (Matsubara et al., 2011). The amniotic membranes may be intact and inside the uterus (Abdalla et al., 2015). Gueye et al. reported protrusion of the fetus with intact membranes outside the uterus into the abdominal cavity (Gueye et al., 2012). The membranes can be ruptured with catastrophic expulsion of the fetus outside the uterus (Gurudut et al., 2011). Noh et al. reported rupture of an unscarred uterus in a primigravida in the 2nd trimester of a twin pregnancy with expulsion of only one fetus outside the uterus just adjacent to the inferior border of the liver (Noh et al., 2013). Occlusion of the defect with extrusion of the fetal legs has been reported (Blihovde et al., 2010). The rupture defect can be single or multiple (Misra et al., 2013; Leroux et al., 2014; Ble et al., 2011). Rupture of the uterus can be as small as 5 mm and can cause hemorrhagic shock at the same time (Cash et al., 2011). The defect can also be large, measuring several centimeters (Abdalla et al., 2015). The site of the uterine rupture may be related to the presence of a scar. A study by Chuni revealed that the anterior wall was the most common site of uterine rupture among scarred uterus cases. Lateral wall rupture accounted for 71.3% of unscarred uterine rupture cases (Chuni, 2006). Unscarred uterine rupture may occur at the fundus, anterior or posterior wall, or corneal region (LeMaire et al., 2001; Uzun et al., 2010; Abdalla et al., 2015; Mizutamari et al., 2014). In a study by Ofir et al., cervical involvement was significantly more common among patients without a previous uterine scar (Ofir et al., 2004). Posterior wall rupture is very rare (Abdalla et al., 2015). Hematoma of the parametrium has been reported (Dane et al., 2009; Abdalla et al., 2015). The defect can be vertical, transverse, or annular (Manouana et al., 1995; Faria et al., 2012; Malhotra et al., 2007). The maternal and fetal prognosis is relatively poor when the uterine rupture is longitudinal (Golan et al., 1980).

## 5.  Clinical features

Unscarred uterine rupture may occur during labor or even during pregnancy (Cash et al., 2011; Abdalla et al., 2015). Rupture can occur during the first, second, or third trimesters (Esmans et al., 2004; Ble et al., 2011; Blihovde et al., 2010). To our knowledge, the earliest spontaneous rupture of an unscarred uterus was documented at the 8th–10th week of pregnancy in a multiparous patient without evident risk factors (Singh et al., 2000). The onset of pain may be gradual or acute (Abdalla et al., 2015; Agarwal et al., 2011). Most cases occur in multiparous patients (Bretones et al., 1997). The presentation of uterine rupture may differ between cases with scarred and unscarred uteri. In a study by Chuni et al., the most common presentation of women with uterine rupture of an unscarred uterus was hypotension and intrauterine death, accounting for 89.1% of cases, while the most common presentation among patients with scarred uteri was abdominal tenderness (76% of cases) and fetal distress (64%) (Chuni, 2006). Noh et al. reported accidental ultrasonography diagnosis of unscarred uterine rupture in the second trimester of a twin pregnancy 3 weeks after multiple syncopes. The patient was asymptomatic, although one of the fetuses was displaced outside the uterus and embedded in the omentum (Noh et al., 2013). Atypical epigastric pain with or without vomiting has also been reported (Sakr et al., 2007). Sun et al. reported a silent rupture of an unscarred uterus, which was diagnosed due to the presence of a pelvic abscess 20 days after vaginal delivery (Sun et al., 2005).

The findings on clinical examination differ depending on the severity of the case. In extreme cases, the patient will present with signs of shock, i.e., increased heart rate, decreased blood pressure, and increased respiratory rate (Agarwal et al., 2011). Surprisingly, a good general condition and normal vital signs have been reported in cases of uterine rupture (Al-Hussaini., 2001). A typical history begins with mild abdominal pain and mild vaginal bleeding. A sudden increase to sharp pain may indicate uterine rupture (Al-Hussaini, 2001). Abdominal pain can be masked by regional analgesia (Faria et al., 2012). Shoulder tip pain is caused by irritation of the peritoneum by intraperitoneal bleeding (Langton et al., 1997). The amount of vaginal bleeding is not always correlated with blood loss, as bleeding into the peritoneal cavity may occur, or blood may collect in the broad ligament and extra-peritoneal space (Dane et al., 2009). Matsubara et al. reported an incomplete unscarred uterine rupture, which presented as a palpable abdominal mass without abdominal pain (Matsubara et al., 2011). Kurdoglu et al. reported postural hypotension as a postpartum sign of unscarred uterine rupture without abdominal pain and abnormal vaginal bleeding (Kurdoglu et al., 2009). Abdominal tenderness, abdominal guarding, and sings of peritoneal irritation may develop (Baruah et al., 2004). In complete rupture cases with dislocation of the fetus outside the uterus, the uterine contour will not be discernable, the fetal parts can be felt separately from the uterus, and, on percussion, a fluid thrill can be elicited (Agarwal et al., 2011). On vaginal examination, in these cases, the presenting part cannot be felt (Al-Hussaini., 2001). However, digital palpation of fetal parts through the cervix does not preclude the diagnosis of fetal extrusion secondary to uterine rupture (Dickinson et al., 1986). Atypical presentations with a lack of abdominal pain and clinical findings of peritoneal irritation have been reported. Cash et al. reported the postnatal diagnosis of uterine rupture after a patient who had a normal vaginal delivery presented with shortness of breath and chest pain (Cash et al., 2011). Cuellar Torriente reported a silent uterine rupture with the use of misoprostol for second trimester pregnancy termination (Cuellar Torriente, 2011). Gurudut et al. reported rupture of the posterior wall of an unscarred uterus as a cause of sudden death in a pregnant patient (Gurudut et al., 2011). Hruska et al. reported an unscarred uterine rupture diagnosed several days after a normal vaginal delivery. The patient presented with abdominal pain since delivery that worsened with time, as well as fever, chills, and dysuria (Hruska et al., 2006). Uterine contractions after labor may have a tamponade-like effect, which may delay immediate hemorrhage from the rupture site (Okano et al., 2015).

# 6.  Diagnosis

The diagnosis of unscarred uterine rupture is difficult and may be delayed up to the time of laparotomy (Mourad et al., 2015). Diagnostic difficulties can be attributed to the fact that there are no specific clinical features of the disease and that the disease entity is very rare and may not be considered in the differential diagnosis. The absence of a caesarean section in the past obstetrical history may further decrease the likelihood that clinicians will consider uterine rupture during interpretation of the clinical data (Abdalla et al., 2015). A carefully collected history of the patient should be performed to detect all possible risk factors. An assessment of the consciousness of the patient, heart rate, blood pressure, and respiratory rate can identify patients who need immediate resuscitation (Agarwal et al., 2011). The diagnosis of rupture may be established after delivery. Rapid deterioration of the mother after vaginal delivery with clinical features of shock together with hemoperitoneum should alert physicians to the possibility of uterine rupture (Leung et al., 2009). The final confirmation of the diagnosis is typically established at the time of laparotomy, where the defect is evident with or without expulsion of the fetus (Faria et al., 2012). The final diagnosis has also been reported to be established by autopsy in cases where the uterine rupture was the cause of sudden maternal death (Gurudut et al., 2011). The differential diagnosis includes obstetrical and non-obstetrical causes of abdominal pain and intraperitoneal hemorrhage. Obstetrical causes include placental abruption, intra-amniotic infection, and liver rupture (Faria et al., 2012).

## 6.1.  Full blood count

Uterine rupture may result in anemia. An acute decline in the hemoglobin and hematocrit may indicate bleeding from the rupture site (Abdalla et al., 2015).

## 6.2.  Ultrasound

Ultrasound examination can be used for an initial assessment of fetal wellbeing as well as to detect complications. Repeated ultrasound examinations may be recommended when there is a doubt about the cause of abdominal pain. Ultrasound examinations may reveal no changes in the beginning. Hemoperitoneum may develop gradually, and intraabdominal free fluid can only be seen after several hours. Non-vascularized masses in the Pouch of Douglas should raise the suspicion of clot formation (Abdalla N. et al., 2015). Uterine rupture is not always associated with hemoperitoneum (Al-Hussaini., 2001). An assessment of the placenta and its pathologies is essential. A retroplacental hematoma may provide a similar clinical picture. Placenta percreta is one of the risk factors for unscarred uterine rupture and should be investigated in patients with risk factors for this pathology, i.e., placenta previa, history of manual placental extraction, multiple pregnancies, dilatation and curettage, high parity, and advanced maternal age (Esmans et al., 2004). In cases of complete rupture of the uterus with expulsion of the fetus to the abdominal cavity, the ultrasound will show an empty uterus with or without a placenta, with a fetus beside the uterus (Al-Hussaini, 2001). In extreme cases, intrauterine fetal death can be diagnosed by ultrasound (Misra et al., 2013). Amniocele is rare and can be diagnosed by ultrasound. It can be seen as a bulging cystic lesion communicating with the intrauterine cavity (Mizutamari et al., 2014). Jo et al. reported the use of a 3D ultrasound to visualize herniation of the amniotic sac through a uterine defect at 23 weeks of gestation in a multiparous patient (Jo et al., 2012). Rana et al. reported an ultrasound diagnosis of an intact amniotic sac extrusion with a dead fetus inside (Rana et al., 2009). An ultrasound can misdiagnose the expulsion of the fetus outside the uterus in the first trimester as an ectopic pregnancy. In cases of visualization of the fetus within the tuboovarian area with free fluid in the pouch of Douglas in the first trimester, uterine rupture should be included in the differential diagnosis (Tola, 2014).

## 6.3.  Other imaging techniques

Magnetic resonance imaging (MRI) and computed tomography (CT) are of limited value because of the emergency presentation of uterine rupture. MRI has been reported to diagnose uterine rupture in a gravid uterus with non- specific signs on ultrasound examination (Hamrick-Turner et al., 1995). MRI and CT scans were also reported in the postpartum diagnosis of atypical cases of spontaneous unscarred uterine ruptures (Hruska et al., 2006; Catry et al., 2004; Mavromatidis et al., 2015). In the reported case of uterine rupture by Hruska et al., a small amount of non-specific free fluid was found in the pelvis. The MRI showed an oblong signal abnormality representing extension from the endometrial cavity through the myometrium, indicating the presence of blood within the uterine defect or a tear, which is a direct sign of spontaneous uterine rupture (Hruska et al., 2006). MRI is less operator-dependent and provides visualization with a larger field of view. MRI is also less uncomfortable for patients with a tender abdomen, does not expose the patient and fetus to radiation, and allows better evaluation of the soft tissues (Hruska et al., 2006). Arteriography can be used to identify arteriovenous malformations when there are symptoms suggesting malformations, such as an abnormal menstrual pattern or uterine atony after delivery (Langton et al., 1997).

## 6.4.  Cardiotocography

Fetal cardiotocography (CTG) is essential for assessing fetal wellbeing and uterine contractions, which may be caused by uterine rupture (Abdalla et al., 2015). An absent fetal heart rate indicates intrauterine death (Agarwal et al., 2011). Sings of fetal distress should alert the physician to a possible uterine rupture (Bank et al., 2011). The most common abnormality on CTG is fetal bradycardia, followed by variable or late decelerations (Faria et al., 2012). Fetal bradycardia may result from cord compression within the uterine rupture, loss of uterine perfusion, or placental abruption (Matsuo et al., 2008). Loss of uterine contractions is thought to be characteristic of uterine rupture. Recent evidence, however, shows that the uterine contraction pattern is not associated with uterine rupture (Matsuo et al., 2008).

## 6.5.  Histopathological assessment of the uterus

A histopathological assessment of the uterus after hysterectomy or biopsy of the defect area can be considered because it may reveal uterine diseases (Abdalla et al., 2015). Placental abnormalities, such as placenta increta and percreta, can be diagnosed (Baruah et al., 2004). Adenomyosis should be investigated, as it has been reported as a possible cause of uterine rupture (Nikolaou et al., 2013).

# 7.  Complications

Hemoperitoneum as a result of uterine rupture has been reported (Abdalla et al., 2015), and patients may present with hemorrhagic shock. Unscarred uterine rupture can cause maternal and/or fetal death. Survivors are left with morbidities, such as severe anemia, septicemia, obstetric fistulae, psychological trauma, and a prolonged recovery. Impaired reproductive functions that result from surgical management may predispose patients to marital disharmony (Eze et al., 2010). A study by Gibbins et al. compared 20 cases of unscarred uterine rupture with 126 control cases with scarred uterine rupture. Patients with uterine rupture had a higher mean estimated blood loss (2644 vs 981 ml), had a higher rate of blood transfusion (68% vs 17%), and were more likely to have a hysterectomy (35% vs 2.4%). The rate of major adverse neonatal neurological outcomes, including intraventricular hemorrhage, periventricular leukomalacia, seizures, and death, among uterine rupture cases was higher than that among control cases (40% vs 12%). Neonatal intensive care unit admissions were also more frequent (58% vs 34%) (Gibbins et al., 2015).

# 8.  Treatment

The management of an unscarred gravid uterine rupture depends mainly on the clinical features. When the patient is in shock, resuscitation should be performed immediately, and an immediate laparotomy should be offered. Further surgical management depends on the extent of uterine rupture, the clinical state of the mother and fetus, and the presence of uterine atony. Some of the procedures discussed below can be performed together. When the clinical picture is vague and the onset is not acute, referral from the district hospital to a tertiary-level hospital may be a choice for preterm pregnancies (Abdalla et al., 2015; Padhye, 2007). If possible, the diagnosis, possible complications, and type of surgery planned should be discussed with the patient (Punguyire et al., 2011).

## 8.1.  Resuscitation

Resuscitation is the initial management for all patients with shock. The main steps include airway securing, oxygen administration, and correction of hypovolemia. Multiple, preferably large-bore, intravenous accesses should be placed. Vigorous fluid resuscitation and blood product replacement should be started immediately (Dane et al., 2009).

## 8.2.  Uterotonic agents and uterine B-Lynch

Administration of uterotonic agents should be performed immediately when uterine atony is present. The successful use of a B-Lynch compression suturing technique has been reported in the management of severe uterine atony following a caesarean section and uterine rupture repair (Bank et al., 2011).

## 8.3.  Caesarean section

A Caesarean section should be performed when there is extensive uterine rupture that is unlikely to be successfully sutured or when there is bleeding (Abdalla et al., 2015). The amniotic membranes may be intact inside the uterus (Abdalla et al., 2015). The fetus and placenta can be delivered through a typical lower segment incision or, when the rupture is extensive, can be delivered through the rupture itself (Abdalla et al., 2015; de Nully et al., 1990).

## 8.4.  Local surgical repair

Local surgical repair may be a choice for preterm pregnancies with a small defect in the uterine wall without extensive bleeding and without membrane rupture. This procedure should always be considered whenever possible to maintain the woman's future child-bearing capacity (Deka et al., 2011; Smith et al., 1994). In a study by Ahmadi et al., local surgical repair was performed in most (67.9%) of the 28 unscarred uterine rupture cases (Ahmadi et al., 2003). Uterine contractions may occur after local surgical repair and need to be controlled with tocolytic medications until the pregnancy reaches term (Chen, 2007). Sterilization can be performed at the same time to prevent pregnancy complications in the future. A study by Ekpo showed that sterilization accompanied uterine repair in 42.7% of cases (Ekpo, 2000). A questionnaire administered by Kapoor et al. to fellows at the Royal College of Obstetricians and Gynecologist revealed that 80.8% of the physicians would choose uterine repair, 48% felt that in-patient management was indicated in subsequent pregnancies, and 91% would perform an elective caesarean section in subsequent pregnancies (Kapoor et al., 2003). The location of the uterine rupture may be related to the choice of management. Mokgokong et al. suggested a simple repair for defects that are small, transverse, and in the lower segment when there is no sign of infection. For ruptures in the lateral aspects of the lower and upper segments, total hysterectomy seems to be the best choice (Mokgokong et al., 1976).

## 8.5. Hysterectomy

Hysterectomy is the best choice in cases of extensive rupture, extensive necrosis of the rupture margins, uterine atony, or severe bleeding that cannot be stopped by other methods (Abdalla et al., 2015; Agarwal et al., 2011). Peripartum hysterectomy is associated with severe morbidity and should be performed by an experienced gynecologist. The hysterectomy can be total or subtotal depending on the clinical state of the patient, location of the rupture, and the gynecologist's experience. It may be technically easier and safer to perform a subtotal hysterectomy. Total hysterectomy should be considered when the placenta is located in the lower segment to prevent postpartum hemorrhage (Turner, 2002). The ovaries and tubes can be left if they are intact (Chen et al; 1995; Agarwal et al., 2011). Hematoma collection in the parametrium may extend to include the adnexal region. A unilateral adnexetomy with hysterectomy has been reported (Abdalla et al., 2015). Patients with unscarred uterine rupture delivering vaginally are more likely to undergo a hysterectomy than those delivering by caesarean section (Gibbins et al., 2015). Bladder injury is a well-recognized complication during hysterectomy and needs to be repaired at the time of laparotomy (Rashmi et al., 2001). Ligation of the internal iliac arteries may be needed to control hemorrhage (Rouzi et al., 2003).

## 8.6. Laparoscopy

Laparoscopy has a limited role in the management of unscarred gravid uterine rupture due to the associated life-threatening and unstable maternal hemodynamic condition, hemoperitoneum, and necessity of prompt fetal delivery with an abdominal approach. Sun et al. reported the successful use of laparoscopy in the management of uterine rupture that was diagnosed 20 days after vaginal delivery (Sun e al., 2005). Laparoscopy may be the best choice in first-trimester uterine rupture cases when the patient is hemodynamically stable (Tola, 2014).

## 8.7.  Medical treatment

Steroid administration should be considered between week 24+0 and 34+6 in cases of premature uterine contractions when the diagnosis of unscarred uterine rupture is doubtful and there is no need for immediate laparotomy (Deka et al., 2011).

# 9.  Prevention

In developing countries, health education, the provision of quality obstetric care, improved governance, and monitoring of the activities of TBAs may help reduce the incidence of unscarred uterine rupture (Eze et al., 2010). Efforts should be made to reduce major preventable risk factors, i.e., multiparity, in developing countries (Gurudut et al., 2011). Proper training of TBAs may reduce mortality, as the leading cause of uterine rupture in developing countries is mismanagement by TBAs (Khan et al., 2003). Improving systemic transportation to facilitate access to medical care in developing countries will also help (Punguyire et al., 2011). In developed countries, prevention of preventable risk factors may decrease the incidence of and mortality from uterine rupture. Induction or augmentation of labor with oxytocin should be managed with extreme caution and careful monitoring (Lao et al., 1987). Women should be properly instructed about safe transportation during pregnancy. They should be informed about the safety of different transportation options and instructed on precautions to avoid trauma (Sisay Woldeyes et al., 2015). Because of the rarity of unscarred uterine rupture, there is a lack of prospective studies investigating disease prevention. Unscarred uterine rupture should be kept in mind for every patient with unexplained abdominal pain (Rana et al., 2009). Early intervention by laparotomy and caesarean section can prevent maternal and fetal morbidity and mortality (Thomakos et al., 2009). Incorporating care managers (especially trained nurses) into the health care system can support the general practitioners and specialists in the management of patients (Ciccone et al., 2010).

# 10.  Prognosis

Uterine rupture is associated with worse outcomes in patients without a history of caesarean section in the past obstetrical history (Appleton et al., 2000; Rahman et al., 1985; Sandhu et al., 2002). The incidence of maternal and fetal morbidity and mortality in cases of unscarred uterine rupture is high. In a study by Ahmadi et al., the incidence of maternal and fetal mortality was 7.1% and 24.1%, respectively, among 28 cases of uterine rupture (Ahmadi et al., 2003). Delivery of a healthy baby 18 months after emergency caesarean section and repair of a uterine rupture has been reported (Bank et al., 2011). In a study by Batra et al. based on 43,886 deliveries in a low-income country, unscarred uterine rupture was confirmed in 0.04% of deliveries. The maternal and fetal mortality rates were 16.6% and 83.3%, respectively (Batra et al., 2015). Causes of maternal death include hemorrhage, shock, sepsis, disseminated intravascular coagulation, pulmonary embolism, paralytic ileus peritonitis, and renal failure (Dane et al., 2009).

# 11. Counseling

Counseling should be offered to patients with a history of uterine rupture who are considering future pregnancies, as pregnancy is not recommended for patients with a previous uterine rupture (Deka et al., 2011). Contraceptive choices should also be discussed with these patients. Risks associated with the next pregnancy should be discussed carefully with patients. Pregnant patients with a previous uterine rupture should be informed about the possible complications during pregnancy and labor as well as the need for hospitalization, careful monitoring, steroid administration, and blood transfusions when needed (Deka et al., 2011). Caesarean sections should be offered to patients with successful local surgical repair of a uterine rupture during pregnancy (Chen, 2007; Faria et al., 2012; Bank et al., 2011). A trial of vaginal delivery is associated with a high risk of rupture. Patients with a previous history of spontaneous rupture should be admitted to a tertiary-level hospital for monitoring. Close monitoring of the patient and fetus enables physicians to interfere at any time if the patient's condition deteriorates (Deka et al., 2011).

# References

Abdalla N, Reinholz-Jaskolska M, Bachanek M, Cendrowski K, Stanczak R, Sawicki W. (2015). Hemoperitoneum in a patient with spontaneous rupture of the posterior wall of an unscarred uterus in the second trimester of pregnancy. BMC Res Notes., 8:603.

Agarwal R, Gupta B, Radhakrishnan G. (2011). Rupture of intrapartum unscarred uterus at the fundus: a complication of passive cocaine abuse? Arch Gynecol Obstet., 283 Suppl 1:53–4.

Ahmadi S, Nouira M, Bibi M, Boughuizane S, Saidi H, Chaib A, Khairi H. (2003). Uterine rupture of the unscarred uterus. About 28 cases. Gynecol Obstet Fertil., 31(9):713–7.

Al-Hussaini TK. (2001). Uterine rupture in second trimester abortion in a grand multiparous woman. A complication of misoprostol and oxytocin. Eur J Obstet Gynecol Reprod Biol., 96(2):218–9.

Appleton B, Targett C, Rasmussen M, Readman E, Sale F, Permezel M. (2000). Vaginal birth after Caesarean section: an Australian multicentre study. VBAC Study Group. Aust N Z J Obstet Gynaecol., 40(1):87–91.

Bank MI, Thisted DL, Krebs L. (2011). Spontaneous rupture in the posterior wall of an unscarred uterus. J Obstet Gynaecol., 31(4):347–8.

Baruah S, Gangopadhyay P, Labib MM. (2004). Spontaneous rupture of unscarred uterus at early mid-trimester due to placenta percreta. J Obstet Gynaecol., 24(6):705.

Batra K, Gaikwad HS, Gutgutia I, Prateek S, Bajaj B. (2015). Determinants of rupture of the unscarred uterus and the related feto-maternal outcome: current scenario in a low-income country. Trop Doct., pii: 0049475515598464. PubMed PMID: 26275978.

Blé RK, Adjoussou S, Doukoure B, Gallot D, Olou N, Koffi A, Fanny M, Koné M. (2011). Placenta percreta: A rare etiology of spontaneous uterine perforation in the second trimester of pregnancy. Gynecol Obstet Fertil., 39(1):e11–4.

Blihovde L, Tawfik J, Hill DA. (2010). Prelabor third-trimester uterine rupture in an unscarred uterus with occlusion by fetal small parts: a case report. J Reprod Med., 55(9–10):437–40.

Bretones S, Cousin C, Gualandi M, Mellier G. (1997). Uterine rupture. A case of spontaneous rupture in a thirty week primiparous gestation. J Gynecol Obstet Biol Reprod (Paris) ., 26(3):324–7.

Cash S, Hodge W, Kuah S. (2011). An unusual clinical presentation of uterine rupture of an unscarred uterus. Aust N Z J Obstet Gynaecol., 51(6):564–5.

Catry F, Geusens E, Vanbeckevoort D, Volders W, Bielen D, Spitz B. (2004). Abdom Imaging., 29(1):120–2. Delivery related rupture of the gravid uterus: imaging findings.

Chen FP. (2007). Term delivery after repair of a uterine rupture during the second trimester in a previously unscarred uterus: a case report. J Reprod Med., 52(10):981–3.

Chen LH, Tan KH, Yeo GS. (1995). A ten-year review of uterine rupture in modern obstetric practice. Ann Acad Med Singapore., 24(6):830–5.

Ciccone MM, Aquilino A, Cortese F, et al. (2010). Feasibility and effectiveness of a disease and care management model in the primary health care system for patients with heart failure and diabetes (Project Leonardo). Vascular Health and Risk Management., 6:297–305.

Cuellar Torriente M. (2011). Silent uterine rupture with the use of misoprostol for second trimester termination of pregnancy : a case report. Obstet Gynecol Int., 584652.

Chuni N. (2006). Analysis of uterine rupture in a tertiary center in Eastern Nepal: lessons for obstetric care. J Obstet Gynaecol Res., 32(6):574–9.

Dane B, Dane C. (2009). Maternal death after uterine rupture in an unscarred uterus: a case report. J Emerg Med., 37(4):393–5.

Deka D, Bahadur A, Dadhwal V, Gurunath S, Vaid A. (2011). Successful outcome in pregnancy complicated by prior uterine rupture: a report of two cases. Arch Gynecol Obstet. 283 Suppl., 1:45–8.

de Nully P, Tobiassen C. (1990). Rupture of the pregnant uterus. Ugeskr Laeger., 152(3):170.

Dickinson JE, Newnham JP, Roberts RV, Reid SE. (1986). Oxytocin induced second trimester uterine rupture. Aust N Z J Obstet Gynaecol., 26(4):251–2.

Ekpo EE. (2000). Uterine rupture as seen in the University of Calabar Teaching Hospital, Nigeria: a five-year review. J Obstet Gynaecol., 20(2):154–6.

Esmans A, Gerris J, Corthout E, Verdonk P, Declercq S. (2004). Placenta percreta causing rupture of an unscarred uterus at the end of the first trimester of pregnancy: case report. Hum Reprod., 19(10):2401–3.

Eze JN, Ibekwe PC. (2010). Uterine rupture at a secondary hospital in Afikpo, Southeast Nigeria. Singapore Med J., 51(6):506–11.

Faria J, Henriques C, Silva Mdo C, Mira R. (2012). Rupture of an unscarred uterus diagnosed in the puerperium: a rare occurrence. BMJ Case Rep., pii: bcr2012006372.

Fatfouta I, Villeroy de Galhau S, Dietsch J, Eicher E, Perrin D. (2008). Spontaneous uterine rupture of an unscarred uterus during labor: case report and review of the literature]. J Gynecol Obstet Biol Reprod (Paris) ., 37(2):200–3.

Fox NS, Rebarber A, Bender S, Saltzman DH. (2009). Labor outcomes after Shirodkar cerclage. J Reprod Med., 54(6):361–5.

Gherman RB, Lockrow EG, Flemming DJ, Satin AJ. (2004). Conservative management of spontaneous *uterine perforation associated with placenta accreta: a case report. J Reprod Med., 49(3):210–3.*

Gibbins KJ, Weber T, Holmgren CM, Porter TF, Varner MW, Manuck TA. (2015). *Maternal and fetal morbidity associated with uterine rupture of the unscarred uterus. Am J Obstet Gynecol., 213(3):382.e1–6.*

Golan A, Sandbank O, Rubin A. (1980). *Rupture of the pregnant uterus. Obstet Gynecol., 56(5):549–54.*

Gonsoulin W, Borge D, Moise KJ Jr. (1990). *Rupture of unscarred uterus in primigravid woman in association with cocaine abuse. Am J Obstet Gynecol., 163(2):526–7.*

Gowda M, Garcia L, Maxwell E, Malik R, Gulyaeva L, Tsai MC. (2010). *Spontaneous uterine rupture in a nulligravida female presenting with unexplained recurrent hematometra. Clin Exp Obstet Gynecol., 37(1):60–2.*

Guèye M, Mbaye M, Ndiaye-Guèye MD, Kane-Guèye SM, Diouf AA, Niang MM, Diaw H, Moreau JC. (2012). *Spontaneous Uterine Rupture of an Unscarred Uterus before Labour. Case Rep Obstet Gynecol., 598356.*

Gurudut KS, Gouda HS, Aramani SC, Patil RH. (2011). *Spontaneous rupture of unscarred gravid uterus. J Forensic Sci., 56 Suppl 1:S263–5.*

Haakman O, Ambrose D, Katopodis C, Altman AD. (2015). *Spontaneous Rupture of an Unscarred Uterus Diagnosed Postpartum: A Case Report. J Obstet Gynaecol Can., 37(11):1021–4.*

Hamrick-Turner JE, Cranston PE, Lantrip BS. (1995). *Gravid uterine dehiscence: MR findings. Abdom Imaging., 20(5):486–8.*

Heckel S, Ohl J, Dellenbach P. (1993). *Rupture of an unscarred uterus at full term after an intracervical application of dinoprostone (Prepidil) gel. Rev Fr Gynecol Obstet., 88(3):162–4.*

Hruska KM, Coughlin BF, Coggins AA, Wiczyk HP. (2006). *MRI diagnosis of spontaneous uterine rupture of an unscarred uterus. Emerg Radiol., 12(4):186–8.*

Jo YS, Kim MJ, Lee GS, Kim SJ. (2012). *A large amniocele with protruded umbilical cord diagnosed by 3D ultrasound. Int J Med Sci., 9(5):387–90.*

Kapoor DS, Sharma SD, Alfirevic Z. (2003). *Management of unscarred ruptured uterus. J Perinat Med., 31(4):337–9.*

Rouzi AA, Hawaswi AA, Aboalazm M, Hassanain F, Sindi O. (2003). *Uterine rupture incidence, risk factors, and outcome. Saudi Med J., 24(1):37–9.*

Khabbaz AY, Usta IM, El-Hajj MI, Abu-Musa A, Seoud M, Nassar AH. (2001). *Rupture of an unscarred uterus with misoprostol induction: case report and review of the literature. J Matern Fetal Med, 10(2):141–5.*

Khan NH. (1993). *Rupture of the uterus. J Pak Med Assoc., 43(9):174–6.*

Khan S, Parveen Z, Begum S, Alam I. (2003). *Uterine rupture: a review of 34 cases at Ayub Teaching Hospital Abbottabad. J Ayub Med Coll Abbottabad., 15(4):50–2.*

Kurdoglu M, Kolusari A, Yildizhan R, Adali E, Sahin HG. (2009). *Delayed diagnosis of an atypical rupture of an unscarred uterus due to assisted fundal pressure: a case report. Cases J., 2:7966.*

Langton J, Fishwick K, Kumar B, Nwosu EC. (1997). *Spontaneous rupture of an unscarred gravid uterus at 32 weeks gestation. Hum Reprod., 12(9):2066–7.*

Lao TT, Leung BF. (1987). *Rupture of the gravid uterus. Eur J Obstet Gynecol Reprod Biol., 25(3):175–80.*

LeMaire WJ, Louisy C, Dalessandri K, Muschenheim F. (2001). *Placenta percreta with spontaneous rupture of an unscarred uterus in the second trimester. Obstet Gynecol., 98(5 Pt 2):927–9. PubMed PMID: 11704207.*

*Leung F, Courtois L, Aouar Z, Bourtembourg A, Eckman A, Terzibachian JJ, Maillet R, Riethmuller D. (2009). Spontaneous rupture of the unscarred uterus during labor. Case report. Gynecol Obstet Fertil., 37(4):342–5.*

*Leroux M, Coatleven F, Faure M, Horovitz J. (2014). Bilateral uterine rupture of an unscarred gravid uterus before labor. Gynecol Obstet Fertil., 42(6):454–7.*

*Malhotra N, Chanana C. (2007). Silent rupture of unscarred uterus: an unusual presentation at second trimester abortion. Arch Gynecol Obstet., 275(4):283–5.*

*Manouana M, Louis O, Lorgeron P, Pettini R, Lameyre D, Meynieu F. (1995). Spontaneous rupture of an unscarred uterus during labor and epidural anesthesia. J Gynecol Obstet Biol Reprod (Paris)., 24(5):557–60.*

*Matsubara S, Shimada K, Kuwata T, Usui R, Suzuki M. (2011). Thin anterior uterine wall with incomplete uterine rupture in a primigravida detected by palpation and ultrasound: a case report. J Med Case Rep., 5:14.*

*Matsuo K, Scanlon JT, Atlas RO, Kopelman JN. (2008). Staircase sign: a newly described uterine contraction pattern seen in rupture of unscarred gravid uterus. J Obstet Gynaecol Res., 34(1):100–4.*

*Mavromatidis G, Karavas G, Margioula-Siarkou C, Petousis S, Kalogiannidis I, Mamopoulos A, Rousso D. (2015). Spontaneous postpartum rupture of an intact uterus: a case report. J Clin Med Res., 7(1):56–8.*

*Misra M, Roychowdhury R, Sarkar NC, Koley MM. (2013). The spontaneous prelabour rupture of anunscarred uterus at 34 weeks of pregnancy. J Clin Diagn Res., 7(3):548–9.*

*Mizutamari E, Honda T, Ohba T, Katabuchi H. (2014). Spontaneous rupture of an unscarred gravid uterus in a primigravid woman at 32 weeks of gestation. Case Rep Obstet Gynecol., 2014:209585.*

*Mokgokong ET, Marivate M. (1976). Treatment of the ruptured uterus. S Afr Med J., 50(41):1621–4.*

*Mourad WS, Bersano DJ, Greenspan PB, Harper DM. (2015). Spontaneous rupture of unscarred uterus in a primigravida with preterm prelabour rupture of membranes. BMJ Case Rep., pii: bcr2014207321.*

*Musson FA. (1977). Nine-week survival of the fetus following spontaneous mid-trimester rupture of an unscarred uterus. Proc R Soc Med., 70(8):533–4.*

*Nikolaou M, Kourea HP, Antonopoulos K, Geronatsiou K, Adonakis G, Decavalas G. (2013). Spontaneous uterine rupture in a primigravid woman in the early third trimester attributed to adenomyosis: a case report and review of the literature. J Obstet Gynaecol Res.. 39(3):727–32.*

*Nkwabong E, Kouam L, Takang W. (2007) Spontaneous uterine rupture during pregnancy: case report and review of literature. Afr J Reprod Health., 11(2):107–12.*

*Noh JJ, Park CH, Jo MH, Kwon JY. (2013). Rupture of an unscarred uterus in a woman with long-term steroid treatment for systemic lupus erythematosus. Obstet Gynecol., 122(2 Pt 2):472–5.*

*Ofir K, Sheiner E, Levy A, Katz M, Mazor M. (2004). Uterine rupture: differences between a scarred and an unscarred uterus. Am J Obstet Gynecol., 191(2):425–9.*

*Okano S, Erfan I, Eskandar O. (2015). Postpartum uterine rupture in an unscarred uterus. J Obstet Gynaecol., 15:1–2.*

*Ozdemir A, Ertas IE, Gungorduk K, Kaya C, Solmaz U, Yildirim G. (2014). Uterine preservation in* placenta percreta complicated by unscarred uterine rupture at second trimester in a patient with repeated molar pregnancies: a case report and brief review of the literature. Clin Exp Obstet Gynecol., 41(5):590–2.

Padhye SM. (2007). Rupture uterus in primigravida: morbidity and mortality. Kathmandu Univ Med J (KUMJ)., 5(4):492–6.

Palmer JM, Indermaur MD, Tebes CC, Spellacy WN. (2008). Placenta increta and cocaine abuse in a grand multipara leading to a second trimester rupture of an unscarred uterus: a case report. South Med J., 101(8):834–5.

Pan HS, Huang LW, Hwang JL, Lee CY, Tsai YL, Cheng WC. (2002). Uterine rupture in an unscarred uterus after application of fundal pressure. A case report. J Reprod Med., 47(12):1044–6. PubMed PMID: 12516327.

Pierzynski P, Laudanski P, Lemancewicz A, Sulkowski S, Laudanski T. (2012). Spontaneous rupture of unscarred uterus in the early second trimester: a case report of placenta percreta. Ginekol Pol., 83(8):626–9.

Porcu G, Courbière B, Sakr R, Carcopino X, Gamerre M. (2003). Spontaneous rupture of a first-trimester gravid uterus in a woman exposed to diethylstilbestrol in utero. A case report. J Reprod Med., 48(9):744–6.

Punguyire D, Iserson KV. (2011). A ruptured uterus in a pregnant woman not in labor. Pan Afr Med J., 8:2.

Rahman J, Al-Sibai MH, Rahman MS. (1985). Rupture of the uterus in labor. A review of 96 cases. Acta Obstet Gynecol Scand., 64(4):311–5.

Rana R, Puri M. (2009). Pre-labor silent rupture of unscarred uterus at 32 weeks with intact amniotic sac extrusion: a case report. Cases J., 2:7095.

Rashmi, Radhakrisknan G, Vaid NB, Agarwal N. (2001). Rupture uterus — changing Indian scenario. J Indian Med Assoc., 99(11):634–7.

Rouzi AA, Hawaswi AA, Aboalazm M, Hassanain F, Sindi O. (2003). Uterine rupture incidence, risk factors, and outcome. Saudi Med J., 24(1):37–9.

Sakr R, Berkane N, Barranger E, Dubernard G, Daraï E, Uzan S. (2007). Unscarred uterine rupture — case report and literature review. Clin Exp Obstet Gynecol., 34(3):190–2.

Samuels TA, Awonuga A. (2005). Second-trimester rudimentary uterine horn pregnancy: rupture after labor induction with misoprostol. Obstet Gynecol., 106(5 Pt 2):1160–2.

Sandhu AK, Al-Jufairi ZA. (2002). A comparative analysis of uterine rupture in 2 decades. Saudi Med J., 23(12):1466–9.

Singh A, Jain S. (2000). Spontaneous rupture of unscarred uterus in early pregnancy—a rare entity. Acta Obstet Gynecol Scand., 79(5):431–2.

Sisay Woldeyes W, Amenu D, Segni H. (2015). Uterine Rupture in Pregnancy following Fall from a Motorcycle: A Horrid Accident in Pregnancy-A Case Report and Review of the Literature. Case Rep Obstet Gynecol., 2015:715180. doi:10.1155/2015/715180.

Smith AJ, LeMire WA 3rd, Hurd WW, (1994). Pearlman M. Repair of the traumatically ruptured gravid uterus. A report of two cases resulting in viable pregnancies. J Reprod Med., 39(10):825–8.

Sun CH, Liao CI, Kan YY. (2005). "Silent" rupture of unscarred gravid uterus with subsequent pelvic abscess: successful laparoscopic management. J Minim Invasive Gynecol., 12(6):519–21.

Sun HD, Su WH, Chang WH, Wen L, Huang BS, Wang PH. (2012). *Rupture of a pregnant unscarred uterus in an early secondary trimester: a case report and brief review.* J Obstet Gynaecol Res., 38(2):442–5.

Syed S, Noreen H, Kahloon LE, Chaudhri R. (2011). *Uterine rupture associated with the use of intra-vaginal misoprostol during second-trimester pregnancy termination.* J Pak Med Assoc, 61(4):399–401. PubMed PMID: 21465985.

Tarney CM, Whitecar P, Sewell M, Grubish L, Hope E. (2013). *Rupture of an unscarred uterus in a quadruplet pregnancy.* Obstet Gynecol., 121(2 Pt 2 Suppl 1):483–5.

Thomakos N, Kallianidis K, Voulgaris Z, Drakakis P, Arefetz N, Antsaklis A. (2009). *Extrauterine pregnancy resulting from late spontaneous rupture of an unscarred gravid uterus: case report.* Clin Exp Obstet Gynecol., 36(3):192–3.

Tola EN. (2014). *First trimester spontaneous uterine rupture in a young woman with uterine anomaly.* Case Rep Obstet Gynecol., 2014:967386.

Turner MJ. (2002). *Uterine rupture.* Best Pract Res Clin Obstet Gynaecol., 16(1):69–79.

Uzun I, Yildirim A, Kalelioglu I, Has R. (2010). *Spontaneous rupture of unscarred uterus at 27 weeks of gestation.* Arch Gynecol Obstet., 281(6):999–1001.

# Chapter 11

# Serum Magnesium Levels and Cardiovascular Outcome in Patients with Advanced Chronic Kidney Disease

Olimpia Ortega[1]

## 1  Introduction

The kidney has a vital role in magnesium homeostasis and thus impairment in renal function has long been recognized as a frequent prerequisite for the development of hypermagnesemia. Traditionally, it has been recommended to avoid oral magnesium supplementation among patients with chronic kidney disease to prevent hypermagnesemia. However, Mg has beneficial effects on cardiovascular system and, in the last years, several authors highlighted the association between lower serum Mg levels and vascular calcification, cardiovascular events and mortality in patients with end-stage renal disease (Kanbay et al., 2010; Massy & Drüeke, 2012; Spiegel, 2011). These findings allow speculating on the possible salutary role of increasing plasma levels of Mg using Mg-based compounds as phosphate binders, to facilitate the healing of vascular injuries. Although a small nonrandomized study suggests minimal progression of vascular calcification in magnesium-supplemented dialysis patients (Spiegel & Farmer, 2009), the long-term effects on both the inhibition of vascular calcification or changes in bone morphology have not been adequately investigated. Otherwise, another relative small prospective study failed to show any association between serum magnesium and mortality or future cardiovascular events among patients with advanced chronic kidney disease not yet on dialysis (Ortega et al., 2013) and more recently, the lowest Mg levels were observed in malnourished and inflamed dialysis patients with cardiac damage (Kurita et al., 2015). These findings may suggest that hypomagnesemia could be a mere marker of illness condition

---

[1] Department of Nephrology, Hospital Severo Ochoa, Leganés, Madrid, Spain.

among patients with end-stage renal disease rather than an active participant in cardio-vascular damage.

In this chapter, we try to analyze the results of some reports to support or to do not support the possible implication of magnesium in cardiovascular damage and cardiovas-cular outcome among patients with advanced chronic kidney disease.

## 2   Magnesium Physiology

Magnesium (Mg) is the 2nd most abundant intracellular divalent cation and functions as a modulator of several enzymes (Wolf & Cittadini, 1999). The total body amount is ap-proximately 25 g: 66% of it is stored in bone, 33% is intracellular and only 1% is extracel-lular; thus, serum magnesium concentration does not reflect total body magnesium con-tent. Normal serum Mg values range from 1.8 to 3 mg/dl (Fox et al., 2001).

Magnesium homeostasis in humans depends on the balance between intestinal up-take and renal excretion (Figure 1). Principal dietary sources of magnesium include green vegetables, seafood, meats, grains and nuts (Spiegel, 2010). The control of body Mg ho-meostasis resides primarily in the kidney tubules. Renal tubular reabsorption is increased by extracellular volume contraction, hypomagnesemia and a high serum of PTH level (Moe, 2005).

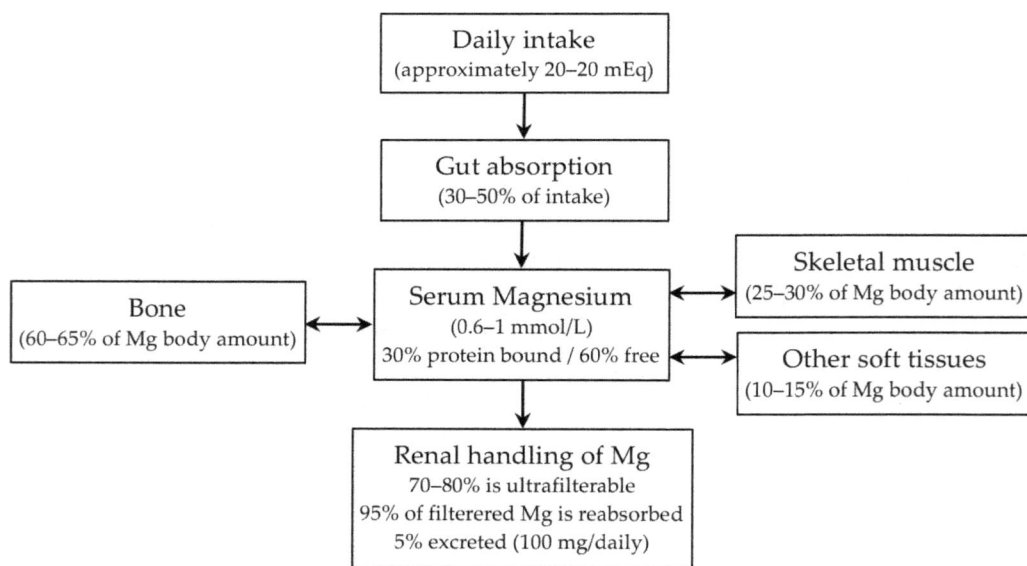

**Figure 1:** Magnesium homeostasis.

## 3   Magnesium Balance in End-stage Renal Disease Patients

Chronic kidney disease (CKD) is the most common cause of hypermagnesemia which is usually mild and asymptomatic. When CKD progresses, urinary Mg excretion may be insufficient to balance intestinal Mg absorption, and serum Mg increases. At this point, dietary Mg intake becomes a major determinant of serum and total body Mg levels (Navarro-Gonzalez et al., 2009). Vitamin D has an important role in absorption of Mg in the jejunum in healthy subjects and in patients with end-stage renal disease (Schmulen et al., 1980). Gastrointestinal magnesium absorption is felt to be normal in patients with CKD although one small study suggested it was decreased compared to normal controls, possibly due to low 1,25 dihydroxy-vitamin D levels (Branan et al., 1976)

In CKD patients, administration of Mg-containing drugs (e.g. antiacids and laxatives) and high Mg concentrations of dialysate may provoke severe or even fatal hypermagnesemia (Fox et al., 2001). PTH can also contribute to hypermagnesemia in CKD patients by increasing gastrointestinal absorption, bone resorption and renal reabsorption. On the other hand, hypermagnesemia inhibits PTH secretion (Cholst et al., 1984; Navarro et al., 1997).

However, even in CKD patients some conditions can lead to negative Mg balance, such as excessive intake of diuretics, reduced gastrointestinal uptake and a low concentration in the dialysate (Truttmann et al., 2002).

## 4    The Beneficial Effect of Mg in the General Population

There is strong evidence suggesting that hypomagnesemia play a significant role in the development of cardiovascular (CV) disease in the general population (Liao et al., 1998; Ma et al., 1995) and some studies provide further evidence that intake of dietary Mg is associated with reduced risk of coronary heart disease (Abott et al., 2003). Low Mg intake may also exacerbate metabolic abnormalities and depression in elderly diabetic patients and may reduce physical performance (Huang et al., 2012).

The benefits of Mg on CV outcome could be explained by its effect on CV system. Mg reduces total peripheral resistance by stimulation of nitric oxide synthesis (Zheng et al., 2001) and in a small trial, it was observed that oral administration of magnesium for a 6-month period improved flow-mediated vasodilatation and exercise tolerance in patients with stable coronary artery disease (Shechter et al., 2000). Magnesium is also a potent inhibitor of vascular calcification (Kircelli et al., 2012; Salem et al., 2012). Magnesium depletion has also been implicated in ventricular arrhythmias and has been associated with a prolonged QT interval (Seelig, 1969). Moreover, Mg deficiency has been reported to promote inflammation and it decreases the specific immune response (Mazur et al., 2007). Experimental findings in animal models suggest that inflammation is the missing link to explain the role of Mg in many pathological conditions (Kanbay et al., 2010).

## 5    Magnesium and Cardiovascular Outcome in Patients with Chronic Kidney Disease

Cardiovascular disease is the leading cause of mortality and morbidity in patients with

CKD. Several traditional and non-traditional risk factors have been identified as predictors of increased mortality in end-stage-renal- disease patients. Accelerated atherosclerosis associated with vascular calcification of intima and media layers and arterial stiffness are frequent findings in these patients (Scholze et al., 2007) and it is a strong risk factor for increased morbidity and mortality (Blacher et al., 2001; Goodman et al., 2000).

In hemodialysis patients, an inverse association between serum Mg and the common carotid intima-media thickness has been observed (Turgut et al., 2008; Tzanikis et al., 2004). The pathogenesis of vascular calcification in CKD is likely to be multifactorial. It appears to be a process that closely resembles the formation of normal bone tissue as some factors act upon the vascular smooth muscle cells influencing their conversion into osteoblast-like cells (Giachelli et al., 2001; Schoppet et al., 2008; Speer & Giachelli, 2004). It has been observed in vitro that Mg prevents this conversion and also increased the expression of anti-calcification proteins (Montezano et al., 2010) (Figure 2).

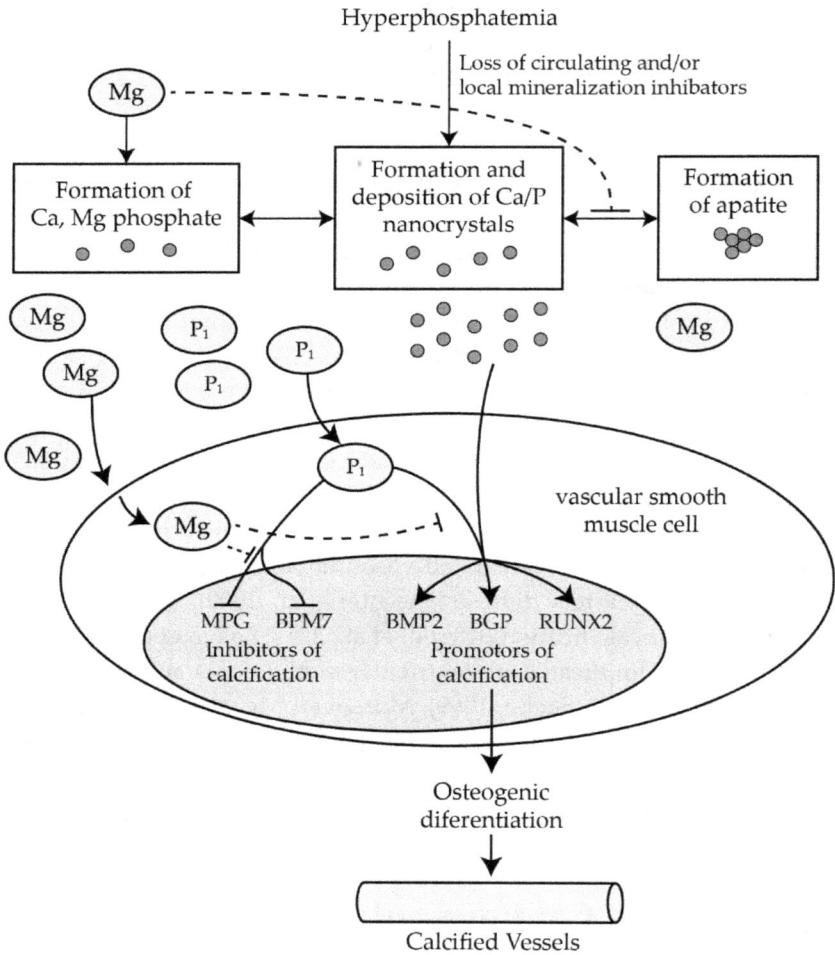

**Figure 2:** The protective roles of magnesium in the course of vascular calcification (modified from Massy & Drüeke, 2012).

Otherwise, hypermagnesemia inhibits PTH secretion and PTH has been reported to play a predominant role in the initiation and progression of vascular calcification (Ganesh et al., 2001). However, some authors suggest that the potential effect of Mg on PTH constitute indirect evidence and does not permit to draw firm conclusions (Cunningham et al., 2012).

Some observational studies have detected an association of low serum Mg concentration and all-cause mortality and cardiovascular mortality even after adjustment for known confounders (Ishimura et al., 2007; Sakaguchi et al., 2014). Recently, a "U shaped" association between serum magnesium and all-cause death has been observed in dialysis patients (Kurita et al., 2015). In this study, patients with the lowest Mg levels tended to be older and had a higher likelihood of diabetic nephropathy, atrial fibrillation and heart failure. These patients showed lower serum phosphorus, potassium and albumin and high serum ferritin and CRP levels. These findings suggest that lower serum Mg may be associated with higher comorbidities, malnutrition and inflammation. The association between lower serum Mg and cardiovascular mortality has also been observed in patients with advanced renal failure not yet on dialysis (Kanbay et al., 2012).

All these findings, added to the beneficial effect of Mg in the reduction of vascular calcification, support its usage as phosphate binder in patients with CKD. Several authors have analyzed the effect of using Mg-based compounds as phosphate binders (Delmez et al., 1996; Spiegel et al., 2007; Tzanakis et al., 2008). All of them concluded that Mg can be administered to many patients without acute adverse side effects and can help to reduce the total calcium intake when substituted for phosphate binder in patients with end-stage renal disease. Serum levels of Mg should always be measured to avoid potential toxicity. However, the long-term effects on both the inhibition of vascular calcification or changes in bone morphology have not been adequately investigated.

In the last years our group has evaluated whether serum Mg level could be an independent predictor of mortality and future cardiovascular (CV) events in patients with advanced CKD not yet on dialysis (Ortega et al., 2013). Seventy patients with CKD stages 4 and 5 (mean creatinine clearance -CrC- at the start $20\pm7$ ml/min) were included. After a single measurement of serum Mg level, patients were followed-up for time-to-event. Primary end-point was all-cause mortality and secondary end-point was the development of fatal or non-fatal CV event. Patients who initiated dialysis during the study period were not censored and were followed until death or until the end of the study. Mean follow-up in this first study was $11\pm2.8$ months.

Mean serum magnesium level was within normal range in our patients ($2.1\pm0.4$ mg/dl), was lower in men ($2.04\pm0.3$ vs. $2.3\pm0.3$ mg/dl in women; p=0.008) and in diabetic patients ($1.98\pm0.3$ vs. $2.2\pm0.3$ in non-diabetic patients; p=0.002). We found no significant differences in Mg levels between patients with and without clinical evident cardiopathy or between patients with and without peripheral vascular disease.

At baseline, serum magnesium did not correlate significantly with patient's age, and with bone and mineral metabolism parameters included PTH levels (p=0.4). No relationship between serum magnesium and basal creatinine clearance was found (r=–0.09; p=0.46). We also found no significant correlation between serum Mg and nutritional data, inflammatory (CRP) and cardiac (NT-proBNP) biomarkers. Serum Mg did not correlate with blood hemoglobin or with the weekly dose of erythropoiesis stimulating agents. On the contrary, serum Mg correlated inversely with the daily dose of loop diuretics although the correlation did not achieved statistical signification (r=–0.23; p=0.052). Serum Mg was slightly higher although no significant, in those patients who did not use diuretics (2.16±0,4 vs. 2.06 ±0.8; p=0.057).

During follow-up, serum Mg did not predict all-cause death and was not an independent predictor of CV events either in univariate or in multivariate analysis. More recently, we have extended the follow-up period (Table 1–2; Figure 3–4) of the same patients to 39±13 months (author's unpublished data). During this period, 11 patients (14%) died, 22 patients (33%) suffered a fatal or non-fatal cardiovascular event and 32 patients (46%) initiated renal replacement therapy. These patients who initiated dialysis were not censored at initiation and were followed until death, transplantation or until the end of the study. Again serum Magnesium at baseline was not associated with overall mortality or with the development of CV events either in univariate or in multivariate Cox proportion analysis. The independent predictors of death in our patients are expressed in Table 1; multivariate analysis showed that only patient's age and renal function (CrC) at baseline were associated with all-cause mortality in our study.

Figure 3 shows the Kaplan Meyer curves of all cause mortality according to median baseline serum Mg levels (<2.1 mg/dl or >2.1 mg/dl); there were no significant differences in both survival curves (p=0.4 by the log-rank test). The factors associated with the development of fatal or non-fatal CV events are expressed in Table2. The multivariate Cox analysis demonstrated that diabetes, the presence of peripheral vascular disease and proteinuria were predictors of cardiovascular events.

Figure 4 expresses the Kaplan-Meier development of fatal and nonfatal cardiovascular events curves according to median baseline serum magnesium levels (<2.1 mg/dl or>2.1 mg/dl). There were no significant differences in both curves (p= 0.7 by the log-rank test). As serum Mg was slightly higher in patients who did not use diuretics, we conducted the same analysis excluding those patients and the results were very similar. Newly serum Mg was not associated with mortality (HR: 1.5; 95% CI: 0.15-14.7; p>0.05) or cardiovascular events (HR: 0.4; 95% CI: 0.08-25; p>0.05). Nevertheless, the proportion of patients without diuretics in our study was very low (9%).

Our results are not consistent with those reported by other authors who suggest a survival advantage in patients with slightly elevated serum Mg concentration. Probably, the smaller sample size in our study is one of our mayor limitations, although the follow-up period was long (more than 3 years) in its second part. In a similar study performed also in patients with advanced CKD not yet on dialysis (Kanbay et al., 2012) the authors found that serum Mg may be an independent predictor of future cardiovascular outcome. Surprisingly, no patient in that study received diuretics while most of our pre-dialysis patients used loop diuretics at different doses as part of our strategy of strict volume control. Since, as expected, we found an inverse correlation between serum Mg and the daily dose of loop diuretics, we could hypothesize that serum Mg levels could be modified by the use of diuretics and hence changing the effect of serum magnesium on cardiovascular outcome in our patients. However, serum Mg did not predict death or cardiovascular events after excluding patients without diuretic therapy. Otherwise, some authors have

| Items | Univariate Analysis | | | Multivariate Analysis | | |
|---|---|---|---|---|---|---|
| | HR | 95%CI | P | HR | 95%CI | P |
| Age (years) | 1.09 | 1.03–1.16 | 0.003 | 1.09 | 1.02–1.17 | 0.004 |
| Diabetes (y/n) | 1.67 | 0.53–5.3 | 0.38 | | | |
| Cardiopathy (y/n) | 1.6 | 0.49–4.9 | 0.4 | | | |
| Peripheral vasc. dis. (y/n) | 3.3 | 1.05–10.2 | 0.04 | | | |
| Serum Mg (mg/dL) | 1.7 | 0.29–9.8 | 0.56 | | | |
| Calcium (mg/dL) | 1.97 | 0.76–5.1 | 0.16 | | | |
| Phosphate (mg/dL) | 0.98 | 0.53–1.8 | 0.94 | | | |
| PTH (pg/mL) | 1.001 | 0.99–1.003 | 0.21 | | | |
| 25 OH vit D (ng/mL) | 0.98 | 0.91–1.07 | 0.7 | | | |
| Serum Albumin (g/dL) | 0.65 | 0.17–2.39 | 0.49 | | | |
| Transferrin (mg/dL) | 0.98 | 0.97–1.00 | 0.052 | | | |
| Proteinuria (g/24h) | 0.92 | 0.66–1.27 | 0.6 | | | |
| CrC (mL/min) | 0.89 | 0.8–0.97 | 0.009 | 0.88 | 0.78–0.99 | 0.036 |
| Hemoglobin (g/dL) | 0.79 | 0.54–1.15 | 0.2 | | | |
| CRP (mg/L) | 1.06 | 0.95–1.08 | 0.65 | | | |

**Table 1**: Predictors of overall mortality. Cox analysis.

| Items | Univariate Analysis | | | Multivariate Analysis | | |
|---|---|---|---|---|---|---|
| | HR | 95%CI | P | HR | 95%CI | P |
| Age (years) | 1.035 | 1.001–1.07 | 0.046 | | | |
| Diabetes (y/n) | 7.6 | 2.94–19.7 | <0.001 | 9.6 | 3.02–30.2 | <0.001 |
| Cardiopathy (y/n) | 5.2 | 2.07–12.7 | <0.001 | | | |
| Peripheral vasc. dis. (y/n) | 8.3 | 3.4–20.3 | <0.001 | 9.6 | 3.02–30.2 | <0.001 |
| Serum Mg (mg/dL) | 1.3 | 0.37–4.8 | 0.66 | | | |
| Calcium (mg/dL) | 0.75 | 0.37–1.5 | 0.43 | | | |
| Phosphate (mg/dL) | 1.1 | 0.75–1.65 | 0.6 | | | |
| PTH (pg/mL) | 0.99 | 0.98–1.001 | 0.51 | | | |
| 25 OH vit D (ng/mL) | 1.007 | 0.96–1.05 | 0.75 | | | |
| Serum Albumin (g/dL) | 0.26 | 0.13–0.56 | 0.001 | | | |
| Transferrin (mg/dL) | 0.99 | 0.98–1.003 | 0.14 | | | |
| Proteinuria (g/24h) | 1.11 | 0.99–1.25 | 0.06 | 1.23 | 1.06–1.4 | 0.007 |
| CrC (mL/min) | 0.99 | 0.93–1.05 | 0.65 | | | |
| Hemoglobin (g/dL) | 0.96 | 0.73–1.27 | 0.79 | | | |
| CRP (mg/L) | 1.05 | 1.01-1.098 | 0.012 | | | |

**Table 2:** Predictors of fatal and non-fatal cardiovascular events. Cox analysis.

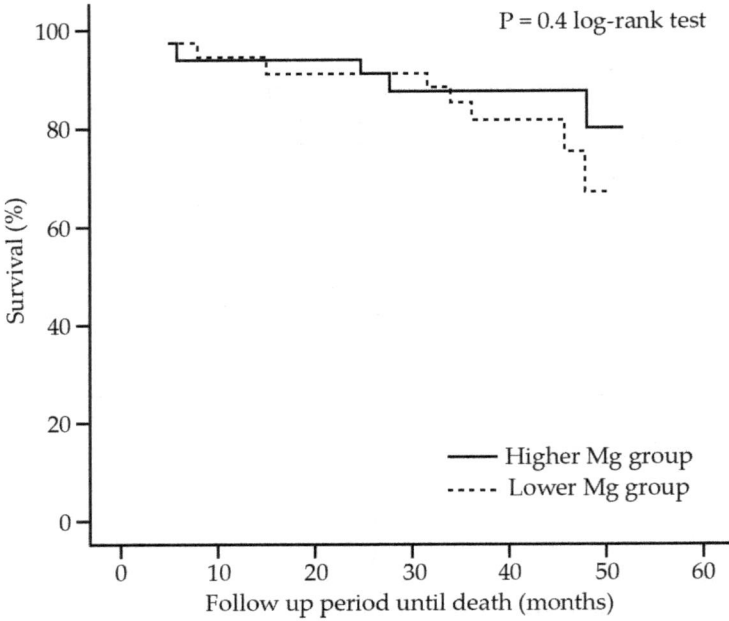

**Figure 3:** Kaplan-Meier survival curves according to median serum magnesium levels (<2.1 mg/dL or ≥ 2.1 mg/dL).

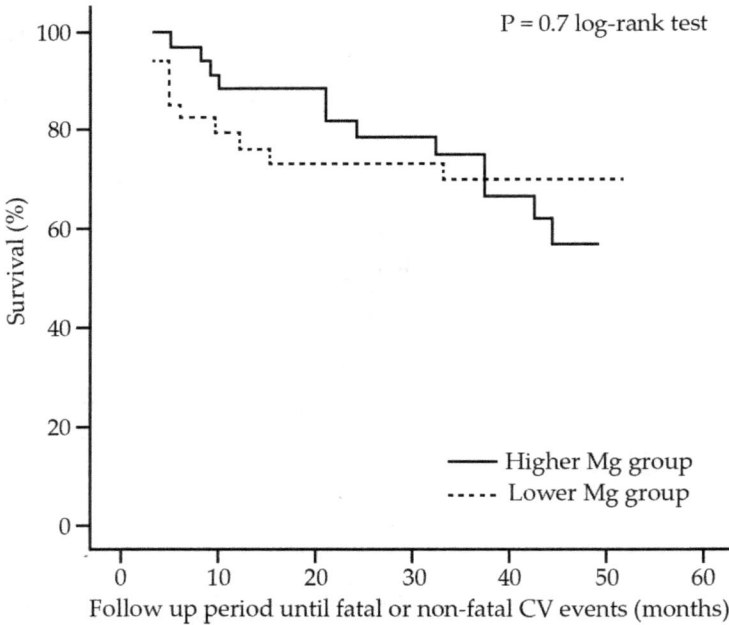

**Figure 4:** Kaplan-Meier development of cardiovascular events according to median serum magnesium levels (<2.1 mg/dL or ≥ 2.1 mg/dL).

observed that the lowest magnesium levels are present in inflamed and malnourished patients with cardiac comorbidities (Kurita et al., 2015) suggesting that hypomagnesemia could also be a marker of the bad health of these patients with worse prognosis in terms of mortality and future cardiovascular events. Nowadays, it is known that malnutrition and inflammation are associated with overhydration in patients with chronic kidney disease (Jacobs et al., 2010; Woodrow, 2006) and that correction of volume overload can improve inflammatory biomarkers over time (Ortega et al., 2009). In our pre-dialysis unit, control of fluid overload has been prioritized for many years. This strategy consists on a low sodium diet prescription in all patients plus the rational use of loop diuretics at increasing doses in those patients with persistent signs of overhydration. Using multifrequency bioelectrical impedance for analyzing body composition in our population, we observed that practically normohydration was achieved in most of our patients using this strategy of strict volume control (unpublished data). Thus, we could hypothesize that our just-about–normovolemic patients with advanced chronic kidney disease constitutes a special population and in this setting, the effect of serum Mg on cardiovascular outcome could be modified.

## 6  Summary

In the last years, several studies support a possible detrimental effect of lower serum magnesium levels on mortality and cardiovascular outcome among patients with advanced CKD, although a prospective smaller simple size study (Ortega et al., 2013) failed to detect this association. Otherwise, the lowest serum Mg levels was observed in inflamed, malnourish patients with cardiovascular comorbidities (Kurita et al 2015) suggesting that serum Mg could be a marker of malnutrition and inflammation and that inflammation could be the underlying factor explained the high mortality in these patients with low serum Mg.

Nowadays, the potential benefits of increasing serum Mg using Mg containing phosphate binders in patients with end-stage renal disease are unknown. All authors agree that prospective randomized trials are needed to confirm this hypothesis.

## References

Abbott RD, Ando F, Masaki KH, Tung KH, Rodriguez BL, Petrovitch , Jano K, Curb JD (2003). *Dietary magnesium intake and the future risk of coronary heart disease (The Honolulu Heart Program). Am J Cardiol 92:665–669.*

Blacher J, Guerin P, Pannier B, Marchais SJ, London GM (2001). *Arterial calcification, arterial stiffness and cardiovascular risk in end-stage renal disease. Hypertension 38:938–942.*

Branan PG, Vergne-Marini P, Park CY, Hull AR, Fordtran JS (1976). *Magnesium absorption in the human small intestine: results in normal subjects, patients with chronic renal disease, and patients with absorptive hypercalciuria. J Clin Invest 57:1412–1418*

Cholst IN, Steinberg SF, Tropper PJ, Fox HE, Segre GV, Bilezikian JP (1984). *The influence of hyper-*

*magnesemia on serum calcium and parathyroid hormone levels in human subject. N Eng J Med 310:1221–1225*

Cunningham J, Rodriguez M, Messa P (2012). *Magnesium in chronic kidney disease stages 3 and 4 and in diálisis patients. Clin Kidney J 5 (suppl 1):i39–i51*

Delmez JA, Kelber J, Norword KY, Giles KS, Slatopolsky E (1996). *Magnesium carbonate as phosphorous binder: a prospective, controlled, crossover study. Kidney Int 49:163–167*

Fox C, Ramsoomair D, Carter C (2001). *Magnesium: its proven and potencial clinical significance. South Med J 94:1195–1201*

Ganesh SK, Stack AG, Levin NW, Hulbert-Shearon T, Port FK (2001). *Association of elevated serum PO(4), Ca×PO(4) product and parathyroid hormone with cardiac mortality risk in chronic hemodialysis patients. J Am Soc Nephrol 12:2131–2138.*

Giachelli CM, Jono S, Shioi A, Nishizawa Y, Mori K, Morii H (2001). *Vascular calcification and inorganic phosphate. Am J Kidney Dis 38:S34–S37*

Goodman WG, Goldin J, Kuizon BD, Yoon C, Gales B, Sider D, Wang Y, Chung J, Emerick A, Greaser L, Elashoff RM, Salusky IB (2000). *Coronary-artery calcification in young adults with end-stage renal disease who are undergoing dialysis. N Eng J Med 342:1478–1483*

Huang JH, Lu YF, Chen FC, Lee JN, Tsai LC (2012) *Correlation of magnesium intake with metabolic parameters, depression and physical activity in elderly type 2 diabetes patients: a cross-sectional study. Nutr J 11:41*

Ishimura E, Okuno S, Yamakawa T, Inaba M, Nishizawa Y (2007). *Serum magnesium concentration is a significant predictor of mortality in maintenance hemodialysis patients. Magnes Res 20:237–244*

Jacobs LH, van de Kerkhof JJ, Mingels AM, Passos VL, Kleijnen VW, Mazairac AH, van der Sande FM, Wodzig WK, Konings CJ, Leunissen KM, van Dieijen-Visser MP, Kooman JP (2010). *Inflammation, overhydration and cardiac biomarkers in haemodialysis patients: a longitudinal study. Nephrol Dial Transplant 25:243–248*

Kanbay M, Goldsmith D, Uyar ME, Turgut F, Covic A (2010). *Magnesium in chronic kidney disease: challenges and opportunities. Blood Purif 29:280–292*

Kanbay M, Yilmaz MI, Apetrii M, Saglam M, Yaman H, Unal HU, Gok M, Caglar K, Oguz Y, Yenicesu M, Cetinkaya H, Eyileten T, Acikel C, Vural A, Covic A (2012) *Relationship between serum magnesium levels and cardiovascular events in chronic kidney disease patients. Am J Nephrol 36:228–237*

Kircelli F, Peter ME, Sevinc Ok E, Celenk FG, Yilmaz M, Steppan S, Asci G, Ok E, Passlick-Deetjen J (2012) *Magnesium reduces calcification in bovine vascular smooth muscle cells in a dose-dependent manner. Nephrol Dial Transplant 27:514–521*

Kurita N, Akizawa T, Fukagawa M ,Onishi Y, Kurokawa K, Fukuhara S (2015). *Contribution of dysregulated magnesium to mortality in hemodialysis patients with secondary hyperparathyroidism: a 3-year cohort study. Clin Kidney J 8:744–752*

Liao F, Folsom AR, Brancati FL (1998) *Is low magnesium concentration a risk factor for coronary heart disease? The Atherosclerosis Risk in Communities (ARIC) Study. Am Heart J 136:480–490*

Ma J, Folsom AR, Melnick SL, Eckfeldt JH, Sharrett AR, Nabulsi AA, Hutchinson RG, Metcalf PA (1995) *Association of serum and dietary magnesium with cardiovascular disease, hypertension, diabetes, insulin and carotid arterial wall thickness: the ARIC study. Atherosclerosis Risk in Communities Study. J Clin Epidemiol 48:927–940*

*Massy ZA, Drüeke TB (2012). Magnesium and outcomes in patients with chronic kidney disease: focus on vascular calcification, atherosclerosis and survival.Clin Kidney J 5:i52–i61*

*Mazur A, Maier JA, Rock E, Gueux E, Nowacki W, Rayssiguier Y (2007). Magnesium and the inflammatory response: potential physiopathological implications. Arch Biochem Biophys 458:48–56*

*Moe SM (2005). Disorders of calcium, phosphorus and magnesium. Am J Kidney Dis 45:213–218*

*Montezano AC, Zimmerman D, Ysuf H, Burger D, Chignalia AZ, Wadhera V, van Leeuwen FN, Touyz RM (2010). Vascular smooth muscle cell differentiation to an osteogenic phenotype involves TRPM7 modulation by magnesium. Hypertension 56:453–462*

*Navarro-Gonzalez JF, Mora-Fernandez C, García-Perez J (2009). Clinical implications of disordered magnesium homeostasis in chronic renal failure and dialysis. Seminars in Dialysis 22:37–44*

*Navarro JF, Macia ML, Gallego E, Mendez ML, Chahin J, Garcia-Nieto V, Garcia JJ (1997). Serum magnesium concentration and PTH levels. Is long-term chronic hypermagnesemia a risk factor for adynamic bone disease? Scand J Urol Nephrol 31:275–280*

*Ortega O, Rodriguez I, Gracia C, Sanchez M, Lentisco C, Mon C, Gallar P, Ortiz M, Herrero JC, Olet A, Vigil A (2009). Strict volume control and longitudinal changes in cardiac biomarker levels in hemodialysis patients. Nephron Clin Pract 113:c96–c103*

*Ortega O, Rodriguez I, Cobo G, Hinostroza J, Gallar P, Mon C, Ortiz M, Herrero JC, Di Gioia C, Oliet A, Vigil A (2013). Lack of influence of serum magnesium levels on overall mortality and cardiovascular outcomes in patients with advanced chronic kidney disease. ISRN Nephrol 2013:191786*

*Salem S, Bruck H, Bahlmann FH, Peter M, Passlick-Deetjen J, Kretschmer A, Steppan S, Volsek M, Kribben A, Nierhaus M, Jankowski V, Zidek W, Jankowski J (2012). Relationship between magnesium and clinical biomarkers on inhibition of vascular calcification. Am J Nephrol 35:31–39*

*Sakaguchi Y, Fujii N, Shoji T, Hayashi T, Rakugi H, Isaka Y (2014). Hypomagnesemia is a significant predictor of cardiovascular and non-cardiovascular mortality in patients undergoing hemodialysis. Kidney Int 85:174–181*

*Shechter M, Sharir M, Labrador MJ, Forrester J, Silver B, Bairey Merz CN (2000). Oral magnesium therapy improved endothelial function in patients with coronary artery disease. Circulation 102:2353–2358*

*Schmulen AC, Lerman M, Pak CY, Zerwekh J, Morawski S, Fordtran JS, Vergne-Marini P (1980). Effect of 1,25 dihydroxyvitamin D3 on jejunal absorption of magnesium in patients with chronic renal disease. Am J Physiol 238:G349–G352*

*Scholze A, Jankowsky V, Henning L, Haass W, Wittstock A, Suvd-Erdene S, Zidek W, Tepel M, Jankowski J (2007) Phenylacetic acid and arterial vascular properties in patients with chronic kidney disease stage 5 on hemodialysis therapy. Nephron Clin Pract 107:c1–c6*

*Schoppet M, Shroff RC, Hofbauer LC, Shanahan CM (2008). Exploring the biology of vascular calcification in chronic kidney disease: what's circulating? Kidney Int 73:384–390*

*Seelig MS (1969) Electrocardiographic patterns of magnesium depletion appearing in alcoholic heart disease. Ann N Y Acad Sci 162:906–917*

*Speer MY, Giachelli CM (2004). Regulation of vascular calcification. Cardiovasc Pathol 13:63–70*

*Spiegel DM, Farmer B, Smits G, Chonchol M (2007). Magnesium carbonate is an effective phosphate binder for chronic hemodialysis patients: a pilot study. J Ren Nutr 17:416–422*

*Spiegel DM, Farmer B (2009). Long-term effects of magnesium carbonate on coronary artery calcification and bone mineral density in hemodialysis patients: a pilot study. Hemodial Int 13:453–459*

Spiegel DM (2010). Normal and abnormal magnesium metabolism; in Schrier RW (ed): Renal and Electrolyte Disorders, ed 7. Philadelphia, Lippincott Williams & Wilkins, pp:229–250

Spiegel DM (2011). Magnesium in chronic kidney disease: unanswered questions. Blood Purif 31:172–176

Truttmann AC, Faraone R, Von Vigier RO, Nuoffer JM, Pfister R, Bianchetti MG (2002). Maintenance hemodialysis and circulating ionized magnesium. Nephron 92:616–621

Turgut F, Kanbay M, Metin MR, Uz E, Akcay A, Covic A (2008). Magnesium supplementation helps to improve carotid intima media thickness in patients on hemodialysis. Int Urol Nephrol 40:1075–1082

Tzanakis I, Virvidakis K, Tsomi A, Mantakas E, Girousis N, Karefyllakis N, Papadaki A, Kallivretakis N, Mountokalakis T (2004) Intra- and extracellular magnesium levels and atheromatosis in hemodialysis patients. Magnes Res 17:102–108

Tzanakis IP, Papadaki AN, Wei M, Kagia S, Spadidakis VV, Kallivretakis NE, Oreopuolos DG (2008) Magnesium carbonate for phosphate control in patients on hemodialysis. A randomized controlled trial. Int Urol Nephrol 40:193–201

Wolf FI, Cittadini A (1999). Magnesium in cell proliferation and differentiation. Front Biosci 4:D607–617

Woodrow G (2006). Extracellular water expansion: part of the malnutrition-inflammation-atherosclerosis syndrome? Perit Dial Int 26:566–570

Zheng D, Upton RN, Ludbrook GL, Martinez A (2001). Acute cardiovascular effects of magnesium and their relationship to systemic and myocardial magnesium concentrations after short infusion in awake sheep. J Pharmacol Exp Ther 297:1176–1183

# Chapter 12

# Fluid Therapy: Analysis of the Components for a Rational Fluid Management

Juan C. Grignola[1], Juan P. Bouchacourt[2]

## 1   Importance and Goals of Fluid Therapy

Decisions regarding fluid therapy, whether this is in the operating room (patients undergoing high-risk surgery), intensive care unit (ICU), or emergency department, remain a highly challenged tasks that clinicians must face daily to maintain adequate oxygen delivery ($DO_2$) and prevent tissue hypoperfusion and fluid overload. $DO_2$ is determined by cardiac output (CO) and the oxygen content of arterial blood. So, after correction of hypoxemia and anemia, maintenance of an adequate CO is the next logical step to improve $DO_2$. Although CO can be monitored (continuous, semi-continuous or intermittent modalities) with reasonable accuracy and precision by different devices, it is difficult to assess the optimal CO for an individual patient. Low CO may be adequate in a context of low global oxygen consumption, especially under sedo-analgesia or general anesthesia and viceversa, a normal CO does not preclude the presence of inadequate microcirculatory perfusion. Adequate fluid management to prevent/treat hypervolemia and hypovolemia and titration of vasoactive drugs are crucial to maintaining adequate $DO_2$ and to improve the outcome of the patients (Navarro et al., 2015). While hypovolemia (under-resuscitation) may lead to reduced CO and $DO_2$, organ hypoperfusion and ischemia, overzealous fluid resuscitation has been associated with increased complications (coagulopathy, organ congestion), increased length of ICU and hospital stay, and increased mortality (Figure 1). Likewise, fluid restriction and diuresis may decrease edema

[1] Department of Pathophysiology, Hospital de Clínicas, School of Medicine, Universidad de la República, Uruguay.
[2] Department of Anesthesiology, Hospital de Clínicas, School of Medicine, Universidad de la República, Uruguay.

in patients with poor ventricular function but concomitantly, may also increase the incidence of acute kidney injury. Also, uncorrected hypovolemia, leading to inappropriate infusions of vasopressors agents may increase organ hypoperfusion and ischemia.

Finally, fluid management goals is a dynamic process depending on the phase of acute illness: during the *rescue and optimization phases*, we should focus on achieving and maintaining adequate effective circulating volume; during the *stabilization phase* the goal is to minimize complications and during *de-escalation phase* the focus is to restore a more normal fluid balance (Raghunathan et al., 2014). It is the purpose of this chapter to provide an overview of the components of a rational fluid management in acute illness.

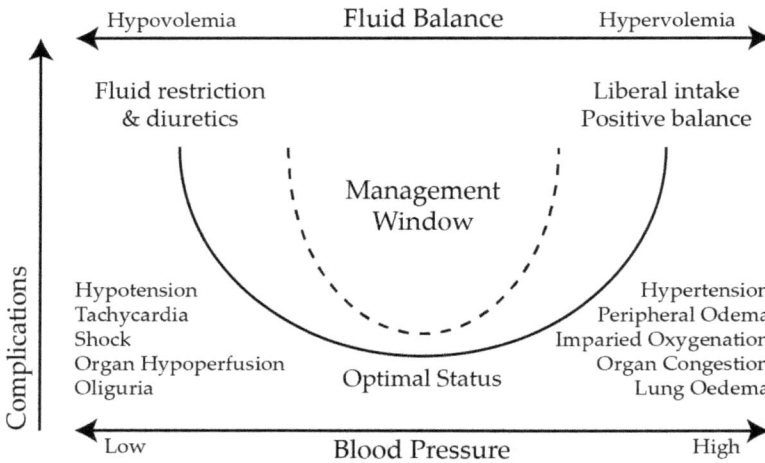

**Figure 1:** Both hypo- and hypervolemia are associated with more complications. (dotted line: reduction of the management window associated with heart and/or kidney dysfunction).

# 2   Fluid Management: Quantitative Aspects

In order to minimize the under or over fluid administration, we should ask the following main questions: when fluid therapy should be considered? When fluid therapy should be started? And when fluid therapy should be stopped? (Figure 2).

Although fluid therapy should be considered when a patient is both in need of enhanced blood flow and are fluid responsive, we must first to assess the benefit/risk ratio of fluid administration patient per patient.

The clinical decision to administer i.v. fluids in acute illness is following by decisions on the amount and type of fluid to be infused. The therapeutic effect of intravenous fluids depends not only on quantitative and qualitative aspects, but also on the clinical setting. Fluid therapy acts by increasing the intravascular volume, thereby increasing venous return and cardiac preload, improving global and regional perfusion, $DO_2$ and tissue oxygenation. Critically ill patients and patients undergoing high-risk surgery often

Decisions in Fluid Therapy

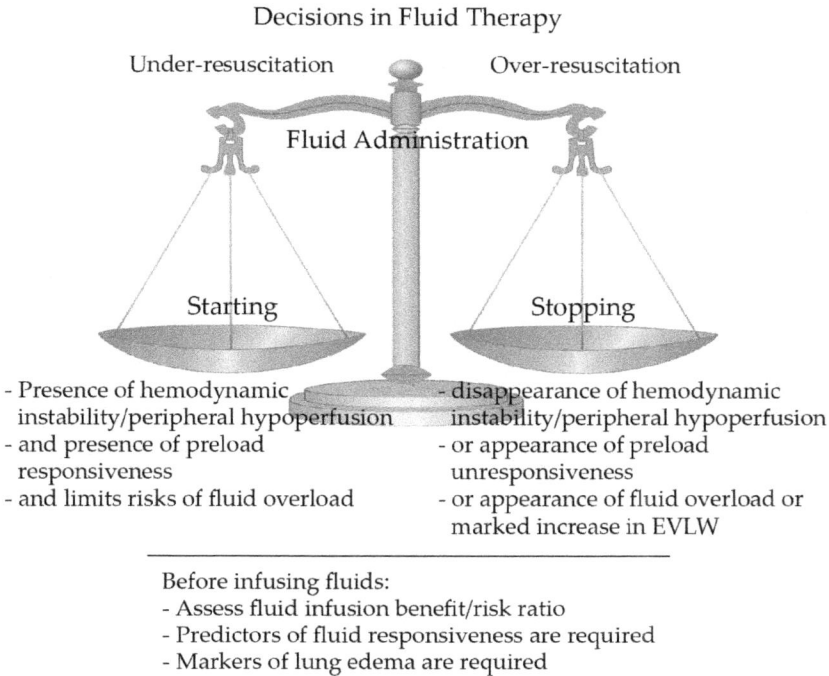

**Figure 2:** Decisions in fluid therapy (EVLW: extravascular lung water).

experience hemodynamic instability and clinicians are tempted to fluid administration to restore adequate hemodynamic conditions. However, these changes are profoundly influenced by the patient's cardiovascular status (Chawla et al., 2014). The blind administration of fluids or the use of vasopressors without knowing the patient's cardiovascular reserve, the certainty of fluid responsiveness and/or the patients were already fluid-resuscitated, is discouraged. The same fluid management can have profoundly different and occasionally opposite changes in cardiovascular state. Being a fluid responder is not equal to being hypovolemic and to benefit from the infusion of fluids. This suggests that not all patients who are "volume responsive" do not necessarily require volume expansion.

A concomitant analysis of the Frank-Starling and extra-vascular lung water (EVLW) curves illustrates that when patients are on the steep part of their Frank-Starling curve they are likely to have a significant increase in stroke volume (SV) with a small increase in lung water (Figure 3). However, when patients are close to the flat part of their Frank-Starling curve, they are likely to have a small or no increase in SV with a substantial increase in lung water. This process is accentuated in patients with endothelial damage (sepsis, ARDS, pancreatitis, burns) (Marik et al., 2014; Marik et al., 2011). It is therefore essential that in all hemodynamically unstable patients, the clinician could estimate the position of their Frank-Starling and Marik-Phillips curves, to give the correct amount of the appropriate fluid promptly with not produce lung edema and tissue swelling. Only patients who are likely to show a significant increase in SV with a fluid challenge and in

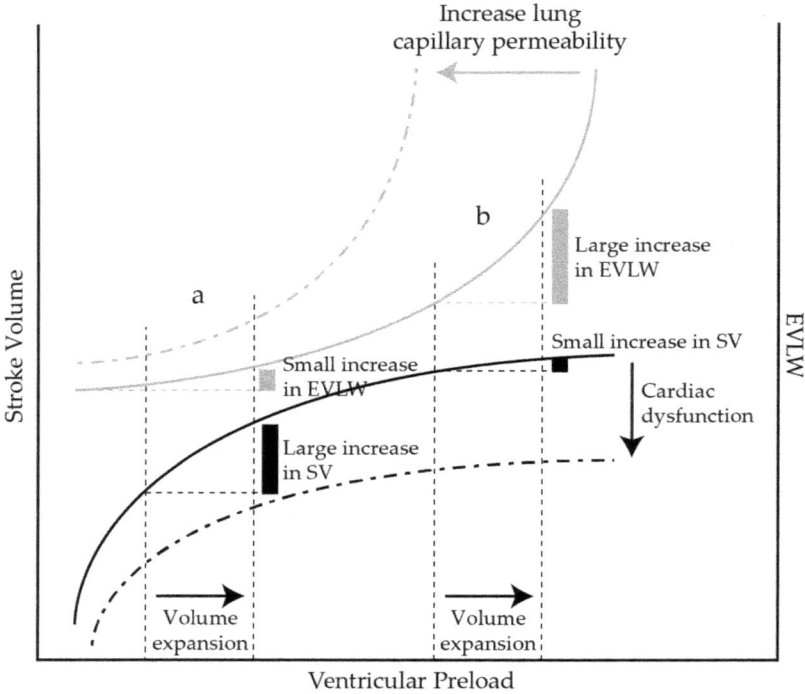

**Figure 3:** Superimposition of the Frank-Starling (black) and Marik-Phillips (red) curves demonstrating the effects of increasing preload on SV and lung water in a patient who is preload responsive (a) and non-responsive (b). The higher the lung vascular permeability (red dot and dash lines), the greater the risk of increase in EVLW during volume expansion. The lower cardiac pump function (black dot and dash lines), the lower increase of SV during volume expansion. EVLW: extravascular lung water, SV: stroke volume (modified from Marik PE & Lemson J, 2014; (Marik et al., 2014).

whom the increased SV is considered to be beneficial should be given a fluid challenge. Thus, two considerations may help to take the correct decision about to start, to stop or to desist for fluid administration in a patient with circulatory failure and lung impairment: to predict fluid responsiveness and to estimate EVLW and pulmonary vascular permeability index (PVPI) (Jozwiak et al., 2015).

Among the different hemodynamic parameters or techniques for predicting fluid responsiveness and guiding fluid therapy in acute illness, we can recognize three groups with different reliability and confounding factors (Table 1) (Marik et al., 2014).

## 2.1    Static Pressure and Volume Parameters (ROC ~ 0.5–0.6)

The origin for using central venous pressure (CVP) and pulmonary artery occlusion pressure (PAOP) to guide fluid management comes from the idea that they truly reflect intra-

| Static pressure and volume parameters (ROC ~ 0.5–0.6) | CVP (central venous pressure) |
|---|---|
| | PAOP (pulmonary artery occlusion pressure) |
| | IVC/SVC diameter (inferior/superior vena cava) |
| | FTc (Flow corrected time) |
| | Right ventricular end-diastolic volume |
| | Left ventricular end-diastolic volume |
| Dynamic techniques based on heart-lung interactions during mechanical ventilation (ROC ~ 0.7–0.8) | PPV (pulse pressure variation) |
| | SVV (stroke volume variation) |
| | Pleth variability index |
| | Aortic blood flow (echocardiography-Doppler) |
| Techniques based on fluid challenge (ROC ~ 0.9) | PLR (passive leg raising) |
| | Rapid fluid challenge (100–250 cc) |

**Table 1:** Techniques assessing fluid responsiveness (ROC: receiver operating curve).

vascular volume. Although numerous experimental and clinical studies have demonstrated that they reflect cardiac filling pressures, they cannot adequately indicate changes in preload or predict fluid responsiveness. Several studies have demonstrated that CVP and PAOP are not significantly different between responders and non-responders before volume expansion and did not correlate with the volume expansion-induced changes in CO across a broad spectrum of clinical conditions (Renner et al., 2009). The ROC values are unacceptable for the decision-making process regarding volume expansion in patients with hemodynamic instability (Osman et al., 2007).

Filling pressures are highly dependent on ventricular compliance that is frequently altered in critical ill patients. Neither absolute values of filling pressures nor their changes are associated with a specific end-diastolic volume or its changes.

Besides, according to the Frank-Starling curve, a given value of preload can be associated with fluid responsiveness in the case of a normal cardiac function (steep part of the curve), but in the case of a failing heart can be associated with fluid unresponsiveness (flat part of the curve) (Figure 3). So, static cardiac filling pressures are not appropriate to assess intravascular volume status and are not reliable predictors of fluid responsiveness (Marik et al., 2008).

Preload is defined as the myocardial fibre length at end diastole. Therefore, left and right ventricular end-diastolic volumes obtained by echocardiography have been introduced as a clinical variable to assess preload (Schober et al., 2009). However, it has been shown that left ventricular end-diastolic area/volume obtained by trans-oesophageal echocardiography (TOE) fail to predict fluid responsiveness. Although measuring aortic diameter improves accuracy of esophageal Doppler in assessing fluid responsiveness, the angle of insonation (known and constant), the kind of blood flow (laminar or turbulent) and the distribution of flow between supra-aortic vessels and descending aorta introduce a considerable potential for erroneous assessments of CO as from aortic blood flow (Monnet et al., 2007; Schober et al., 2009).

In contrast to TOE, trans-oesophageal doppler (TOD) does not allow direct visual estimation of ventricular filling, contractility or valvular function. With TOD, the descending aortic flow velocity is calculated on the Doppler equation. The systolic portion of the aortic blood is typically triangular, and the base of the triangle represents the systolic ejection time, referred as flow time (FT) (Schober et al., 2009). Because FT depends on the heart rate, it is usually corrected by a the square root of the period (FTc). The FTc is often claimed to indicate preload and allows the assessment of fluid responsiveness in hypovolemic patients (Lee et al., 2007). However, because FTc is inversely related to systemic vascular resistance (afterload), a shortened FTc may also indicate an increase in afterload. Very recently, Guinot et al. showed that FTc did not predict haemodynamic response to fluid infusion in ninety patients undergoing surgery. Baseline FTc was not statistically different between responders and nonresponders. They concluded that FTc is a complex static indicator influenced by preload, afterload and inotropic state that limit its accuracy (Guinot et al., 2013).

## 2.2   Dynamic Techniques Based on Heart-lung Interactions During Mechanical Ventilation (ROC ~ 0.7–0.8)

Nowadays dynamic indices based in heart-lung interaction are commonly used in clinical setting to predict fluid responsiveness (Michard, 2005). The dynamic parameters of fluid responsiveness are related to cardiopulmonary interactions in patients under general anesthesia with mechanical ventilation (Cannesson et al., 2011). Observing and analysing the respiratory variation of haemodynamic variables such as systolic pressure (systolic pressure variation, SPV), pulse pressure (pulse pressure variation, PPV), stroke volume (stroke volume variation, SVV) and the plethysmographic waveform (plethysmographic variability index, PVI) is the main concept of what is known as functional haemodynamic monitoring (Renner et al., 2009). The higher the preinfusion value of all these dynamic variables, the more pronounced the increase in SV in response to fluid administration will be. This is due to the cyclic changes in RV and LV SV are greater when the ventricles operate on the steep rather the flat portion of the Frank-Starling curve (Marik et al., 2011). Among the different dynamic parameters and since Michard et al. (Michard et al., 2000) demonstrated that PPV was superior to SPV, PPV is the most commonly used index. Accordingly, Marik et al. reported from a systematic review that the area under the curve is 0.94 (0.93–0.95) for PPV versus 0.86 (0.82–0.90) and 0.84 (0.78–0.88) for SPV and SVV, respectively (Marik et al., 2009).

The clinical utility of dynamic parameters is limited by many confounding factors that must be clearly understood and respected to be able to predict fluid responsiveness accurately (sensitivity 88%, specificity 89%). The most common physiological limitations to the use of PPV is summarized in Table 2.

- *Cardiac rhythm.* In patients with cardiac arrhythmias, the beat-to-beat variation of SV and PP may no longer reflect the effects of mechanical ventilation. This is particularly true in patients with atrial fibrillation or frequent extrasystoles. Besides, both heart rate (HR) and HR variability may affect the magnitude of the respiratory variation in arterial pressure. A decrease or an increase in HR variability may reduce the respirator

|  | False Positive | False Negative |
|---|:---:|:---:|
| Low HR/RR Ratio |  | √ |
| Irregular Heart Beats | √ |  |
| Mechanical Ventilation (Low Vt) |  | √ |
| Increased abdominal Pressure | √ |  |
| Thorax Open |  | √ |
| Spontaneous Breathing | √ | √ |

**Table 2:** Limitations to the use of pulse pressure variation can be summarized as 'LIMITS'. False positive: significant PPV not related to fluid responsiveness; False negative: low PPV despite fluid responsiveness. (HR/RR: heart rate/respiratory rate, Vt: tidal volume).

variation in arterial pressure (Michard, 2005). Nodal rhythm may increase the size of respiratory-induced dynamic parameters by effectively decreasing preload due to the loss of the atrial kick (Perel et al., 2013).

- *Small variations in pleural and transpulmonary pressures.* If changes in pleural and transpulmonary pressure are small over a single respiratory cycle, inspiration does not induce any significant change in pulmonary arterial and aorta flows, even during hypovolemic conditions.

De Backer et al. have reported that PPV is a very effective predictor of fluid responsiveness in patients with mechanical ventilation provided that the tidal volume ($V_t$) is greater than 8 mL/kg (De Backer et al., 2005). High $V_t$ can generate high intrathoracic pressures creating higher variation in SV. When low $V_t$ is used, changes in intrathoracic pressure may be insufficient to generate changes in preload even in responder patients. The predictive value of PPV in septic patients with ALI/ARDS under protective ventilation (Vt ≈ 6 mL/kg) can identify responders if the cut-off is decreased to 8%. Because of this, some authors suggest that when $V_t$ is less than 8 ml/Kg the cut-off of PPV should be lowered than 8%, knowing that the predictive value of this index decreases, not being even better than classic preload indices (De Backer et al., 2005). More recently, Vistisen et al. have showed that PPV increased significantly with increasing Vt at different volemic levels, proposing that dynamic parameters are improved by indexing to Vt (Vistisen et al., 2010). Under normovolemia and moderate hemorrhage (15% of volemia), dynamic parameters were not influenced by the ventilatory modalities (either pressure- or volume-controlled). However, in more severe hemorrhage (30% of volemia) volume-controlled ventilation determines higher value of PPV when compared to pressure-controlled ventilation (Fonseca et al., 2008).

Applications of incremental PEEP levels are often limited by a reduction in SV, as a result of the increase in lung volume, the increase in intrathoracic pressure, increased right ventricular afterload and increased pulmonary vascular resistance and decreased LV preload. It has been shown by Kubitz et al. that increasing PEEP levels increased both PPV and SVV (false positive) (Kubitz et al., 2006). At PEEP not greater than 5 cmH$_2$O, SVV and PPV can identify responder patients with acceptable specificity and sensitivity. When PEEP increases to 10 or more cmH$_2$O, PPV lost its ability to predict fluid responsiveness and SVV requires a higher threshold value to identify responders (Renner et al., 2008).

- *Intra-abdominal pressure.* Intra-abdominal pressure (IAP) is frequently increased in critically ill patients, and a sustained intra-abdominal hypertension (IAH) has been claimed to induce multiple organ failure and death. IAH is associated with a mechanical impairment of venous return as the result of inferior vena cava compression and may mask hypovolemia. Several authors have showed that in intra-abdominal hypertension, threshold values discriminating responders and non-responders might be significantly higher than during normal IAP (Jacques et al., 2011; Mahjoub et al., 2010). Accordingly, Mahjoub et al. noticed that among 41 mechanically ventilated patients with IAH and a PPV >12%, 10 (24.4%) were not fluid responders (false positives) (Mahjoub et al., 2010). Although SVV and PPV remain indicative of fluid responsiveness, threshold values identifying responders and non-responders might be higher than during normal IAP.

- *Open chest.* The cyclic changes in intrathoracic pressure during positive pressure ventilation should be decreased if the chest is opened, and consequently, the effect on dynamic variables of fluid responsiveness should be less pronounced (Rex et al., 2007).

- *Spontaneous breathing.* Several studies have failed to demonstrate the ability to predict response to volume administration for PPV, SVV and PVI in spontaneous breathing, being this one of the most important limitations. When a patient has some respiratory effort or not being mechanically ventilated, the variation in intrathoracic pressure is not regular, nor in frequency nor in intensity, so that the change in stroke volume may not be related to preload dependence of the CO. During spontaneous tidal volume ventilation PPV not only fails to reliably identify responders to fluid challenge, but their predictive value is even lower than the cardiac filling pressures in these conditions (Maguire et al., 2011).

Other limitations include:

- *Technical factors,* such as the fluid filled catheters (presence of air bubbles, kinks, clot formation, compliant tubing, excessive tubing length) may affect the dynamic response of the monitoring system (Michard, 2005). The site of arterial pressure monitoring can also impact the observed pressures, with significant differences between central and peripheral pulse pressure.

    Studies differed on the threshold values of dynamic indices depending on automatically versus manually measured. They also differed on the fluid challenge performed (a bolus of 500 mL, 20 mL/kg in 20 min) and the definition of responder and non-responder (SV variation of 5, 12 and 25%), adding uncertainty of the cut-off values of the dynamic parameters (Renner et al., 2009).

- *Vasomotor tone.* It has been suggested that vasopressors might exert a direct effect on regional vascular capacitance and they would alter PPV and SVV and interfere with their ability to predict fluid responsiveness. Nouira et al. (Nouira et al., 2005) have showed that norepinephrine (NE) induces a significant increase in CO and SV during severe hypovolemia with a concomitant decrease in PPV and SPV. They proposed that both effects were related to the shift of blood from unstressed to stressed blood volume. This is in accordance to Renner et al. (Renner et al., 2009) data on an animal hemorrhage model. However, on account of the global end-diastolic volume (PiCCO) remained unchanged, they proposed the effects of NE administration beyond shifting blood from unstressed to stressed blood volume.

To clarify the effects of vasopressors on the dynamic parameters predictability of fluid responsiveness, we analyzed in a separate manner the direct effects of a pure vasopressor versus the indirect effects of the change in arterial pressure on the arterial wall viscoelastic properties (Santana et al., 2005). In a rabbit hemorrhage model, we demonstrated that the infusion of phenylephrine (a pure α1-receptor agonist) blunts the dynamic preload indexes increase after bleeding. This effect is mainly due to an acute increase of vasomotor tone without any apparent change of the effective intra-vascular volume. This result may suggest the limitation of dynamic indexes in predicting fluid responsiveness in routine clinical practice during hypovolemia and vasopressor drug administration (Bouchacourt et al., 2013).

- *Right ventricular dysfunction/pulmonary hypertension.* In the presence of RV failure and normovolemia, PPV and SVV are mainly related to an inspiratory increase in RV afterload (and not to a decrease in RV preload), they are falsely elevated and cannot serve as indicators of fluid responsiveness (Michard, 2005). Therefore, the presence of RV failure should be suspected when a patient has large variations of SV or PP but does not respond to fluids (Perel et al., 2013). In a cohort of thirty-five mechanically ventilated patients with a PPV > 12%, Majhoub et al. reported that those patients without increase of 15% of LV SV after volume expansion can be caused by RV dysfunction (i.e. false-positive) (Mahjoub et al., 2009). They hypothesized that in the nonresponder group the failing RV becomes more sensitive to afterload increase and is less affected by preload variation. Willer von Ballmoos et al. reported that patients with pulmonary hypertension (cardiac surgery and septic shock) with the risk of acute RV dysfunction respond poorly to fluid administration. High values of PPV cannot be used to predict fluid responsiveness (false-positive) (Wyler Von Ballmoos et al., 2010). The fact that almost half of the nonresponders and none of the responders presented an impaired ejection fraction of RV would suggest that RV dysfunction is in part responsible for the poor predictive value of PPV.

We analyzed the effects of the dysfunction of RV on preload dynamic indices and their ability to predict fluid responsiveness in a rabbit model of pulmonary embolism. We found that RV dysfunction secondary to pulmonary embolism blunts the PPV and SVV increase after bleeding, and it also prevents the fluid responsiveness. We cannot discard the role of a concomitant LV dysfunction secondary to ventricular interdependence (Bouchacourt et al., 2015).

The threshold values of dynamic variables of fluid responsiveness range from 10 to 15% and a change greater than 12 to 13% (cut-off values) is highly predictive of fluid responsiveness.(Cannesson, 2010) Cannesson et al. (Cannesson et al., 2011) and more recently Biais et al. (Biais et al., 2014), have used the "grey zone" approach to investigate the clinical value of PPV. By defining two cut-offs between which the diagnosis of fluid responsiveness remains uncertain; the grey zone corresponds to the zone of uncertainty. It is noteworthy that the patients included in both papers suffer of methodological noise (various methods of CO measurements, with unique errors of measurements and limited clinical agreement between them) and no respect of limitations (wide range of Vt, including low Vt), which makes artificially large grey zone, leading to the wrong conclusion that PPV has limited clinical value (Michard et al., 2015). A recent systematic review and meta-analysis including only mechanically ventilated patients with Vt more than 8 mL/kg and without spontaneous breathing and cardiac arrhythmia (n = 807) reported a pooled sensitivity and specificity of 0.88 and 0.89, respectively, with an AUC of 0.94 (0.91-0.95) (Yang et al., 2014). For these reasons, PPV and its surrogate parameters continues to have clinical utility making more rational and informed decisions when clinicians design a fluid therapy.

Likewise, some authors have analyzed the applicability of PPV in routine clinical practice, since factors including low Vt, cardiac arrhythmias, and the calculation method can substantially reduce their predictive value (Lansdorp et al., 2012). In a recent work, Mahjoub et al. concluded that only 2% of ICU patients satisfied all criteria for valid use of PPV (Mahjoub et al., 2014). However, 49% were not mechanically ventilated, 25% were mechanically ventilated but kept a spontaneous breathing activity, and 12% had cardiac arrhythmias. On the contrary, Benes et al. showed that dynamic parameters were usable in 51% of ICU patients admitted for polytrauma, 37% for sepsis and 33% after surgery (Benes et al., 2014). Assuming the same evaluation had been done in patients undergoing major surgery, we can reasonably assume that PPV can be safely used in around 85% of the cases.

## 2.3    Techniques Based on Fluid Challenge (ROC ~ 0.9)

Ultimately, in all these situations when dynamic parameters cannot be obtained accurately and in case of any doubt about interpretation two other reliable dynamic tests are currently available with a high degree of accuracy, namely passive leg raising (PLR) manoeuvre and rapid fluid challenge (200 mL or 3 mL/kg given in 5' or 100 mL given in 1') (Carsetti et al., 2015; Marik et al., 2011).

PLR causes an "endogenous fluid challenge" transfering of blood from the legs and abdominal compartments and increasing venous return and cardiac preload. Unlike fluid challenge, no fluid is infused, and, the effects are reversible and transient (Monnet et al., 2008). The method for performing PLR is of the utmost importance because it fundamentally affects its hemodynamic effects and reliability. Five rules should be followed: a) check that patient's trunk is of 45°, b) use the bed adjustment to raise the legs and do not touch the patient to avoid adrenergic stimulation (pain, awakening), c) assess PLR effects by directly measuring CO (not with arterial blood pressure only), d) use a real-time measurement of CO and e) re-assess CO in the semi-recumbent position (Monnet et al., 2015). For obvious technical reasons, the rapid fluid challenge technique is preferred during anesthesia in the operating room, while PLR is more frequently used in the ICU and postoperatively (Marik et al., 2014). In a recent meta-analysis, Cavallaro et al. reported that

PLR-induced changes in CO can reliably predict fluid responsiveness regardless of cardiac rhythm and ventilation mode with an AUC of 0.95 (Cavallaro et al., 2010).

It is today acknowledged that the cumulative fluid balance is an independent predictor of mortality in several categories of patients (septic shock, ARDS, acute kidney injury) (Payen et al., 2008; Sakr et al., 2005; Vincent et al., 2006). EVLW and pulmonary vascular permeability (PVP) may be used as criteria indicating the risk of fluid administration (Jozwiak et al., 2015). During the acute phase of resuscitation, high EVLW and PVP may serve as indicators for fluid restriction and promote clinicians to choose alternative interventions for hemodynamic resuscitation. Likewise, after post-resuscitation phase (de-escalation phase), EVLW may be helpful in beginning a controlled fluid removal strategy. Therefore, clinicians can use EVLW and PVP to guide fluid therapy in patients at risk of fluid overload (septic shock and ARDS) (Jozwiak et al., 2015).

EVLW corresponds to the fluid that is accumulated in the interstitial and alveolar spaces. To preserve their function of gas exchange and compliance, the lungs must be kept dry (Miserocchi, 2009). The volume of EVLW is strictly controlled by two main mechanisms: the lymphatic drainage system, which constantly removes fluid from the interstitial tissue to the superior vena cava through the thoracic duct, and the active ion transport that removes excess fluid from the alveoli to the interstitial space across the alveolar epithelial membrane (Matthay et al., 2002). Increased interstitial EVLW can occur either because of increased lung permeability or because of increased hydrostatic pressure and/or decreased oncotic pressure in the pulmonary capillaries. This may be worsen in ARDS since both, the lymphatic network is injured, and alveolar fluid clearance is impaired. The only technique that provides a relatively easy measurement of EVLW at the bedside is transpulmonary thermodilution (Sakka et al., 2012). Various experimental and clinical studies have validated EVLW measurements by thermodilution based on reasonable correlations with gravimetry (experimental gold standard method) or thermo-dye dilution (human being gold standard method) (Jozwiak et al., 2015). Indexed EVLW to predicted body weight (EVLWI) is better correlated with the lung injury score and the oxygenation compared to non-indexed EVLW. It is also a better predictor of mortality of patients with acute lung injury and ARDS (Craig et al., 2010; Phillips et al., 2008).

Transpulmonary thermodilution also provides the PVP index (PVPI), which is an indirect method for estimating the permeability of the pulmonary capillary barrier. It is the ratio between EVLWI and pulmonary blood volume and is automatically provided by the transpulmonary thermodilution system each time a cold bolus injected (Monnet et al., 2007). In patients with pulmonary oedema, a PVPI value of 3 was the best cutoff to distinguish between both forms of pulmonary oedema (Monnet et al., 2007). Both, EVLWI and PVPI predict mortality in different kinds of critically ill patients (severe sepsis, septic shock, burned patients, ARDS) (Bognar et al., 2010; Chung et al., 2010). It is interesting to note that the prediction of mortality in ARDS patients occur in an independent way, suggesting they indicate a different pathophysiological concern of ARDS. PVPI appears to characterize the degree of impairment of the alveolocapillary membrane itself while EVLWI should indicate the severity of the interstitial pulmonary leak resulting from this injury. The normal ranges for cardiopulmonary variables as derived by transpulmonary thermodilution are resumed in Table 3 (Sakka et al., 2012).

| Items | Values |
|---|---|
| CI: cardiac index | 3-5 L/min/m$^2$ |
| ITBVI: intrathoracic blood volume index | 850-1000 mL/m$^2$ |
| GEDVI: global end-diastolic volume index | 680-800 mL/m$^2$ |
| SVRI: systemic vascular resistance index | 1700-2400 dyn.s.m$^2$/cm$^5$ |
| CFI: cardiac function index | 4.5-6.5/min |
| GEF: global ejection fraction | 25-35% |
| EVLWI: extravascular lung water index | < 7mL/kg |
| PVPI: pulmonary vascular permeability index | 1.0-3.0 |

**Table 3:** Normal ranges for the different derived variables from the transpulmonary thermodilution technique.

The current approach focusing primarily on CO and haemodynamic stability can be misleading and lead to excessive volume administration. Taking into account the recent progress of vascular biology and that fluid is a drug, the international Acute Dialysis Quality Initiative (ADQI) proposes four main components that can lead to hypoperfusion at both macro- and microcirculatory level whenever any significant perturbation occurs in any of these domains: vascular content, vascular tone, vascular barrier, and blood flow They have named the vascular component approach for fluid management to the patient with hypoperfusion.

The *vascular content* is represented mainly by the whole blood volume (plasma volume plus volume containing red cells). Clinically, the 'patient's volume status' is an important feature of any clinical assessment. A diminished vascular content establishes an absolute hypovolemia. The administration of fluid during resuscitation may not significantly improve DO$_2$ to the parenchymal cells, since plasma water has <3% oxygen carrying capacity. Blood volume in veins represents more than 60% of the whole blood volume (Figure 4). The two best validated techniques for assessment the whole blood volume utilize indocyanine green and I$_{131}$ (*Recommended methods for measurement of red-cell and plasma volume: International committee for standardization in haematology, 1980*). However, it is time-consuming, expensive and complex for clinical routine. So, the haematocrit dilution technique has emerged as a bedside alternative (Lobo et al., 2010).

The *vascular tone* domain can be estimated by the systemic vascular resistance (steady component) and systemic compliance (pulsatile component) (Bouchacourt et al., 2015). The isobaric analysis can separate a direct from an indirect effect of vasopressors drugs on the vasomotor tone since arterial stiffness depends not only on intravascular pressure (indirect effect) but also on viscoelastic properties of the vascular wall (direct effect) (Santana et al., 2005). Recently, the PPV/SVV ratio has also been proposed as a functional approach to arterial tone assessment (Garcia et al., 2014; Monge Garcia et al., 2011). It is important to point out that vasodilation leads to a relative hypovolemia as a consequence of vascular space increased with vascular content unchanged. In this case, the patient may, in fact, require a drug to restore vasomotor tone instead of volume therapy.

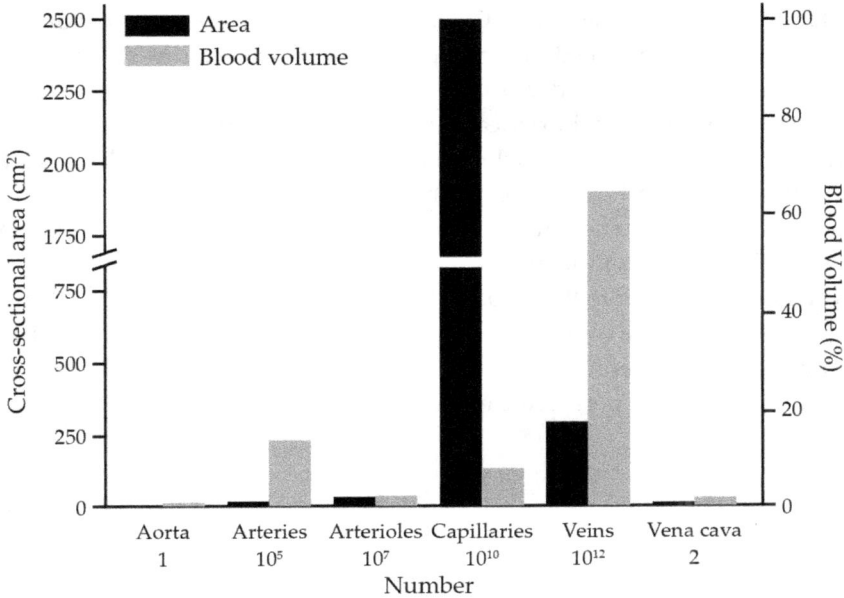

**Figure 4:** Cross-sectional area and blood volume distribution in the systemic circuit.

The endothelial glycocalyx and endothelial cells form the primary constituents of the *vascular barrier* domain (Chawla et al., 2014). The endothelial glycocalyx plays a major role of in regulating vascular permeability. It also participates in other important physiological processes such as preventing adhesion of leukocytes to the vessel wall, transmission of shear stress and modulating inflammatory and haemostatic processes. For this reason, the preservation of the glycocalyx must be considered in any resuscitation strategy (Jacob et al., 2013). The endothelial glycocalyx is composed of membrane-bound glycoproteins and proteoglycans, mainly syndecan and glypican, carrying negatively charged side chains (mainly heparan, but also dermatan and chondroitin sulphates) and hyaluronan which account for much of the biophysical properties. The increased plasma levels of glycocalyx components secondary to the disruption of the glycocalyx is an early manifestation of endothelial injury. The radical oxygen species directly attack the integrity of the glycocalyx and cleave membrane-bound proteoglycans and glycoproteins off the endothelial glycocalyx (Becker et al., 2010). Likewise, excessive volume expansion increases the release of natriuretic peptides, which in turn damages the endothelial glycocalyx, and this is followed by a rapid shift of intravascular fluid into the interstitial space (Bruegger et al., 2011). Avoidance of intravascular hypervolaemia promises to protect a significant part of the vascular barrier (Jacob et al., 2013). The knowledge of how much the vascular barrier is preserved would allow the clinician to select a more appropriate i.v. fluid. Although various biomarkers can be used to assess the integrity of the glycocalyx (most notably syndecan-1, and hyaluronic acid), currently, the assessment of vascular barrier is not objectively determined.

At last, *blood flow* is assessed as CO at a systemic level. Besides, observation of the microcirculation using handheld microscopes gives insight into the nature of shock and the nature of the convective and diffusive defect in hypovolemia, at the bedside (Ince, 2014). These devices, applied in critically ill patients mostly for the observation of the sublingual microcirculation, have included a first- and second-generation OPS (orthogonal polarized spectral) and SDF (sidestream dark field) imaging handheld microscopes using video cameras. Various authors have been proposed a microcirculatory approach that may provide a useful complement to targeting systemic hemodynamic variables during resuscitation. They refer to this approach as functional microcirculatory hemodynamics (FMH) in parallel to the concepts underlying functional hemodynamics. The optimal fluid volume is thereby defined as that needed to achieve normalized convective flow with an optimal density of perfused capillaries (B in figure 5).

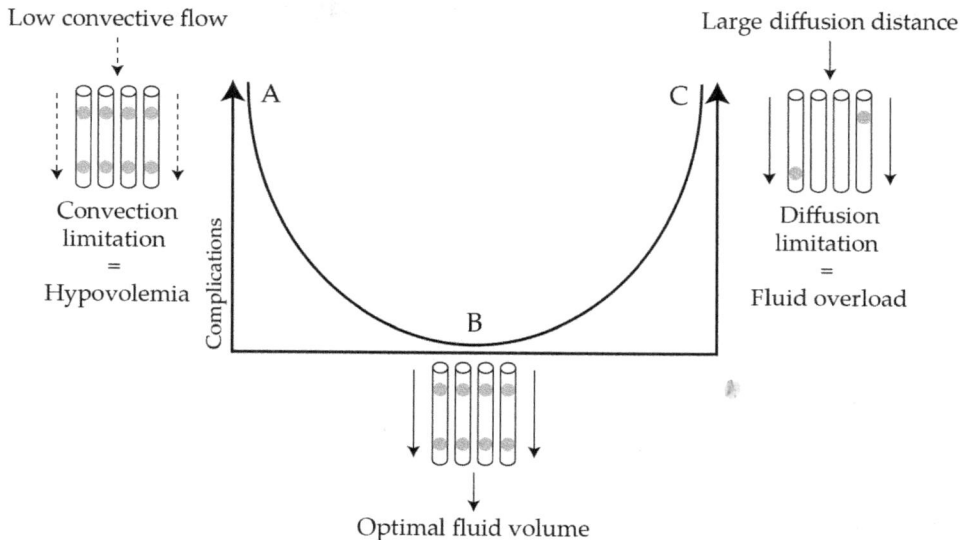

**Figure 5:** Functional microcirculatory hemodynamics approach (modified from Ince, 2014).

We can obtain different microcirculatory parameters from the video clips that provide different aspects of the microcirculatory status. Microvascular density (MVD) was determined as the number of vessels per mm². Flow quantification was performed using a score that distinguishes between no flow (0), intermittent flow (1), sluggish flow (2), and continuous flow (3), assigning a value to each individual vessel. The overall score, i.e., the microvascular flow index (MFI), corresponds to the average of all the individual vessels. To determine perfusion heterogeneity we can calculate the heterogeneity flow index (HFI) as the highest MFI minus the lowest MFI divided by the mean MFI. The proportion of perfused vessels (PPV) was calculated as ((total number of vessels - number of vessels with flow = 0 or 1) / total number of vessels) × 100. Finally, we can estimate the perfused vessel density (PVD) as MVD × PPV. It has been emphasized that the MFI only represents the convective component of tissue perfusion and oxygenation. Because PVD takes into account both MVD and MFI changes, it also represents the diffusive component of tissue oxygenation, resulting in a more integrative variable. Finally, the distribution of micro-vascular blood flow should be taken into account and is represented by the HFI (De Backer et al., 2007; Edul et al., 2012).

In summary, the vascular component approach, including the microcirculatory level, has potential advantages to the current diagnostic system. Targeting systemic he-modynamic targets and/or clinical surrogates of hypovolemia gives inadequate guarantee for the correction of tissue perfusion by fluid therapy especially in conditions of distributive shock as occur in inflammation and sepsis. The new concept of 'volume responsiveness' tends to be focus on the optimization of the microcirculatory determinants of oxygen transport to the tissues in addition to optimizing global systemic hemodynamic variables (Chawla et al., 2014; Ince, 2014; Ostergaard et al., 2015).

## 3   Fluid Management: Qualitative Aspects

Like any other drug used during acute illness, i.v. fluids have not only quantitative but also qualitative potential harmful effects. For this reason, after making the decision to give fluid, the choice of fluid to be given becomes an important decision and should be guided by contextual patient-specific factors (Raghunathan et al., 2014). Classically, fluid categorization focused on the comparison between specific crystalloids and colloids. Crystalloids are electrolyte solutions which are best used to replace extracellular volume losses. Although they increase vascular volume and may improve hemodynamics, the effectiveness is transient due to pass through capillary membranes. Crystalloids can be classified by their composition and osmolality (Table 4).

| Fluid | Osmolality (mOsm/L) | pH | Na$^+$ (mEq/L) | K$^+$ (mEq/L) | Ca$^{++}$ (mEq/L) | Lactate (mEq/L) | Cl$^-$ (mEq/L) | Acetate (mEq/L) |
|---|---|---|---|---|---|---|---|---|
| Plasma | 285 to 295 | 7.4 | 142 | 4 | 5 | 27 | 100 | |
| 0.9% saline | 308 | 5.5 | 154 | | | | 154 | |
| Lactate Ringer's | 273 | 6.5 | 130 | 5.4 | 2.7 | 29 | 109 | |
| Plasma-lyte | 294 | 7.4 | 140 | 5 | | | 98 | 27 |

**Table 4:** Commonly applied crystalloid solutions.

Colloids, which contain macromolecules suspended in sterile electrolyte solutions are expected to distribute largely within intravascular space by exerting a colloid osmotic pressure across the microvascular tissue barrier. Thus, according to Starling's original model, colloids may be expected to have about three-fold greater volume expansion efficacy than crystalloids. However, the recent revised Starling model, which recognizes the vital role in maintaining the vascular integrity of the endothelial glycocalyx has changed this relative advantage of colloids over crystalloids. In systemic inflammatory states such as surgery, sepsis, burns, the vascular barrier is compromised as the integrity of the glycocalyx is lost and all resuscitation fluids can contribute to the formation of interstitial oedema and tissue swelling. Thus, in these conditions, the fluid balance may be more important than fluid type concerning efficacy.

However, differences in safety are significant between them. The recent network meta-analyses are designed to evaluate direct and indirect effects via comparisons of multiple interventions and offer an opportunity to interpret the results of different types of fluids in similar scenarios with common outcomes. This network suggests that bolus of both crystalloid and colloid increased mortality compared with simple triage measures in critical illness, that is, the rate of administration may have greater effects on outcomes rather fluid type. Likewise, the greatest risk of renal replacement therapy (RRT) is conferred by HES (hydroxyethyl starch 6%), the least risk by balanced salt solutions, and both albumin and saline have approximately the same risk of necessitating RRT.

Infusions of moderate to large volumes of 0.9% saline can cause a hyperchloraemic acidosis with respect to balanced crystalloids (which are similar to human plasma in their composition, and strong ion difference). Hyperchloraemia can cause renal vasoconstriction, decreased renal artery flow velocity, blood flow, and reduced glomerular filtration rate, leading to salt and water retention when compared with balanced crystalloids (Chowdhury et al., 2012). A recent observational study of 22851 surgical patients with normal preoperative serum chloride concentration and renal function showed an incidence of acute postoperative hyperchloraemia (serum chloride > 110 meq/L) of 22% (Mccluskey et al., 2013). Patients with hyperchloraemia were found to be at increased risk of 30 day postoperative mortality, have a longer median hospital stay and were more likely to have postoperative renal dysfunction. This suggests that it may be time to reconsider the use of 0.9% saline as the default crystalloid of choice. However, high-quality randomized clinical trials are required (Raghunathan et al., 2014).

In summary, based on the current evidence, the ideal resuscitation fluid or combination of fluids remains undefined in a heterogeneous population of critically ill patients. It would appear that HES does increase the need of RRT, but does not increase mortality. Specific fluids may be superior in certain clinical settings, for example, saline in head injury and balanced fluids when there is risk of renal injury. Balanced salt solutions may reasonable default choice.

# 4   Perioperative versus Critical Ill Patients Fluid Management

Fluid management strategies can be different according to the clinical scenario. The majority of surgical patients receiving fluid therapy are ward patients in a healthy condition (or with little co-morbidity) scheduled to minor or median surgery. Until now, traditional perioperative fluid administration were based by estimates of known or anticipated fluid deficits and by ongoing sensible and insensible intraoperative fluid losses. Fixed perioperative fluid regimens to replace them has mostly been abandoned. Responses to fluid therapy vary widely between patients, and not all patients benefit from fluids (Navarro et al., 2015). Recent approaches are focused in both optimize and individualize perioperative fluid therapy with the application of specific goal-directed fluid therapy (GDT) protocols (Gurgel et al., 2011). To fluid optimization anesthesiologist should care: patient status (health, age and co-morbidities); surgical risk (procedure, approach) and selection of hemodynamic monitoring. GDT has many advantages of these strategies in terms of hemodynamic stability, oxygen transport balance, organ protection, and patient outcomes (Pearse et al., 2014). It includes the type, timing, rate, and amount of fluid being administered and the best measures to both optimize and individualize perioperative fluid therapy. Using specific parameters to identify best hypovolemia and tissue hypoperfusion and target parameters, the anesthesiologist can optimize perioperative fluid administration even in the presence of comorbidities, major surgical procedures, and large fluid shifts. In surgical scenario, dynamic indices should be an integral part of GDT to guide fluid administration since few confounders are usually present.

We recommend crystalloid solutions and the use of ASA standard monitors for routine surgery of short duration (low-risk patients and low-risk surgery). However, in major surgery the use of GDT containing colloid and balanced salt solutions is recommended, increasing the level of hemodynamic monitoring, concomitantly (Navarro et al., 2015). On the other hand, critical ill patients, especially in intensive care unit, hypotension, and inadequate organ perfusion are the most frequent hemodynamic perturbations, more care should be taken with fluid resuscitation. Fluid therapy is commonly the first-line treatment of circulatory failure in critically ill patients, and the ultimate goal is to improve CO and tissue perfusion after fluid challenge. Often these patients were fluid resuscitated for hours or days which imply the potential fluid overload with subsequent risks of complications. In ICU, positive cumulative fluid balance is an independent predictor of death, so conservative fluid strategies are highly recommended. Fluid challenge based on clinical criteria leads to a significant increase in SV and CO in approximately 52% of patients. As we previously mentioned, there are several methods that can be readily used at the bedside to assess the fluid responsiveness such as monitoring dynamic changes in SVV and pressure surrogates. All these methods have their limitations that can reduce their applicability and should be interpreted in the context of the patient. Nowadays, several hemodynamic monitors can calculate SV continuously, providing dynamic parameters such as SVV and PPV. Probably, while the fluid bolus challenge is one of the best tools that the anesthesiologist has for assessing fluid responsiveness, PLR is more common in ICU settings (Marik et al., 2011).

# 5 Conclusion

We recommend that fluid choice and therapy be individualized in unstable patients, either in the emergency department, operating room and ICU, with predefined physiologic targets. Both, quantity and quality of fluid are very important tasks. The final decision to administer fluids must be supported by the need for hemodynamic improvement, the presence of fluid responsiveness and the lack of associated risk.

Nowadays, several parameters are available to assess fluid responsiveness. These methods have evolved from static pressure and volume parameters (which are unable to predict fluid responsiveness), to dynamic indices (which are able to predict fluid responsiveness with a higher degree of accuracy), to those techniques based on either a virtual or a real fluid challenge (which have the higher degree of accuracy in predicting fluid responsiveness). Clinicians need to know all of them, with their limitations, being the final aim of all therapies to improve the microcirculation.

# Acknowledgement

Juan C Grignola is supported by PEDECIBA (Programa de Desarrollo de las Ciencias Básicas) and ANII (Agencia Nacional de Investigación e Innovación).

# References

Becker, B. F., Chappell, D., Jacob, M. (2010). Endothelial glycocalyx and coronary vascular permeability: The fringe benefit. Basic research in cardiology, 105, 687–701.

Benes, J., Zatloukal, J., Kletecka, J., Simanova, A., Haidingerova, L., Pradl, R. (2014). Respiratory induced dynamic variations of stroke volume and its surrogates as predictors of fluid responsiveness: Applicability in the early stages of specific critical states. Journal of clinical monitoring and computing, 28, 225–231.

Biais, M., Ehrmann, S., Mari, A., Conte, B., Mahjoub, Y., Desebbe, O., Pottecher, J., Lakhal, K., Benzekri-Lefevre, D., Molinari, N., Boulain, T., Lefrant, J. Y., Muller, L., AzuRea, G. (2014). Clinical relevance of pulse pressure variations for predicting fluid responsiveness in mechanically ventilated intensive care unit patients: The grey zone approach. Critical care, 18, 587.

Bognar, Z., Foldi, V., Rezman, B., Bogar, L., Csontos, C. (2010). Extravascular lung water index as a sign of developing sepsis in burns. Burns : journal of the International Society for Burn Injuries, 36, 1263–1270.

Bouchacourt, J. P., Riva, J. A., Grignola, J. C. (2013). The increase of vasomotor tone avoids the ability of the dynamic preload indicators to estimate fluid responsiveness. BMC anesthesiology, 13, 41.

Bouchacourt, J. P., Riva, J. A., Grignola, J. C. (2015). Right ventricular dysfunction: Another caution for functional preload parameters to predict volume responsiveness. Anesthesia and analgesia, 120, S360.

Bruegger, D., Schwartz, L., Chappell, D., Jacob, M., Rehm, M., Vogeser, M., Christ, F., Reichart, B., Becker, B. F. (2011). Release of atrial natriuretic peptide precedes shedding of the endothelial glycocalyx equally in patients undergoing on- and off-pump coronary artery bypass surgery. Basic research in cardiology, 106, 1111–1121.

Cannesson, M. (2010). Arterial pressure variation and goal-directed fluid therapy. Journal of cardiothoracic and vascular anesthesia, 24, 487–497.

Cannesson, M., Aboy, M., Hofer, C. K., Rehman, M. (2011). *Pulse pressure variation: Where are we today? Journal of clinical monitoring and computing, 25, 45–56.*

Cannesson, M., Le Manach, Y., Hofer, C. K., Goarin, J. P., Lehot, J. J., Vallet, B., Tavernier, B. (2011). *Assessing the diagnostic accuracy of pulse pressure variations for the prediction of fluid responsiveness: A "gray zone" approach. Anesthesiology, 115, 231–241.*

Carsetti, A., Cecconi, M., Rhodes, A. (2015). *Fluid bolus therapy: Monitoring and predicting fluid responsiveness. Current opinion in critical care, 21, 388–394.*

Cavallaro, F., Sandroni, C., Marano, C., La Torre, G., Mannocci, A., De Waure, C., Bello, G., Maviglia, R., Antonelli, M. (2010). *Diagnostic accuracy of passive leg raising for prediction of fluid responsiveness in adults: Systematic review and meta-analysis of clinical studies. Intensive care medicine, 36, 1475–1483.*

Craig, T. R., Duffy, M. J., Shyamsundar, M., McDowell, C., McLaughlin, B., Elborn, J. S., McAuley, D. F. (2010). *Extravascular lung water indexed to predicted body weight is a novel predictor of intensive care unit mortality in patients with acute lung injury. Critical care medicine, 38, 114–120.*

Chawla, L. S., Ince, C., Chappell, D., Gan, T. J., Kellum, J. A., Mythen, M., Shaw, A. D., Workgroup, A. X. F. (2014). *Vascular content, tone, integrity, and haemodynamics for guiding fluid therapy: A conceptual approach. British journal of anaesthesia, 113, 748–755.*

Chowdhury, A. H., Cox, E. F., Francis, S. T., Lobo, D. N. (2012). *A randomized, controlled, double-blind crossover study on the effects of 2-l infusions of 0.9% saline and plasma-lyte(r) 148 on renal blood flow velocity and renal cortical tissue perfusion in healthy volunteers. Annals of surgery, 256, 18–24.*

Chung, F. T., Lin, H. C., Kuo, C. H., Yu, C. T., Chou, C. L., Lee, K. Y., Kuo, H. P., Lin, S. M. (2010). *Extravascular lung water correlates multiorgan dysfunction syndrome and mortality in sepsis. PloS one, 5, e15265.*

De Backer, D., Heenen, S., Piagnerelli, M., Koch, M., Vincent, J. L. (2005). *Pulse pressure variations to predict fluid responsiveness: Influence of tidal volume. Intensive care medicine, 31, 517–523.*

De Backer, D., Hollenberg, S., Boerma, C., Goedhart, P., Buchele, G., Ospina-Tascon, G., Dobbe, I., Ince, C. (2007). *How to evaluate the microcirculation: Report of a round table conference. Critical care, 11, R101.*

Edul, V. S., Enrico, C., Laviolle, B., Vazquez, A. R., Ince, C., Dubin, A. (2012). *Quantitative assessment of the microcirculation in healthy volunteers and in patients with septic shock. Critical care medicine, 40, 1443–1448.*

Fonseca, E. B., Otsuki, D. A., Fantoni, D. T., Bliacheriene, F., Auler, J. O. (2008). *Comparative study of pressure- and volume-controlled ventilation on pulse pressure variation in a model of hypovolaemia in rabbits. European journal of anaesthesiology, 25, 388–394.*

Garcia, M. I., Romero, M. G., Cano, A. G., Aya, H. D., Rhodes, A., Grounds, R. M., Cecconi, M. (2014). *Dynamic arterial elastance as a predictor of arterial pressure response to fluid administration: A validation study. Critical care, 18, 626.*

Guinot, P. G., de Broca, B., Abou Arab, O., Diouf, M., Badoux, L., Bernard, E., Lorne, E., Dupont, H. (2013). *Ability of stroke volume variation measured by oesophageal doppler monitoring to predict fluid responsiveness during surgery. British journal of anaesthesia, 110, 28–33.*

Gurgel, S. T., do Nascimento, P., Jr. (2011). *Maintaining tissue perfusion in high-risk surgical patients: A systematic review of randomized clinical trials. Anesthesia and analgesia, 112, 1384–1391.*

Ince, C. (2014). *The rationale for microcirculatory guided fluid therapy. Current opinion in critical care, 20,*

*301–308.*

*Jacob, M., Chappell, D. (2013). Reappraising starling: The physiology of the microcirculation. Current opinion in critical care, 19, 282–289.*

*Jacques, D., Bendjelid, K., Duperret, S., Colling, J., Piriou, V., Viale, J. P. (2011). Pulse pressure variation and stroke volume variation during increased intra-abdominal pressure: An experimental study. Critical care, 15, R33.*

*Jozwiak, M., Teboul, J. L., Monnet, X. (2015). Extravascular lung water in critical care: Recent advances and clinical applications. Annals of intensive care, 5, 38.*

*Kubitz, J. C., Annecke, T., Kemming, G. I., Forkl, S., Kronas, N., Goetz, A. E., Reuter, D. A. (2006). The influence of positive end-expiratory pressure on stroke volume variation and central blood volume during open and closed chest conditions. European journal of cardio-thoracic surgery : official journal of the European Association for Cardio-thoracic Surgery, 30, 90–95.*

*Lansdorp, B., Lemson, J., van Putten, M. J., de Keijzer, A., van der Hoeven, J. G., Pickkers, P. (2012). Dynamic indices do not predict volume responsiveness in routine clinical practice. British journal of anaesthesia, 108, 395–401.*

*Lee, J. H., Kim, J. T., Yoon, S. Z., Lim, Y. J., Jeon, Y., Bahk, J. H., Kim, C. S. (2007). Evaluation of corrected flow time in oesophageal doppler as a predictor of fluid responsiveness. British journal of anaesthesia, 99, 343–348.*

*Lobo, D. N., Stanga, Z., Aloysius, M. M., Wicks, C., Nunes, Q. M., Ingram, K. L., Risch, L., Allison, S. P. (2010). Effect of volume loading with 1 liter intravenous infusions of 0.9% saline, 4% succinylated gelatine (gelofusine) and 6% hydroxyethyl starch (voluven) on blood volume and endocrine responses: A randomized, three-way crossover study in healthy volunteers. Critical care medicine, 38, 464–470.*

*Maguire, S., Rinehart, J., Vakharia, S., Cannesson, M. (2011). Technical communication: Respiratory variation in pulse pressure and plethysmographic waveforms: Intraoperative applicability in a north american academic center. Anesthesia and analgesia, 112, 94–96.*

*Mahjoub, Y., Lejeune, V., Muller, L., Perbet, S., Zieleskiewicz, L., Bart, F., Veber, B., Paugam-Burtz, C., Jaber, S., Ayham, A., Zogheib, E., Lasocki, S., Vieillard-Baron, A., Quintard, H., Joannes-Boyau, O., Plantefeve, G., Montravers, P., Duperret, S., Lakhdari, M., Ammenouche, N., Lorne, E., Slama, M., Dupont, H. (2014). Evaluation of pulse pressure variation validity criteria in critically ill patients: A prospective observational multicentre point-prevalence study. British journal of anaesthesia, 112, 681–685.*

*Mahjoub, Y., Pila, C., Friggeri, A., Zogheib, E., Lobjoie, E., Tinturier, F., Galy, C., Slama, M., Dupont, H. (2009). Assessing fluid responsiveness in critically ill patients: False-positive pulse pressure variation is detected by doppler echocardiographic evaluation of the right ventricle. Critical care medicine, 37, 2570–2575.*

*Mahjoub, Y., Touzeau, J., Airapetian, N., Lorne, E., Hijazi, M., Zogheib, E., Tinturier, F., Slama, M., Dupont, H. (2010). The passive leg-raising maneuver cannot accurately predict fluid responsiveness in patients with intra-abdominal hypertension. Critical care medicine, 38, 1824–1829.*

*Marik, P. E., Baram, M., Vahid, B. (2008). Does central venous pressure predict fluid responsiveness? A systematic review of the literature and the tale of seven mares. Chest, 134, 172–178.*

*Marik, P. E., Cavallazzi, R., Vasu, T., Hirani, A. (2009). Dynamic changes in arterial waveform derived variables and fluid responsiveness in mechanically ventilated patients: A systematic review of the literature. Critical care medicine, 37, 2642–2647.*

Marik, P. E., Lemson, J. (2014). Fluid responsiveness: An evolution of our understanding. British journal of anaesthesia, 112, 617–620.

Marik, P. E., Monnet, X., Teboul, J. L. (2011). Hemodynamic parameters to guide fluid therapy. Annals of intensive care, 1, 1.

Matthay, M. A., Folkesson, H. G., Clerici, C. (2002). Lung epithelial fluid transport and the resolution of pulmonary edema. Physiological reviews, 82, 569–600.

McCluskey, S. A., Karkouti, K., Wijeysundera, D., Minkovich, L., Tait, G., Beattie, W. S. (2013). Hyperchloremia after noncardiac surgery is independently associated with increased morbidity and mortality: A propensity-matched cohort study. Anesthesia and analgesia, 117, 412–421.

Michard, F. (2005). Changes in arterial pressure during mechanical ventilation. Anesthesiology, 103, 419-428; quiz 449–415.

Michard, F., Boussat, S., Chemla, D., Anguel, N., Mercat, A., Lecarpentier, Y., Richard, C., Pinsky, M. R., Teboul, J. L. (2000). Relation between respiratory changes in arterial pulse pressure and fluid responsiveness in septic patients with acute circulatory failure. American journal of respiratory and critical care medicine, 162, 134–138.

Michard, F., Chemla, D., Teboul, J. L. (2015). Applicability of pulse pressure variation: How many shades of grey? Critical care, 19, 144.

Miserocchi, G. (2009). Mechanisms controlling the volume of pleural fluid and extravascular lung water. European respiratory review : an official journal of the European Respiratory Society, 18, 244–252.

Monge Garcia, M. I., Gil Cano, A., Gracia Romero, M. (2011). Dynamic arterial elastance to predict arterial pressure response to volume loading in preload-dependent patients. Critical care, 15, R15.

Monnet, X., Anguel, N., Osman, D., Hamzaoui, O., Richard, C., Teboul, J. L. (2007). Assessing pulmonary permeability by transpulmonary thermodilution allows differentiation of hydrostatic pulmonary edema from ali/ards. Intensive care medicine, 33, 448–453.

Monnet, X., Chemla, D., Osman, D., Anguel, N., Richard, C., Pinsky, M. R., Teboul, J. L. (2007). Measuring aortic diameter improves accuracy of esophageal doppler in assessing fluid responsiveness. Critical care medicine, 35, 477–482.

Monnet, X., Teboul, J. L. (2008). Passive leg raising. Intensive care medicine, 34, 659–663.

Monnet, X., Teboul, J. L. (2015). Passive leg raising: Five rules, not a drop of fluid! Critical care, 19, 18.

Navarro, L. H., Bloomstone, J. A., Auler, J. O., Jr., Cannesson, M., Rocca, G. D., Gan, T. J., Kinsky, M., Magder, S., Miller, T. E., Mythen, M., Perel, A., Reuter, D. A., Pinsky, M. R., Kramer, G. C. (2015). Perioperative fluid therapy: A statement from the international fluid optimization group. Perioperative medicine, 4, 3.

Nouira, S., Elatrous, S., Dimassi, S., Besbes, L., Boukef, R., Mohamed, B., Abroug, F. (2005). Effects of norepinephrine on static and dynamic preload indicators in experimental hemorrhagic shock. Critical care medicine, 33, 2339–2343.

Osman, D., Ridel, C., Ray, P., Monnet, X., Anguel, N., Richard, C., Teboul, J. L. (2007). Cardiac filling pressures are not appropriate to predict hemodynamic response to volume challenge. Critical care medicine, 35, 64–68.

Ostergaard, L., Granfeldt, A., Secher, N., Tietze, A., Iversen, N. K., Jensen, M. S., Andersen, K. K., Nagenthiraja, K., Gutierrez-Lizardi, P., Mouridsen, K., Jespersen, S. N., Tonnesen, E. K. (2015). Microcirculatory dysfunction and tissue oxygenation in critical illness. Acta anaesthesiologica

*Scandinavica, 59, 1246–1259.*

Payen, D., de Pont, A. C., Sakr, Y., Spies, C., Reinhart, K., Vincent, J. L., Sepsis Occurrence in Acutely Ill Patients, I. (2008). A positive fluid balance is associated with a worse outcome in patients with acute renal failure. Critical care, 12, R74.

Pearse, R. M., Harrison, D. A., MacDonald, N., Gillies, M. A., Blunt, M., Ackland, G., Grocott, M. P., Ahern, A., Griggs, K., Scott, R., Hinds, C., Rowan, K., Group, O. S. (2014). Effect of a perioperative, cardiac output-guided hemodynamic therapy algorithm on outcomes following major gastrointestinal surgery: A randomized clinical trial and systematic review. Jama, 311, 2181–2190.

Perel, A., Habicher, M., Sander, M. (2013). Bench-to-bedside review: Functional hemodynamics during surgery - should it be used for all high-risk cases? Critical care, 17, 203.

Phillips, C. R., Chesnutt, M. S., Smith, S. M. (2008). Extravascular lung water in sepsis-associated acute respiratory distress syndrome: Indexing with predicted body weight improves correlation with severity of illness and survival. Critical care medicine, 36, 69–73.

Raghunathan, K., Murray, P. T., Beattie, W. S., Lobo, D. N., Myburgh, J., Sladen, R., Kellum, J. A., Mythen, M. G., Shaw, A. D., Group, A. X. I. (2014). Choice of fluid in acute illness: What should be given? An international consensus. British journal of anaesthesia, 113, 772–783.

Recommended methods for measurement of red-cell and plasma volume: International committee for standardization in haematology (1980). Journal of nuclear medicine : official publication, Society of Nuclear Medicine, 21, 793–800.

Renner, J., Gruenewald, M., Meybohm, P., Hedderich, J., Steinfath, M., Scholz, J., Bein, B. (2008). Effect of elevated peep on dynamic variables of fluid responsiveness in a pediatric animal model. Paediatric anaesthesia, 18, 1170–1177.

Renner, J., Meybohm, P., Hanss, R., Gruenewald, M., Scholz, J., Bein, B. (2009). Effects of norepinephrine on dynamic variables of fluid responsiveness during hemorrhage and after resuscitation in a pediatric porcine model. Paediatric anaesthesia, 19, 688–694.

Renner, J., Scholz, J., Bein, B. (2009). Monitoring fluid therapy. Best practice & research. Clinical anaesthesiology, 23, 159–171.

Rex, S., Schalte, G., Schroth, S., de Waal, E. E., Metzelder, S., Overbeck, Y., Rossaint, R., Buhre, W. (2007). Limitations of arterial pulse pressure variation and left ventricular stroke volume variation in estimating cardiac pre-load during open heart surgery. Acta anaesthesiologica Scandinavica, 51, 1258–1267.

Sakka, S. G., Reuter, D. A., Perel, A. (2012). The transpulmonary thermodilution technique. Journal of clinical monitoring and computing, 26, 347–353.

Sakr, Y., Vincent, J. L., Reinhart, K., Groeneveld, J., Michalopoulos, A., Sprung, C. L., Artigas, A., Ranieri, V. M., Sepsis Occurence in Acutely Ill Patients, I. (2005). High tidal volume and positive fluid balance are associated with worse outcome in acute lung injury. Chest, 128, 3098–3108.

Santana, D. B., Barra, J. G., Grignola, J. C., Gines, F. F., Armentano, R. L. (2005). Pulmonary artery smooth muscle activation attenuates arterial dysfunction during acute pulmonary hypertension. Journal of applied physiology, 98, 605–613.

Schober, P., Loer, S. A., Schwarte, L. A. (2009). Perioperative hemodynamic monitoring with transesophageal doppler technology. Anesthesia and analgesia, 109, 340–353.

Schober, P., Loer, S. A., Schwarte, L. A. (2009). Transesophageal doppler devices: A technical review. Journal of clinical monitoring and computing, 23, 391–401.

Vincent, J. L., Pelosi, P., Pearse, R., Payen, D., Perel, A., Hoeft, A., Romagnoli, S., Ranieri, V. M., Ichai, C., Forget, P., Della Rocca, G., Rhodes, A. (2015). *Perioperative cardiovascular monitoring of high-risk patients: A consensus of 12. Critical care, 19, 224.*

Vincent, J. L., Sakr, Y., Sprung, C. L., Ranieri, V. M., Reinhart, K., Gerlach, H., Moreno, R., Carlet, J., Le Gall, J. R., Payen, D., Sepsis Occurrence in Acutely Ill Patients, I. (2006). *Sepsis in european intensive care units: Results of the soap study. Critical care medicine, 34, 344–353.*

Vistisen, S. T., Koefoed-Nielsen, J., Larsson, A. (2010). *Should dynamic parameters for prediction of fluid responsiveness be indexed to the tidal volume? Acta anaesthesiologica Scandinavica, 54, 191–198.*

Wyler von Ballmoos, M., Takala, J., Roeck, M., Porta, F., Tueller, D., Ganter, C. C., Schroder, R., Bracht, H., Baenziger, B., Jakob, S. M. (2010). *Pulse-pressure variation and hemodynamic response in patients with elevated pulmonary artery pressure: A clinical study. Critical care, 14, R111.*

Yang, X., Du, B. (2014). *Does pulse pressure variation predict fluid responsiveness in critically ill patients? A systematic review and meta-analysis. Critical care, 18, 650.*

# Chapter 13

# Sweet Potato: Production Trends And Health Benefits

Lowell Dilworth[1], Dewayne Stennett[2] and Felix Omoruyi[3]

## 1   Introduction

Sweet potato (*Ipomoea batatas (L)* Lam), is a dicotyledonous plant belonging to the family *Convulaceae*, genus *Ipomoea*, and species *batatas*. It is a highly nutritious hardy crop believed to be first cultivated in Central and South America. It is thought to have been taken from the new world to Europe by early explorers and from there, transported to other parts of the world. Although this sequence of events is often disputed, most people seem to agree on the origins of the crop. Historically, it has been produced in various parts of the world where different names including camote, boniato, Kumar, cilera abana, karaimo, among others were ascribed to this single plant (Denham, 2013). It is grown in about one hundred and eleven (111) countries, with 90% of these being classified as developing countries (Philpott et al., 2003). It serves as an important means of income generation for many people from low income backgrounds. Unlike potato which is categorized as a tuber, sweet potato is a storage root with cultivars differing from each other by the color of the skin, which can vary from white, brown, yellow or purple. Color of skin and root tissue itself is due to pigments including carotenoids and phenolic compounds within the plant. These colored compounds are thought to possess beneficial properties and are extracted from sweet potato for utilization in the food industry as natural colorants (Cevallos-Casals and Cisneros-Zevallos, 2004). There are many other commercial applications

---

[1] Department of Pathology, The University of the West Indies, Mona, Jamaica.

[2] Department of Basic Medical Sciences, Biochemistry Section, The University of the West Indies, Mona, Jamaica.

[3] Department of Life Sciences, College of Science and Engineering, Texas A&M University – Corpus Christi, Corpus Christi, Texas, USA.

of sweet potato and its components that remain to be unraveled. However, the crop is still considered exotic in some areas hence the emphasis on its production remains low in many parts of the world.

Data from the food and agriculture organization indicates that sweet potato production in two of the top five producing countries recorded a decline over ten years (as seen in China and Vietnam) while the other nations recorded increased productivity over that timeframe. Production values for North America remained relatively steady within that time where approximately 28,000 tons were produced per annum. Although the United States of American is not in the top five sweet potato producing countries, they have been the top exporters with most of the product destined for the UK market (FAO-STAT, 2013). This trend is thought to be due to the impact of globalization especially with respect to emerging trends in diaspora populations. In the USA, sweet potatoes are mistakenly referred to as yams but this is a misnomer as there are clear distinctions between both. Sweet potatoes belong to the *Convolvulaceae* family and are dicotyledonous plants while yams belong to the *Dioscoreaceae* family and are monocotyledons (Bovell-Benjamin et al., 2007). In addition, the edible portions of yams normally have higher levels of starch, are drier and are true tubers while sweet potatoes are true roots.

Sweet potato is now the fifth most important crop, moving up two places since the early 2000s, with current global production of over 105 million metric tons (The International Potato Center, 2015). Sweet potato is a staple food source for many indigenous populations (Bovell-Benjamin, 2007). Sweet potato cultivars exceed that for yam, cassava or cocoyams. Many of these cultivars are from systematic breeding efforts, while others are through natural hybridization and mutations. Although the crop is vastly important, the botanical origin as well as timing and location(s) of its domestication are still undetermined. However, wild types are thought to have been domesticated in Central and South America such that two gene pools have been identified (Roullier et al., 2013).

Sweet potatoes are generally grown between latitudes 42° N and 35° S, anywhere from sea level up to an altitude of 3000 M with 90 % of worldwide production occurring in China (CIP 2015). In some areas, for example sub-Saharan Africa, sweet potato is one of the main carbohydrate crops that is adaptable to low rainfall and marginal soils resulting in some amount of yield even in drought conditions (Mbanaso et al., 2012). Apart from the nutritional content, this crop is highly favored for its low concentration of antinutrients such as cyanides and oxalates compared to similar crops such as cassava, yams and cocoyams (Nwokocha, 1993). Sweet potato also has a short turn-around time (between 4 to 6 months) from planting to harvesting, thereby making it possible to harvest two to three crops for the year (Mbanaso et al., 2012). Another aspect of this crop which makes it versatile is that the root, stem and leaves are edible; the crop is highly utilized for both human and animal consumption. Per capita production has however fallen to about one-third the levels in 1970s in part due to the decline in demand in China especially for animal feed (FAOSTAT 2013). Nevertheless, worldwide production per hectare is still appreciable at 14.1 t/ha although production tends to be lower in sub-Saharan African countries with an average of 9.53t/ha (FAOSTAT, 2009).

Table 1 shows sweet potato production trends for the top five producing countries over ten years. A decline in production was recorded in China and Vietnam while all other nations on the top five list recorded increased productivity. Although a reduction in production trend is noticed in the main producers such as China, Brazil, Indonesia and the Phillipines, some African countries have recorded increased production with increased harvesting in Uganda — about 2 million Mt in 1999 to 2.83 Mt in 2010 (Scott et al., 1999). Currently, more than 105 million metric tons of sweet potato are produced annually (cipotato.org). These figures may however be grossly underestimated due to the informal nature of sweet potato cultivation that takes place in many low income countries which makes it difficult to gather data. Nonetheless, global projection shows that sweet potato production is expected to increase steadily up to the year 2020 (Scott, 2000).

| Country | Production (Tons) | |
|---|---|---|
| | 2003–2008 | 2009–2013 |
| China | 91,761,833 | 81,104,450 |
| Nigeria | 3,035,500 | 3,216,300 |
| Uganda | 2,642,118 | 2,663,341 |
| Indonesia | 1,894,713 | 2,055,199 |
| Vietnam | 1,459,350 | 1,385,217 |

**Table 1:** Sweet potato production trend in top five producing countries between 2003 and 2013 (Source: FAOSTAT, 2015).

## 2   Nutritional Properties of Sweet Potato

Sweet potatoes are thought to be one of the oldest vegetables known to man and have been consumed since prehistoric times (Murray et al., 2005). The roots are the most used part of this plant species, although the leaves can also be used. The roots are sweet tasting, moist and delicate with a pleasant aromatic smell. They also have high nutritional value (about 50% higher than potato), and plays an important role in the diet of the world's population. The roots display diverse shapes and flesh colors depending on the cultivar (Maloney et al., 2012). They are a staple food source for many indigenous populations in China, Central and South Americas, Ryukyu Island, Africa, the Caribbean, the Maori people, Hawaii, and Papua New Guinea. The sweet potato plant is adaptable to a wide ecological range with relatively short growing seasons and of high yield potential even on infertile soil (Hahn, 1984). The root is prepared for eating after it is boiled in or out of the skin until soft and mealy. The root may also be fried to make chips, baked to make sweet potato pies or puddings or cooked in a variety of other ways to make confectionaries, snacks and drinks.

The sweet potato plant serves both nutritional and medicinal importance in society. Every part of the plant exhibits some beneficial role and is now being recognized as a health food. It has been ranked amongst the vegetable superstars based on nutrient content by the Center for Science in the Public Interest (CSPI). The CSPI gave points for content of dietary fiber, simple sugars and complex carbohydrates, proteins, vitamins and minerals. Points were deducted for fats, particularly saturated fat, sodium, cholesterol, added refined sugars and caffeine. The vegetables with the highest scores were deemed most nutritious.

The main nutritional materials in sweet potato's tubers are carbohydrates, protein, fat and fat soluble vitamins. The peel of the sweet potato root contains potentially valuable proteins that may be beneficial to human health (Maloney et al., 2012). Sweet potato starch is composed of about one quarter amylose and three-quarters amylopectin and most of them are converted to maltose during cooking (Onwueme, 1978). It is a good source of fiber and some important vitamins and minerals. The protein of sweet potato (about 5% on a dry weight basis) consists of about two thirds globulin. The protein contains reasonable amounts of most essential amino acids. However, the levels of tryptophan and other sulphur containing amino acids are slightly low (Onwueme, 1978). The peel of sweet potato is higher in protein, minerals and other non-carbohydrate constituents than the rest of the tuber. The major minerals present in sweet potato tuber include potassium, sodium, calcium, and phosphorous. Other minerals such as zinc, iron and magnesium are also present. Although most of the cultivars are rich in the antioxidant β-carotene, the cultivars with flesh that are orange or yellow in color also contain significant amount of carotene, the vitamin A precursor (Allen et al., 2012) compared to those with white flesh. Sweet potatoes have the ability to raise the blood vitamin A levels and can meet up to 90% of our vitamin A needs. All varieties of sweet potatoes are good sources of vitamins A, C and E as well as dietary fiber, potassium, and iron (Sobukola et al., 2010). The roots are low in fat and cholesterol while serving as a substantial source of dietary fiber. Dietary fiber is the undigested and unabsorbable carbohydrate and lignin components of plants present in the diet (Slavin, 2008). Research has revealed the relationship between dietary fiber intake and the incidence of constipation, obesity, cardiovascular diseases, colon cancer, and diabetes mellitus (Redondo-Cuenca et al., 2006). Crude fiber in the leaves tend to be higher than the tubers making it very important because of its possible role in the prevention and treatment of diseases such as obesity, diabetes, cancer and gastro intestinal disorders (Saldanha, 1995). The table below outlines the nutritional composition of sweet potato roots.

Several epidemiologic studies have shown that higher sodium and lower potassium intake are associated with increased risk of developing cardiovascular diseases and mortality (Yang et al., 2011). Sweet potatoes may therefore be beneficial in reducing the risk of developing cardiovascular diseases due to its high potassium levels. Both the leaves and storage roots of the sweet potato plant contain phytochemicals, such as tannins, oxalates and phytate, which could affect the bioavailability of nutrients to the body (Fleming 1981; Udoessien and Ifon, 1990; Osagie 1998). In our assessment of some tuber crops in the Carribeean, phytic acid level was highest in sweet potato compared to other tuber crops (Omoruyi et al., 2004). Processing and cooking can however be used to reduce the antinutrient content. Some phytochemicals, however, are known to be beneficial to human health. The medicinal properties attributed to sweet potato include anti-diabetic, anti-oxidant and anti-proliferative, anti-inflammatory, anti-bacterial, anti-fungal, anti-viral, anti-ulcer, hepatoprotective, wound healing and immunomodulatory due to the presence of valuable nutritional and mineral components (Parle and Monica,

2015). Furthermore, *Ipomoea batatas* tubers appear to be very beneficial in the diet of diabetics with an insulin resistance due to its low glycemic index (Ludvik et al., 2004; Allen et al., 2012).

While the fleshy portions of most varieties of sweet potatoes range in color from yellow to orange, some varieties have flesh that are purple in color. This occurs as a result of the presence of anthocyanins. They are also responsible for the color of the skin. Anthocyanins have important antioxidant and anti-inflammatory properties and play potentially therapeutic roles in various diseases (Basuny et al., 2012). Anthocyanins and their aglycones exhibit antiproliferative and pro-apoptotic properties in a wide range of cancers (Martin et al., 2003; Shih et al., 2005; Yi et al., 2005). The cytotoxic effects involve induction of apoptosis rather than necrosis through caspase dependent and independent pathways (Reddivari et al., 2007). The anthocyanins have also been shown to possess neuroprotective effects by increasing the activities of mouse brain as well as causing a decrease in production of neuro-inflammatory factors such as nuclear factor-kappa B (NFκB), nitric oxide synthase (iNOS) and cyclooxygenase (COX)-2 (Shan et al., 2009). The sweet potato storage root has a high content of enzymes such as polyphenol oxidase (PPO), catalase (CAT), and superoxide dismutase (SOD) which could possibly be effective in protecting cells against oxidative damage (Teow et al., 2007). Antioxidant properties have also been exhibited by storage proteins in the tubers known as sporamins (Shewry 2003). Other important nutrients present in sweet potato tubers include phytochelatins, which bind toxic heavy metals, and the glycosides batatins and batatosides, both of which possess antibacterial and antifungal properties.

# 3   Industrial Uses of Sweet Potato

Currently, sweet potatoes are utilized in various forms across the globe. In the food industry sweet potato serves as a source of raw materials for products such as flour, which is used for baking purposes. Other food related products created from the sweet potato base materials include beers and beverages, chips, jam, jelly, noodles, canned sweet potato, starch, liquid glucose, high fructose syrup, maltose (Attaluri et al., 2010; Odebode et al., 2008). The animal feed industry utilizes all parts of the plant to prepare compound feed for cattle, poultry and pigs (Attaluri et al., 2010). Reports from the Bureau of Agriculture Research in the Department of Agriculture in the Phillipines have highlighted the use of sweet potatoes in the production of aquafeeds for fishes and crabs. Starch produced from sweet potatoes is also used in the manufacture of a wide variety of products. These include starch syrups, isomerized glucose syrup, lactic acid beverages, bread and other baked goods as well as distilled spirits. In beer production, amylase from sweet potato can be substituted for amylase from barley (Joo Suh et al, 2003). Various studies have shown that the sweet taste developed during the cooking of sweet potato occurs as a result of the action of amylases (Walter et al., 1975). Slow cooking (range 60°C –100°C) increases the susceptibility of the starch towards enzymatic hydrolysis (Walter et al., 1975). Sweet potato processing increases the length of the storage and marketing times. Processing can take place with or without the application of heat. High pressure processing, pulse electric field and electronic beams are all examples of processing without heat. Processing by heat application includes blanching, pasteurisation, sterilization, evaporation, drying, concentration, microwave and infra-red (Oke and Workneh, 2013).

Varieties of sweet potatoes have been created for bioenergy purposes that could serve as a biorenewable alternative for fossil fuels. These varieties are not intended for consumption. To date, the major source of bioethanol production has been sugarcane and grains (Lareo *et al*, 2013). Sweet potato, however, has a higher yield per unit land cultivated than grains and therefore serves as a promising raw material for alcohol fermentation (Lareo et al., 2013). The three main steps involved in the production of fuel ethanol include the liquefaction of starch using amylase, saccharification of the liquefied product to produce glucose and fermentation to ethanol (Sree et al., 2000). The liquefaction or hydrolysis process involves two stages, namely dextrinisation and saccharification. The dextrinisation process employs the use of alpha-amylase enzyme while glucoamylase is used in saccharification. The liquefaction process however requires a preliminary step to be performed, known as gelatinisation, in order to ensure efficient hydrolysis. Yeast is subsequently added to allow for the fermentation of the resulting glucose to ethanol utilizing an anaerobic fermentation process. The resulting fermentation broth then undergoes distillation resulting in the production of ethanol that is 95% pure.

One major setbacks relation to the use of sweet potato tubers in product development is the issue of discoloration upon exposure to air. This problem of browning occurs as a result of the enzymatic oxidative browning caused by polyphenol oxidase. This enzyme catalyzes the reaction involved in the production of
o-quinones from phenols. The resulting o-quinones react with amino acids and proteins to form brown/dark melanin pigments (Severini et al., 2003). These browning reactions can be controlled by the application of aqueous solutions containing antioxidants to freshly cut tubers. Antioxidant solutions most popularly used include sulphites, ascorbic acid and citric acid (Arogundade and Mu, 2012).

# 4   Bioactive Components in Sweet Potato

In addition to vitamins, minerals, carbohydrates and fiber, sweet potatoes are also found to be rich sources of antioxidants, including β-carotene, phenolic acids, anthocyanins and tocopherol (Woolfe, 1993). In our assessment of some tuber crops, phytic acid level was highest in sweet potato and lowest in cocoyam (Omoruyi et al., 2004). While the roots are widely studied, sweet potato leaves are also shown to be highly nutritious as they can serve as dietary source of antioxidants, vitamins, minerals, dietary fiber and essential fatty acids (Johnson and Pace, 2010). Bioactive components are of special interest especially in light of their perceived health benefits. Recent research has focused on the antioxidant activities of these bioactive compounds as a means of improving mammalian health. In this regard, sweet potato has become an area of interest since it has appreciable concentrations of some important bioactive compounds discussed below.

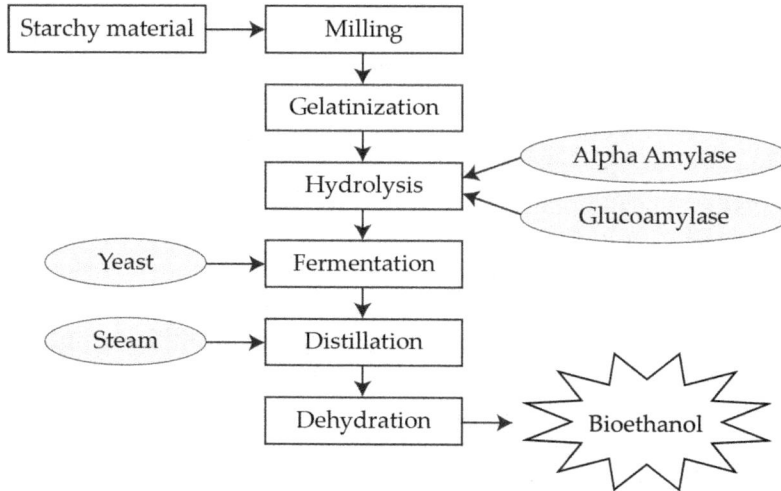

**Figure 1:** Main steps in fuel ethanol production.

# 5   Antocyanins

Anthocyanins belong to the phenolic class of compounds and are considered to be the most important group of flavonoid pigments. They are responsible for the wide variety of intense orange, red and blue pigments observed in leaves, flowers and fruits of many plants including berries (cranberry, gooseberry, blackberry, blueberry, strawberry etc.), grapes, citrus, plums and vegetables (Wu et al., 2006). In some quarters, it is thought that once a fruit is intensely red or purple colored, it is highly likely that the anthocyanin content will be high. From an economic standpoint, it is thought that these intense colors displayed by the crop attracts buyers attention while from an ecological perspective, herbivores are attracted to the plant resulting in increased chance of seed dispersal and plant proliferation. In addition to fruits, some tuber crops including purple yam (*Dioscorea alata*) and some cultivars of sweet potatoes are also shown to have high anthoycyanin concentrations. In fact, studies done on tuber crops have reported that cultivars with more intense colors had higher anthocyanins concentrations and subsequently displayed higher antioxidant activities compared to those with yellow or white tissue (Lubag et al., 2008; Hamouz et al., 2011). Not only do these compounds confer appreciable antioxidant potential to plants but as a result of their intense coloration, they are widely utilized in the food industry as substitutes for synthetic dyes as natural colorants. These natural food additives are thought to be safer than synthethic additives owing to the reduced risk of allergic reactions associated with synthetics (Jansen and Flamme, 2006). Overall, low toxicity, beneficial health properties, desirable colors and water soluble properties make anthocyanins very useful in a wide range of commercial applications. Substitution of the R groups with other functional groups leads to the formation of different anthocyanins.

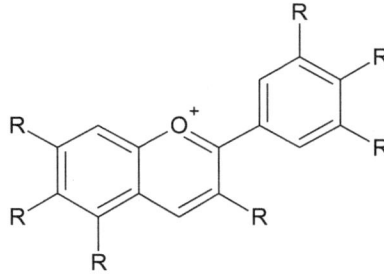

**Figure 2:** General structure of Anthocyanins.

# 6   Anthocyanin Chemistry and Health Benefits

In plants, anthocyanins are thought to play important roles in pollination and seed dispersal by attracting animals, while in storage tissues such as tubers and roots, they are believed to play key roles in plant defense mechanisms and protection from herbivory (Philpott et al., 2004). One reason for these conclusions is the observed upregulation of anthocyanin content of plant tissue following external stress factors that result in generation of reactive oxidative species (Dixon et al., 1994). Anthocyanins are shown to possess free radical scavenging activity ability that gives rise to their antioxidant properties making them useful targets in the treatment of cardiovascular and other diseases including diabetes mellitus and cancers (Castañeda-Ovando et al., 2009).

Even within the same plant species anthocyanins content and concentration differ. The most common ones found in regularly eaten tubers include p-coumaroyl-5-glucoside-3-rhamnoglucosides of pelargonidin, cyanidin, peonidin, delphinidin, petunidin, and malvidin 3,5- diglucoside (Ramos-Escudero, 2010; Hamouz et al., 2011). Interestingly, it was found that there are slight differences in molecular structure of anthocyanins from berries compared to those in tubers. Anthocyanins in sweet potato are normally acylated which may confer greater activity on the molecule (Lim et al., 2013). This along with other factors show that anthocyanins from some sweet potato cultivars display higher antioxidant potential compared to anthocyanins derived from fruits and vegetables. This free radical scavenging ability was demonstrated by reduced parameters of liver damage observed in rats subjected to oxidative damage in the form of carbon tetra chloride followed by subsequent administration of sweet potato anthocyanins (Kano et al., 2005). Further studies on cell viability and cell cycle progression indicate that sweet potato anthocyanins protect against colorectal cancer in mice by inducing cell cycle arrest as well as upregulating other anti-proliferative and apoptotic mechanisms (Lim et al., 2013). Studies in vision research indicate that sweet potato anthocyanins are capable of crossing the blood–retinal barrier thereby accumulating in the eyes and may therefore be beneficial to proliferation and maintenance of cells responsible for sight (Sun et al., 2015). Anthocyanin extracts from sweet potato may also play a role in obesity control. It is thought that the compounds work by inhibiting hepatic lipid accumulation by way of activating adenosine monophosphate–activated protein kinase (AMPK) signaling pathways in both *in vitro* and *in vivo* systems (Hwang et al., 2011).

Numerous other health benefits are attributed to sweet potato anthocyanins extracts in purified or semi-purified forms. *In vivo* and *in vitro* studies indicate that anthocyanins extracted from sweet potatoes possess anti-aging, anti-diabetic properties in addition to anti-tumor properties already discussed (Jang et al., 2013; Zhao, 2013). These extracts are also shown to play a role in modulating cognitive and motor function as well as enhancing memory in part by preventing neural function decline normally associated with the normal ageing process (Lila, 2004). Although anthocyanins have been shown to possess high thermostability, the processing methods that foods undergo may affect anthocyanins content differently. Only marginal reductions in anthocyanins were observed in sweet potato subjected to baking, however, the use of moist heat in the form of steam, reduces anthocyanins content by almost 50% (Kim et al., 2012). Processing methods of foods should therefore be taken into consideration once the goal of preserving anthocyanin integrity becomes important. From a commercial standpoint, purple sweet potatoes are used in the food industry to make food coloring, and in the clothing and textile industry to make dyes (The American Chemical Society, 2013; Peng et al., 2012) due to the high anthocyanin content of the crop.

# 7   Estrigenic Effect of Anthocyanins

Studies on anthocyanins show that some of these compounds play key roles in altering the development of hormone-dependent disease symptoms otherwise referred to as estrogenic properties. It is thought that some anthocyanins react with estrogen receptors owing to some degree of structural homology between the molecules and estrogen. *In vitro* studies on the estrogen-receptor positive cell line MCF-7, shows that some anthocyanins are capable of binding to estrogen receptor-alpha followed by induction of expression of a reporter gene, thereby activating estrogen-independent gene expression (Harris and Go, 2006). The entire mechanism of action is not entirely clear but flow cytometry analysis shows that anthocyanins can manipulate cellular proliferation by reducing the number of cells in the G0/G1 phase and increase the numbers in G2/M phases respectively (Nanashima, 2015). Further work aimed at unraveling the full mechanisms involved is needed. In addition to MCF-7 cell lines, anthocyanins are also shown to display estrogenic effects in BG-1 cell lines but no activity was observed in receptor negative MDA-MB-231 cells (Schmitt et al, 2001). To this end, the estrogenic effects of these compounds are thought to play key roles in development of hormone-dependent cancers involving a mechanism of action similar to that of phytoestrogens (Bandera and Kushi, 2003). Some estrogenic effects of anthocyanins are based on positive effects that they have on arterial walls leading to reduced risk of cardiovascular diseases (Hidalgo et al., 2012). Clinical studies with patients who have a preexisting cardiovascular pathology shows that anthocyanin consumption is positively associated with low incidences of ischemia, blood pressure, inflammatory status and dyslipidemia, all of which contribute to coronary artery diseases (Wallace, 2011). Cardiovascular health may also be positively influenced by anthocyanins by increasing nitric oxide production in endothelial cells via $Er\alpha$ activation

(Chalopin et al., 2010). In one study, the estrogenic properties of anthocyanins were attributed to their ability to modulate neurodegenerative effects of domoic acid. This occurs following binding of sweet potato anthocyanins and subsequent stimulation of estrogen receptor-$\alpha$-mediated mitochondrial biogenesis signaling and by reduced expression of the NADPH oxidase subunits p47phox and gp91phox (Lu et al., 2012). Research indicates that since anthocyanins have an affinity for estrogen receptors, they can potentially act on target genes and tissues leading to beneficial health effects (Hidalgo et al., 2012). Finally, it is believed that estrogenic properties of anthocyanins can be exploited in cases of mammalian estrogen deficiency with research showing improved learning and memory in estrogen deficit rats that are fed anthocyanin supplemented diets (Varadinova et al., 2009).

# 8    Phytates

Phytates are found in tuber crops including sweet potatoes. These compounds are reported to have numerous beneficial properties and have sparked a great amount of research interest. Phyates are formed when phytic acid, myoinositol (1, 2, 3, 4, 5, 6) hexakisphosphoric acid forms salts with divalent cations including calcium, zinc, potassium, iron and magnesium (Raboy, 2002). They are predominantly found in grains, nuts and cereals where they function as the main storage form of phosphorus accounting for 50% to 80% of total phosphorus content of mature seeds (Loewus, 2002; Lin *et al.*, 2005). Phytic acid (IP6) is thought to be responsible for seeds remarkable longevity of up to 400 years (Owen et al., 1996; Lopez, 1998). Roots and tubers also have significant levels of phytic acid. However, the levels of phytic acid in fruits are generally lower than the levels in seeds with the exception of avocado fruit. They are also found in animal tissue and even in soil. In fact, their presence in seeds is thought to be protective against oxidative damage which results in some seeds surviving prolonged storage for many years with viability retention (Doria et al., 2009).

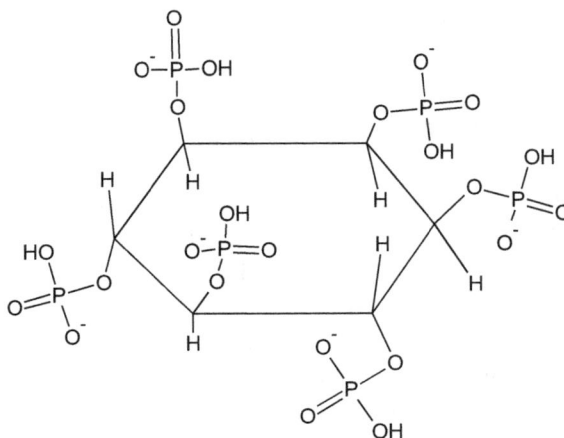

**Figure 3:** General Structure of Phytic acid.

Phosphate groups may chelate divalent cations forming salts. In the past, the chelating ability of the compound has resulted in its classification as an anti-nutrient as it binds to minerals in the gastrointestinal tract making them unavailable for absorption and metabolism (Lonnerdal, 2003). It is also thought that IP6 is capable of binding to some enzymes in the gastrointestinal tract (GIT). This is however thought to be beneficial as it may result in the slow release of digestion products and reduced absorption (Yoon et al., 1983; Omoruyi et al., 2013).

# 9   Beneficial Properties of Phytates

Phytates derived from sweet potato are shown to possess hypoglycemic properties which make them a potential target in the treatment of diabetes mellitus. The mechanism is thought to be related to the ability of sweet potato IP6 to regulate enzymes related to carbohydrate and lipid metabolism (Dilworth et al., 2005). Phytates may also possess cardioprotective properties as seen by its positive effects in controlling dyslipidemia. Animal studies have shown that following the consumption of a diet supplemented with sweet potato IP6 extract, there was observed increase in fecal cholesterol output along with increased serum high density lipoprotein (Dilworth et al., 2015). These effects are thought to be in part due to upregulation of intestinal lipase by IP6 extract. Other studies corroborate this data as reduced serum triglycerides and increased HDL were observed in animals that consumed phytate supplemented diets (Omoruyi et al., 2013). It is also thought that phytates elicit hypoglycemic properties due to their ability to enhance insulin activity thereby reduced glycated hemoglobin (HBA1c) in the long term (Lee et al., 2006). Still, other studies indicate that the hypoglycemic properties of phytates are in part due to their ability to modulate serum amylase activity thereby reducing the rate of release of simple sugars into the blood while simultaneously reducing damage that are normally observed with inflammatory disorders (Kunyanga et al., 2011). There is good evidence for the utilization of sweet potato phytates in the treatment of metabolic disorders including diabetes mellitus and dyslipidemias as these compounds are able to modulate enzymes and metabolites involved in carbohydrate and lipid metabolism.

# 10   Anticancer Properties of Phytates

Phytates are known to possess anticancer properties. As a natural antioxidant, they are capable of lowering the incidence of diseases caused by free radicals and lipid peroxidation products (Zajdel et al., 2013). This makes phytates suitable candidates for use in the prevention of cancers that may arise from free radical activities. Once ingested, the highest IP6 analogues are degraded to lower analogues that interfere with signal transduction mechanisms while initiating cell cycle arrest (Vicenik and Shamsuddin, 2003). Phytic acid has been reported to reduce tumor incidence and tumor load in rodent mammary tumors (Shamsuddin and Ullah, 1989; Shamsuddin et al, 1989; Ullah and Shamsuddin, 1990; Pretlow et al., 1992; Vucenik et al., 1995, 1997; Challa, 1997; Shamsuddin and Vucenik,

1999). Graf and Eaton (1990) suggested that phytic acid could reduce the active oxygen species-mediated carcinogenesis and cell injury through its anti-oxidative function. Minihane and Rimbach (2002) reported that high levels of dietary phytate may reduce iron-induced oxidative injury and reverse iron dependent augmentation of colorectal tumorigenesis. Vital cellular functions such as signal transduction, cell proliferation and differentiation are believed to be regulated by phytic acid (Vucenik and Shamsuddin, 2006). Phytic acid inhibition of cancer has been reported to be through the control of cell division. Phytic acid has been shown to reduce the rate of cellular proliferation both *in vivo* and *in vitro* (Shamsuddin, 2002). Norazalina, et al., (2010) reported decrease in the incidence and multiplicity of total tumors by phytic acid supplementation. They specifically demonstrated the potential value of phytic acid in reducing colon cancer risk in rats. Phytic acid has also been shown to inhibit tumor blood vessel growth in a number of studies and in the process starve cancer cells of oxygen and essential nutrients (Vucenik et al., 2004). Phytate chelating ability may also explain the role of the compound in the prevention, inhibition and the cure of some cancers by depriving those cells of minerals such as iron that they require for reproduction, or chelation of free radicals that are produced when some minerals, for example iron, are in excess. Raina et al., (2008) reported that oral phytates suppress prostate tumor growth and progression at the neoplastic stage and reduce the incidence of adenocarcinoma through its antiproliferative and proapoptotic effects. Other suggested health benefits of phytate include the prevention of pathological calcification and kidney stone formation, reduction of serum cholesterol and pathological platelet activity (Vucenik and Shamsuddin, 2006). Phytic acid has also been shown to have other significant benefits including antioxidant properties (Kunyanga et al., 2011), nutritional effects (Tran et al., 2011), food preservative for fruits and vegetables (Zhang et al., 2013), and as an important nutritional substance to support the early stages of growth in seedlings (Tran et al., 2011). Phytic acid potent antioxidant properties may protect tissues against oxidative damage to DNA that may reduce mutation and cancerous cell production. Other studies indicate that the anticancer effects of phytates are due to their ability to increase DNA fragmentation as well as other mechanisms detrimental to cellular proliferation resulting in induction of apoptosis (Verghese et al., 2006). It is also thought that protective outcomes may be related to the ability of phytates to reduce β-catenin and COX-2 expression in tumors (Shafie et al., 2013).

# 11    Antidiabetic Properties of Phytates

Diabetes mellitus is a global epidemic which significantly contributes to increasing mortality associated with non-communicable diseases worldwide. Diabetic patients have problems with the uptake of glucose into the cells. A reduction in glucose movement into the cells will result in a deficiency of inositol because glucose is a precursor for inositol in the cells. Interestingly, while glucose requires insulin to enter into the cell, inositol and phytic acid do not. The involvement of phosphorylated inositols ($IP_1$ to $IP_6$), especially $IP_6$ in insulin secretion has been reported (Vanderlinden and Vucenik, 2004). Phytic acid extract from the skin of sweet potato has been shown to aid in the control of type II diabetes by reducing insulin resistance (Ludvik et al., 2003). Elevated intracellular level of D-*myo*-inositol 1,2,3,4,5,6-hexakisphosphate (IP6) in cells that are involved in insulin secretion and several other cell types has been reported (French et al., 1991, Jackson et al., 1987 and Li et al., 1992). There is a general belief that phosphorylated inositol, especially phytic acids have roles in the secretion of insulin by the beta cells of pancreas. Efanov et al., (1997) reported the intracellular variation of the levels of inositol polyphosphates in cells and their high levels in insulin-secreting cells. The changes in the rates of phytic acid synthesis and conversion and the subsequent attainment of a physiological concentration range is thought to play important roles in the regulation of vesicle trafficking and recycling as well as endocytosis and exocytosis in insulin-secreting cells (Sasakawa et al., 1995; Efanov et al., 1997). The effects of phytic acid are dependent on the activation of protein kinase C which suggests a linkage of the role of inositol polyphosphates as that of signaling molecules in stimulus-secretion coupling in pancreatic beta-cells (Efanov et al., 1997). Ammala et al., (1994) and Zaitsev et al., (1995) reported the role of protein phosphorylation in the regulation of exocytosis in the pancreatic beta-cells. An increase in cellular phosporylation through the inhibition of protein dephosprylation by IP6 has been proposed as the probable regulatory mechanism linking glucose stimulated polyphosphoinositide formation to insulin exocytosis in insulin-secreting cells (Lehtihet et al., 2004). We recently reported that the antidiabetic function of phytic acid supplementation may be through the decrease in the activity of intestinal amylase which is indicative of lesser products of carbohydrate digestion formation and subsequently absorption, leading to a decreased percentage spike in blood glucose (Omoruyi et al., 2013 and Dilworth et al. 2005).

## 12    Phytates and Cardiovascular Disease

There is a large body of evidence showing that the major risk factors for cardiovascular disease are triglyceride, cholesterol and LDL-cholesterol, while HDL-cholesterol level has inverse correlation with such a risk. The therapeutic approach is to control the levels of serum lipids. Elevated cholesterol level is a risk factor that can lead to the blockage of arteries. The blockage of arteries begins with the formation of plaques which are essentially composed of cholesterol and other lipids, inflammatory cells and calcium deposits. Plaque formation can activate the clotting process of blood which may lead to the blockage of blood flow in the artery resulting in strokes. Therapeutic decrease of LDL-cholesterol and increase HDL-cholesterol reduces the development of atherosclerosis and stabilizes the atherosclerotic plaques and their partial regression (Kanjuh et al., 2009). Manktelow and Potter (2009) reported that interventions which reduce total and LDL cholesterol levels also reduce coronary heart disease and stroke events in patients with a history of coronary heart disease. Katayama (1997) showed that dietary phytates lowered hepatic weight, total lipids and triglyceride levels in rats fed sucrose, and suggested that dietary myo-inositol or phytate effect on fatty liver in rats caused by sucrose feeding may be at least in part mediated through the depression of hepatic lipogenesis. We also reported that the elevated liver weight seen in diabetic rats which may be indicative of the presence of liver disease was ameliorated by phytic acid supplementation (Omoruyi et al. 2013). Phytic acid has been suggested to inhibit the initiation of plaque formation (Vanderlinden and Vucenik, 2004) and lower serum cholesterol and triglycerides (Zhou and Erdman, 1995). Supplementation of phytic acid extract from sweet potatoes decreased blood cholesterol and increased HDL-cholesterol. We recently reported the association between decreased body weight and increased HDL level in the serum of rats fed phytic acid supplement, indicating that decrease in body weight due to phytic acid supplementation may be sensitive to elevated serum HDL cholesterol (Omoruyi et al, 2013). Faergeman et al., (2009) reported that a slight increase in triglycerides levels is associated with higher risk for the recurrence of cardiovascular events in statin-treated patients and they recommended that it be considered as a useful risk marker. Phytic acid has also been suggested to inhibit the initiation of plaque formation (Vanderlinden and Vucenik, 2004) and lower serum cholesterol and triglycerides (Vanderlinden and Vucenik, 2004). Grases et al., (2008) reported that phytic acid supplementation reduces age related aorta calcification suggesting the involvement of this compound in the protection of the arteries against hardening. However, the strong correlation between systemic inflammation with a low degree of plaque stability points to the reduction of the breaking up of plague that blocks blood flow by decreased inflammation and phytic acid has been shown to reduce inflammation and also inhibit platelet aggregation (Sudheer, et al., 2004; Kamp, et al., 1995; Vanderlinden and Vucenik, 2004). It is believed that the presence of antioxidants in the pigment of red wine reduces the prevalence of heart disease among red wine users (Vanderlinden and Vucenik, 2004). These findings support the use of phytic acid, a physiological antioxidant, in the reduction of heart disease (Omoruyi, 2010).

# 13   Carotenoids

Carotenoids are organic macromolecuels that fall under the terpenoid group of compounds. They consist of eight isoprenoid units and are widely distributed compounds responsible for the pigments in flowers, roots, leaves and even some animals (Kammona et al., 2015). The beneficial effects of carotenoids are thought to be due to their antioxidant activities with the most widely studied ones being beta-carotene, lycopene, lutein and zeaxanthin (Johnson, 2002).

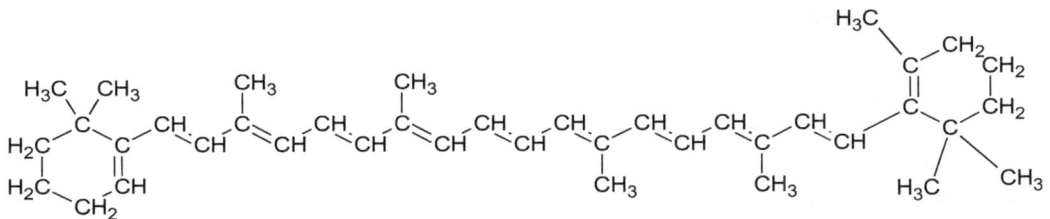

**Figure 4:** Structure of β-carotene.

Carotenoids are thought to enhance immune system function, reduce the risk of cardiovascular diseases, age-related muscular degeneration, and are important in the prevention of some cancers (Byers and Perry 1992; Kammona et al., 2015). They are also important contributors to mammalian nutrition as about fifty of these compounds serve as important precursors of vitamin A (Lee et al., 1989). Of this number however, only a few of these, namely β-carotene, α-carotene and β-cryptoxanthin, are important precursors of vitamin A in humans (Jaarsveld et al., 2005). These carotenoids are important because vitamin A deficiency is a recognized public health problem in many countries especially in developing countries where over 250 million persons may be affected (Underwood and Arthur, 1996). In south Asia, fifty percent of preschool children may be at risk while there is a prevalence of sixty one percent in preteens in Ethiopia (Mitra et al., 1998; Kassaye et al., 2001). Vitamin A is important in maintaining healthy cells within the retina of the eye to the extent that low intake is a risk factor for night blindness. Vitamin A is also important in maintaining connective tissues as well as mucosal membranes in the body such that impaired growth and development and susceptibility to infections are observed in vitamin A deficient individuals. Sweet potato carotenoids therefore have an important role to play in addressing the problem of vitamin A deficiency. To this end, flesh color of sweet potato varieties may serve as an indicator of higher carotenoid content with lower levels of provitamin A present in white fleshed varieties (Ameny and Wilson, 1997). Sweet potato breeding programs and agricultural practices in these vulnerable areas should therefore be geared at producing yellow and orange varieties that contain high levels of beta carotene.

Another method of improving beta carotene intake involves processing method that sweet potato undergoes prior to consumption. Since the tuber has to be processed prior to consumption, consideration has to be given to the fact that degradation of bioactive compounds will vary based on the type of processing methods employed. The percentage loss during processing is thought to vary between 0 to 12 % while higher percentage losses are thought to occur following dehydration (Burri, 2011). It is thought that oven drying results in the highest retention of carotenoids followed by boiling, frying and sun drying (Vimala et al., 2011). Loss is thought to occur through oxygen, UV and thermal exposure during processing (Fonseca et al., 2008). In this light, food products including juice and salads made from fresh tubers are thought to contain highest concentrations of beta carotene.

# 14   Flavonoids

Sweet potato flavonoids may soon play a role in the sports industry as novel anti-fatigue properties of these compounds have been recorded. The molecules are shown to help in muscle recovery post exercise by reducing fatigue that arises from muscular exertion. This is important especially for elite athletes who compete regularly and to whom muscle recovery in the shortest possible time is of great importance. Animal studies indicate that rats given flavonoid supplements showed improvements in exercise endurance over those not given the supplements. In these studies, muscle performance was also shown to increase with increasing flavonoid concentration. The mechanism points to a direct relationship between flavonoid consumption and reduced serum lactic acid as well as blood urea nitrogen (Li and Zhang, 2013). High serum lactate and urea nitrogen are thought to be directly related to increased muscular fatigability (Xiuhong et al., 2015). In this study, the observation of increased hepatic and muscular glycogen stores indicates sufficient availability of substrate required for aerobic respiration. It will then become less likely that anaerobic respiration leading to lactate production will predominate. Flavonoids may therefore be considered anti-fatigue agents as their consumption is expected to significantly improved muscle endurance by lowering serum urea and lactic acid while increasing glycogen availability.

In addition to anti-fatigue properties, several studies show that sweet potato flavonoids possess potent hypolipidemic and hypoglycemic properties (Li et al., 2009; Zhao et al., 2013). These properties are significant with respect to treatment of metabolic diseases involving disorders of glucose and lipid metabolism as seen diabetes mellitus. There is heightened focus on this disease as it is expected that over 592 million adults are predicted to become diabetic by 2035 due to a myriad of factors including prevalence of obesity, aging and population growth (International Diabetes Federation, 2014). There appears to be complex mechanisms contributing to the antidiabetic properties of flavonoids. Currently it is thought that the compounds are capable of enhancing insulin secretion, promoting pancreatic beta cell development and promoting translocation of GLUT-4 receptors via PI3K/AKT and AMPK pathways (Vinayagam and Xu, 2015). Other studies also show that flavonoids upregulate expression of GLUT-2 glucose transporters in pancreatic beta cells and upregulation of GLUT-4 transporter proteins via pathways mentioned above in addition to the CAP/Cb1/TC10 pathway (Hajiaghaalipour et al., 2015). Glucose metabolism may therefore be modulated by flavonoids through various pathways that involve insulin secretion and sensitivity that in turn dictate the outcome of metabolic processes involving carbohydrates and lipids.

The antioxidant and anti-inflammatory properties of flavonoids are widely thought to contribute to the beneficial properties of sweet potatoes. These properties of flavonoids along with their mineral-chelating activities may also enhance mammalian immune system thereby affording protection against heart disease, cancers and other inflammatory disorders (Monhanraj and Sivasankar, 2014). Other properties ascribed to sweet potato flavonoids include antibacterial, antiviral, anti-allergic, anti-oesteoporotic and anti-tumor activities (Anthoney and Omwenga 2014). Interestingly, high flavonoid content of some sweet potato cultivars has increased the scope for marketing those cultivars as healthy alternatives to synthetic antioxidant agents.

# 15   Changes in Bioactive and Chemical Components of Sweet Potato due to Storage

Production of sweet potatoes in most countries is highly seasonal which necessitates conducting extensive research to determine the effects of long term storage and preservation.

| Component | Therapeutic effects |
|---|---|
| Anthocyanins | Estrogenic effects: Including reduction of cognitive defects. Stimulates estrogen receptors leading to reduced rates of some hormone dependent pathologies (Lu et al., 2012; Harris & Go, 2006). |
| | Antioxidant, anti-ageing and anti-diabetic properties (Hamouz et al., 2011; Lila, 2004; Jang et al., 2013; Zhao et al., 2013; Nizamutdinova et al., 2009). |
| | Anti-cancer, radical scavenging properties (Lim et al., 2013). |
| Phytates | Hypolipidemic effects: Promote cholesterol metabolism and excretion (Dilworth, 2015; Omoruyi et al., 2013). |
| | Anticancer properties: Reduce free radical formation, removal of lipid peroxidation products, initiation of cell cycle arrest, and suppress expression of tumor promoting proteins (Zajdel et al., 2013; Shafie et al., 2013). |
| | Anti-diabetic effects: Enhance insulin activity (Lee et al., 2006). |
| Carotenoids | Anticancer and free radical scavenger properties (Mohanraj & Sivasankar, 2014. Jin et al., 2007) |
| | Hypolipidemic properties: Decrease cholesterol absorption in the intestine while increasing its excretion (Silva et al., 2013). |
| Flavonoids | Anti-fatigue agent: Promotes muscle health and improve recovery post exercise (Li & Zhang, 2013). |
| | Display anti-diabetic properties highlighted by hypolipidemic and hypoglycemic properties (Vinayagam & Xu, 2015; Li et al., 2009; Zhao et al., 2013). |
| | Antioxidant activities: Suppress free radical formation rates and serve as free radical scavengers (Hajiaghaalipour et al., 2015; Monhanraj & Sivasankar, 2014) |
| | Antibacterial, antifungal and antiviral activities (Orhan et al., 2010). |

**Table 2:** Showing some bioactive components in sweet potato and their therapeutic effects.

The bulky and perishable nature of this root crop affects its quality and ability to be transported economically over long distances. In temperate growing regions such as the United States, the tubers are held in a properly ventilated facility, where temperature and humidity are regulated (about 29°C, 85–90% relative humidity) for about a week to prolong integrity (Edmunds et al., 2008). The content and stability of nutrients and phytochemicals in sweet potatoes are also affected by post-harvest storage conditions and environmental factors such as temperature, light exposure, humidity and farming site (Grace et al., 2014). Post-harvest storage affects different sweet potato varieties in different ways. In a study carried out by Grace et al (2014) on four different varieties, curing and storage for up to 8 months did not have an effect on the total phenolic content of three of the varieties, however in one variety, referred to as NCPUR06-020, total phenolic content was reduced. This was attributed to anthocyanin degradation during storage. Enzymes such as glycosidases (anthocyanases), polyphenol oxidases and peroxidases can degrade anthocyanins in plant tissues (Shi et al., 1992). Other plant chemicals significantly affected by post-harvest storage in this study include ascorbic acid and carotenoids. There was an overall decrease in the ascorbic acid concentration for all varieties of sweet potatoes studied, whereas the effects on carotenoids were genotype dependent. Changes in antioxidant activity varied according to the curing and storage methods utilized. For tubers that were cured at 29°C and 85% relative humidity, there was a gradual decline over time (Grace et al., 2014). Storage of the roots at 5°C however resulted in an increase in the antioxidant activity after 3 weeks (Padda and Picha, 2008). In a study carried out by Zhang et al (2002), starch content decreased slightly in all but one genotype studied, where there was a dramatic decrease. Carbohydrate content plays an important role in eating quality and processing traits, and contributes significantly to product firmness. The longer the storage time, the less firm the products will be. The genotype that showed the most dramatic decrease in starch content also showed the most significant increase in $\alpha$-amylase activity during storage. Zhang et al (2002), also reported that storage had little effect on trypsin inhibitor activity; total sugars were increased early in storage and remained constant subsequently. This is of interest as trypsin inhibitors reduce the availability of proteins and are therefore considered to be an undesirable component of foods.

# 16   Conclusion

Sweet potato is known to be a nutritious crop that is widely utilized and cultivated throughout many regions of the world. Because of its ease of cultivation, increased production is thought to play a significant role in alleviating world hunger especially in vulnerable societies. With respect to this crop, there are untapped resources still to be unveiled especially as it relates to utilization of different parts of the plant for consumption. This is of significance since the leaves are thought to be highly nutritious but heavily underutilized in modern societies. The bioactive compounds in sweet potatoes are numerous and coverage of all of them is beyond the scope of this chapter. However, an attempt was made at assessing some of the most prominent ones that are associated with reported health benefits. Antioxidant and anticancer properties are observed in specific components including anthocyanins, phytates, flavonoids and carotenoids. Interestingly, the antineoplastic properties of these compounds are achieved via different mechanisms including free radical scavenging and mineral chelation as well as modulation of enzymes and proteins that are important in free radical formation. These bioactive compounds are also important agents that may be utilized for treating diabetes mellitus and associated complications including dyslipidemia and microvascular damage. Antidiabetic properties are thought to be due to the ability of bioactive compounds to modulate enzymes that play key roles in glycolysis and lipogenesis. Estrogenic properties of anthocyanins are well recognized and thought to occur following their binding to estrogen receptors followed by modulation of hormone induced cellular proliferation. Estrogenic properties of anthocyanins are also related to improvement in neuronal functioning and memory in the estrogen deficiency state. While studies have alluded to numerous nutraceutical benefits to be derived from bioactive compounds in sweet potatoes, it is imperative that new research be directed at unraveling the mechanism of action of these bioactive components on mammalian cells. While some mechanisms are known, much is still left to be uncovered for example the roles of bioactive compounds in regulating some genes involved in cell cycle regulation. Such studies will direct the way forward regarding the use and validation of use of different parts of the sweet potato plant and/or its components as nutraceuticals against common metabolic disorders. In light of positive results to date, further research into the efficacy of these compounds is needed as we continue to seek solutions for some of the most devastating maladies that affect humans. Evidence therefore points to increased cultivation and utilization of this crop for sustainable development of modern societies.

# References

Allen, J.C., Corbitt, A.D., Maloney, K.P., Butt, M.S. & Truong, V.D. (2012). Glycemic index of sweet potato as affected by cooking methods. The Open Nutrition Journal, 6, 1–11.

Ammala, C., Eliasson, L., Bokvist, K., Berggren, P. O., Honkanen, R. E., Sjoholm, Å. & Rorsman, P. (1994). Activation of protein kinases and inhibition of protein phosphatases play a central role in the regulation of exocytosis in mouse pancreatic beta cells. Proceedings of the National Academy of Sciences USA, 91(10), 4343–4347.

Ameny, M.A. & Wilson, P.W. (1997). Relationship between the hunter colour values and beta carotene contents in white-fleshed African sweet potatoes (Ipomoea batatas Lam). Journal of the Science of Food and Agriculture, 73, 301–306.

Anthoney, S. T. & Omwenga, J. (2014). Analysis of phytochemical composition of white and purple sweet potato (Ipomoea batatas [L.] Lam) root. Indian Journal of Advances in Plant Research (IJAPR), 1(3), 19–22.

Arogundadea, L.A. & Mu, T. (2012). Influence of oxidative browning inhibitors and isolation techniques on sweet potato protein recovery and composition. Food Chemistry, 134(3), 1374–1384.

Attaluri, S., Janardhan, K.V. & Light, A. ed. (2010). Sustainable sweet potato production & utilization in Orissa, India. Proceedings of a workshop and training held in Bhubaneswar, Orissa, India, 17–18 March 2010. Bhudaneswar, India. International Potato Center (CIP).

Bandera, E.V. & Kushi, L.H. (2003). Phytoestrogens in the prevention and prognosis of female hormonal cancers. In: Preedy, V. R.;Watson, R. R. (eds). Reviews in food and nutrition toxicology, 1, 63–87.

Basuny, A.M.M., Arafat, S.M. & El-Marzooq, M.A. (2012). Antioxidant and Antihyperlipidemic activities of anthocyanins from eggplant peels. Journal of Pharma Research and Reviews, 2(3), 50–57.

Bovell-Benjamin, A. C. (2007). Sweet potato: a review of its past, present, and future role in human nutrition. Advances in Food and Nutrition Research, 52, 1–59.

Burri, B.J. (2011). Evaluating sweet potato as an intervention food to prevent vitamin A deficiency. Comprehensive Reviews in Food Science and Food Safety, 10, 118–130.

Byers, T., & Perry, G. (1992). Dietary carotenes, vitamin C and vitamin E as protective antioxidants in *human cancers. Annual Review of Nutrition, 12, 139–159.*

*Castañeda-Ovando, A., Pacheco-Hernández, l., Páez-Hernández, E., Rodríguez, J. & Galán-Vidal, C.A. (2009). Chemical studies of anthocyanins: A review. Food chemistry, 113 (4), 859–871.*

*Cevallos-Casals, B.A. & Cisneros-Zevallos, L. (2004). Stability of anthocyanin-based aqueous extracts of Andean purple corn and red-fleshed sweet potato compared to synthetic and natural colorants. Food Chemistry, 86(1), 69–77.*

*Challa, A., Rao, D. R. & Reddy, B. S. (1997). Interactive suppression of aberrant crypt foci induced by azoxymethane in rat colon by phytic acid and green tea. Carcinogenesis, 18, 2023–2026.*

*Chalopin, M., Tesse, A., Martı́nez, M.C., Rognan, D., Arnal, J.F. & Andriantsitohaina, R. (2010). Estrogen receptor alpha as a key target of red wine polyphenols action on the endothelium. PLoS One, 5(1):e8554.*

*CIP — Centro Internacional de la Papa (2015). Sweet potato I. http://www.cipotato.org/sweetpotato (September 11, 2015).*

*Denham, T. (2013). Ancient and historic dispersals of sweet potato in Oceania. Proceedings of the National Academy of Sciences of the United States of America, 110(6), 1982–1983.*

*Dilworth, L.L., Omoruyi, F.O., Simon, O.R., Morrison, E.Y. & Asemota, H.N. (2005). The effect of phytic acid on the levels of blood glucose and some enzymes of carbohydrate and lipid metabolism. West Indian Medical Journal, 54(2), 102–106.*

*Dilworth, L. Omoruyi, F. & Asemota, H. (2015). Effects of IP6 and sweet potato (Ipomoea batatas) phytate on serum, liver and faecal lipids in rats. International Journal of Food Science and Nutrition Engineering, 5(1), 53–58.*

*Dixon, R.A., Harrison, M.J. & Lamb, C.J. (1994). Early events in the activation of plant defence responses. Annual Review of Phytopathology, 32, 479–501.*

*Doria, E., Galleschi, L., Calucci, L., Pinzino, C., Pilu, R., Cassani, E. & Nielsen, E. (2009). Phytic acid prevents oxidative stress in seeds: evidence from a maize (Zea mays L.) low phytic acid mutant. Journal of Experimental Botany, 60(3), 967–978.*

*Edmunds, B., Boyette, M., Clark, C., Ferrin, D., Smith, T., & Holmes, G. (2008). Postharvest handling of sweetpotatoes. North Carolina Cooperative Extension Service, pp. 53.*

*Efanov, A. M., Zaitsev, S. V. & Berggren, P. (1997). Inositol hexakisphosphate stimulates non Ca2+-mediated and primes Ca2+- mediatedexocytosis of insulin by activation of protein kinase C. Proceedings of the National Academy of Sciences, 94, 4435–4439.*

*Faergeman, O., Holme, I., Fayyard, R., Bhatia, S., Grundy, S. M., Kastelein, J. J., LaRosa, J. C., Larsen, M. L., Lindahl, C., Olsson, A. G.,Tikkanen, M. J., Waters, D. O., Pedersen, T. R. & Steering Committees of IDEAL and TNT Trials (2009). Plasmatriglycerides and cardiovascular events in the Treating to New Targets and Incremental Decrease in End-Points through aggressive lipid lowering trials of statins in patients with coronary artery disease. American Journal of Cardiology, 104(4), 459–463.*

*FAOSTAT (2009). FAO Statistics. http://faostat.fao.org/site/567/default.aspx#ancor. Accessed September 20, 2015*

*FAOSTAT (2013). http://issuu.com/faooftheun/docs/syb2013issuu/154. Accessed September 15, 2015.*

*FAOSTAT (2015). http://faostat3.fao.org/browse/Q/QC/E-Accessed September 25, 2015.*

*Fleming, S.F. (1981). A study of relationships between flatus potential and carbohydrate distribution in legume seeds. Journal of Food Science, 106, 779–803.*

Fonseca, Marcos José de O, Soares, Antonio G, Freire Junior, Murillo, Almeida, Dejair L de & Ascheri, José Luiz R. (2008). *Effect of extrusion-cooking in total carotenoids content in cream and orange flesh sweet potato cultivars. Horticultura brasileira, 26(1), 112–115.*

French, P. J., Bunce, C. M., Stephence, L. R., Lord, J. M., McConnell, F. M., Brown, G., Creba, J. A. & Michell, R. H. (1991). *Changes in the levels of inositol lipids and phosphates during the differentiation of HL60 promyelocytic cells towards neutrophils or monocytes. Proceedings Biological Sciences, 245 (1314), 193–201.*

Graf, E. & Eaton, J. W. (1990). *Antioxidant function of phytic acid. Free Radicals in Biology and Medicine, 8, 61–69.*

Grace, M.H. Yousef G.G., Gustafson S.J., Truong, V., Yencho, C. & Lila, M.A. (2014). *Phytochemical changes in phenolics, anthocyanins, ascorbic acid, and carotenoids associated with sweet potato storage and impacts on bioactive properties. Food Chemistry, 145, 717–724.*

Grases, F., Sanchis, P., Perello, J., Isern, B., Prieto, R. M., Fernandez-Palomegue, C. & Saus, C. (2008). *Phytate reduces age-related cardiovascular calcification. Frontiers in Bioscience, 13, 7115–7122.*

Hahn, S.K. (1984). *Tropical root crop their improvement and utilization IITA conference paper 2– 28.*

Hajiaghaalipour, F., Khalilpourfarshbafi, M. & Aditya Arya, A. (2015). *Modulation of Glucose Transporter Protein by Dietary Flavonoids in Type 2 Diabetes Mellitus. International Journal of Biological Sciences, 11(5), 508–524.*

Hamouz, K., Lachman, J., Pazderů, K., Tomášek, J., Hejtmánková, K. & Pivec, V. (2011). *Differences in anthocyanin content and antioxidant activity of potato tubers with different flesh colour. Plant, Soil and Environment, 57(10), 478–485.*

Harris, D.M., & Go. V.L. (2006). *How dietary components protect from cancer. In: Awad, AB and Bradford P.G. (eds). Nutrition and Cancer Prevention. CRC Press, Boca Raton, Florida, pp 27–58.*

Hidalgo M, Martin-Santamaria S, Recio I, Sanchez-Moreno C, de Pascual-Teresa B, Rimbach G, & de Pascual-Teresa S. (2012). *Potential anti-inflammatory, anti-adhesive, anti/estrogenic, and angiotensin-converting enzyme inhibitory activities of anthocyanins and their gut metabolites. Genes and Nutrition, 7, 295–306.*

http://cipotato.org/sweetpotato/facts-2-Accessed March 7, 2016

Hwang, Y.P., Choi, J.H., Han, E.H., Kim, H.G., Wee, J., Jung, K.O., Jung, K.H., Kwon, K., Jeong, T.C., Chung, Y.C. & Jeong, H.G. (2011). *Purple sweet potato anthocyanins attenuate hepatic lipid accumulation through activating adenosine monophosphate–activated protein kinase in human HepG2 cells and obese mice. Nutrition Research, 31(12), 896–906.*

International Diabetes Federation (2014). *Sixth edition.*

Jaarsveld, P.J., Faber, M., Tanumihardjo, S.A., Nestel, P., Lombard, C.J. & Benadé, A.J. (2005). *β-carotene-rich orange fleshed sweet potato improves the vitamin A status of primary school children assessed with the modified-relative-dose response test. American Journal of Clinical Nutrition, 81, 1080–1087.*

Jackson, T. R., Hallam, T. J., Downes, C. P. & Hanley, M. R. (1987). *Receptor coupled events in bradykinin action: rapid production of inositol phosphates and regulation of cytosolic free Ca2+ in a neural cell line. EMBO Journal, 6 (1), 49–54.*

Jang, H.H., Kim, S.M., Kim, S.H., Kim, J.B & Lee, Y.M. (2013). *Anti-diabetic effects of anthocyanins isolated from Korean purple sweet potato, "Shinzami". The FASEB Journal, 27, 630.21.*

Jansen, G. & Flamme, W. (2006). *Coloured potatoes (Solanum Tuberosum L.) – anthocyanin content and tuber quality. Genetic Resources and Crop Evolution, 53(7), 1321–1331.*

Jin, Y.R., Lee, M.S., Lee, J.H., Hsu, H.K., Lu, J.Y., Chao, S.S., Chen, K.T, Liou, S.H. & Ger, L.P. (2007). *Intake of vitamin A-rich foods and lung cancer risk in Taiwan: with special reference to garland chrysanthemum and sweet potato leaf consumption. Asia Pacific Journal of Clinical Nutrition, 16(3):477–488.*

Johnson, E.J. (2002). *The role of carotenoids in human health. Nutrition in Clinical Care, 5(2), 56–65.*

Johnson, M. & Pace, R.D. (2010). *Sweet potato leaves: properties and synergistic interactions that promote health and prevent disease. Nutrition Reviews, 68(10), 604–615.*

Joo Suh, H., Man Kim, J. & Moon Choi, Y. (2003). *The incorporation of sweet potato application in the preparation of a rice beverage. International Journal of Food Science & Technology, 38, 145–151.*

Katayama, T. (1997). *Effects of dietary myo-inositol or phytic acid on hepatic concentrations of lipids and hepatic activities of lipogenic enzymes in rats fed on corn starch or sucrose. Nutrition Research, 17 (4), 721–728.*

Kammona, S., Othman, R., Jaswir, I. & Jamal, P. (2015). *Characterisation of carotenoid content in diverse local sweet potato (Ipomoea batatas) flesh tubers. International Journal of Pharmacy and Pharmaceutical Sciences, 7(2), 347–351.*

Kamp, D. W., Israbian, V. A., Yeldandi, A. V., Panos, R. J., Graceffa, P. & Weitzman, S. A. (1995). *Phytic acid, an iron chelator, attenuates pulmonary inflammation and fibrosis in rats after intratracheal instillation of asbestos. Toxicologic Pathology, 23(6), 689–695.*

Kanjuh, V., Ostojic, M., Lalic, N., Stokic, E., Adic-Cemerlic, N. & Gojkovic-Bukarica, (2009). *Low and high density lipoprotein-cholesterol and coronary atherothrombosis. Medicinski Pregled, 62 Suppl, 3, 7–14.*

Kano, M., Takayanagi, T., Harada, K., Makino, K., & Ishikawa, F. (2005). *Antioxidative activity of anthocyanins from purple sweet potato, Ipomoea batatas cultivar Ayamurasaki. Bioscience, Biotechnology, and Biochemistry, 69(5), 979–988.*

Kassaye, T., Receveur, O., Johns, T. & Becklake, M.R. (2001). *Prevalence of vitamin A deficiency in children aged 6–9 years in Wukro, northern Ethiopia. Bulletin of the World Health Organization, 79(5), 415–422.*

Kim, H.W., Kim, J.B., Cho, S.M., Chung, M.N., Lee, Y.M., Chu, S.M., Che, J.H., Kim, S.N., Kim, S.Y., Cho, Y.S., Kim, J.H., Park, H.J. & Lee, D.J. (2012). *Anthocyanin changes in the Korean purple-fleshed sweet potato, Shinzami, as affected by steaming and baking. Food Chemistry, 130(4), 966–972.*

Kunyanga, C.N., Imungia, J.K., Okotha, M.W., Biesalskib, H.K. & Vadivel, V. (2011). *Antioxidant and type 2 diabetes related functional properties of phytic acid extract from Kenyan local food ingredients: Effects of traditional processing methods. Ecology of Food and Nutrition, 50(5), 452–471.*

Lareo, C., Ferrari, M. D., Guigou, M., Fajardo, L., Larnaudie, V., Ramírez, M. B. & Martínez-Garreiro, J. (2013). *Evaluation of sweet potato for fuel bioethanol production: hydrolysis and fermentation. Springerplus, 2, 493.*

Lee, C.Y., Simpson, K.L. & Gerber, L. (1989). *Vegetables as a major vitamin A source in our diet. New York's Food and Life Sciences Bulletin, 126.*

Lee, S.H., Park, H.J., Cho, S.Y., Cho, S.M. & Lillehoj, H.S. (2006). *Dietary phytic acid lowers the blood glucose level in diabetic KK mice. Nutrition Research, 26, 474–479.*

Lehtihet, M., Honkanen, R. E. & Sjoholm, A. (2004). *Inositol hexakisphosphate and sulfonylureas regulate beta-cell protein phosphatases. Biochemical Biophysical Research Communications, 316, 893–897.*

Li, G., Pralong, W. F., Pittet, D., Mayr, G. W., Schlegel, W. & Wollheim, C. B. (1992). Inositol tetrakisphosphate isomers and elevation of cytosolic Ca2+ in vasopressin-stimulated insulin secreting RINm5F cells. Journal of Biological Chemistry, 267 (7), 4349–4356.

Li, C.G. & Zhang, L.Y. (2013). In vivo anti-fatigue activity of total flavonoids from sweet potato (Ipomoea batatas L.) leaf in mice. Indian Journal of Biochemistry Biophysics, 50(4), 326–329.

Li, F., Li, Q., Gao, D. & Peng, Y. (2009). The Optimal Extraction Parameters and Anti-Diabetic Activity of Flavonoids from Ipomoea batatas Leaf. African Journal of Traditional, Complementary, and Alternative Medicines, 6(2): 195–202.

Lila, M.A. (2004). Anthocyanins and human health: An in vitro investigative approach. Journal of Biomedicine and Biotechnology, 2004(5), 306–313.

Lim, S. Xu, J., Kim, J. Chen, T., Su, X., Standard, J., Carey, E., Griffin, J., Herndon, B., Katz, B. Tomich, J. & Wang, W. (2013). Role of anthocyanin-enriched purple-fleshed sweet potato P40 in colorectal cancer prevention. Molecular Nutrition and Food Research, 57(11), 1908–1917.

Lin, L., Ockenden, I. & Lott, J.N.A. (2005). The concentrations and distribution of phytic acid-phosphorus and other mineral nutrients in wild-type and low phytic acid1-1 (lpa1-1) corn (Zea mays L.) grains and grain parts. Canadian Journal of Botany, 83, 131–141.

Loewus, F.A. (2002). Biosynthesis of phytate in food grains and seeds. In: Reddy NR, Sathe SK (Eds.). Food Phytates. CRC Press, Boca Raton Florida, 53–61.

Lonnerdal, B. (2003). Genetically modified plants improved trace element nutrition. Journal of Nutrition, 133, 1490S–1493S.

Lopez, H. W., Coudray, C., Bellanger, J., Younes, H., Demigne, C. & Remesy, C. (1998). Intestinal fermentation lessens the inhibitory effects of phytic acid on mineral utilization in rats, Journal of Nutrition, 128 (7), 1192–1198.

Lu, J., Wu, D., Zheng, Y., Hu, B., Cheng, W. & Zhang, Z. (2012). Purple sweet potato color attenuates domoic acid-induced cognitive deficits by promoting estrogen receptor-α-mediated mitochondrial biogenesis signaling in mice. Free Radical Biology and Medicine, 52, 646–659.

Lubag, A.J.M., Laurena, A.C. & Tecson-Mendoza, E.M. (2008). Antioxidants of purple and white greater yam (Dioscorea alata L.) varieties from the Philippines. Philippine Journal of Science, 137(1), 61–67.

Ludvik, B., Neuffer, B. & Pacini, G. (2004). Efficacy of Ipomoea batatas (Caiapo) on diabetes control in type 2 diabetic subject treated with diet. Diabetes Care, 27, 436–440.

Ludvik, B., Waldhausl, W., Prager, R., Kautzy-Miller, A. & Pacini, G. (2003) Mode of action of Ipomoea batatas (Caiapo) in type 2 diabetic patients. Metabolism, 52 (7), 875–880.

Manktelow, B.N. & Potter, J.F. (2009). Interventions in the management of serum lipids for preventing stroke recurrence. Cochrane Database Systematic Reviews, (3), CD002091.

Maloney, K., Truong, V.D. & Allen, J.C. (2012). Chemical Optimization of Protein Extraction from Sweet Potato (Ipomoea batatas) Peel. Journal of Food Science, 77, 306–312.

Martin,S., Favot, L., Matz, R., Lugnier, C. & Andriantsitohaina, R. (2003). Delphinidin inhibits endothelial cell proliferation and cell cycle progression through a transient activation of ERK-1/-2. Biochemical Pharmacology, 65, 669–675.

Mbanaso, E.O., Agwu, A.E., Anyanwu, A.C. & Asumugha, G.N. (2012). Assessment of the extent of adoption of sweet potato production technology by farmers in the southeast agro-ecological zone of Nigeria. Journal of Agriculture and Social Research, 12(1), 124–136.

Minihane, A. M. & Rimbach, G. (2002). Iron absorption and the iron binding and anti-oxidant properties of phytic acid. International Journal of Food Science and Technology, 37, 741–748.

Mitra, A.K., Alvarez, J.O., Guay-Woodford, L., Fuchs, G.J., Wahed, M.A. & Stephensen, C.B. (1998). Urinary retinol excretion and kidney function in children with shigellosis. American Journal of Clinical Nutrition, 68, 1095–1103.

Mohanraj, R & Sivasankar, S. (2014). Sweet Potato (Ipomoea batatas [L.] Lam) — A Valuable Medicinal Food: A Review. Journal of Medicinal food, 17(7), 733–741.

Murray, M. T., Pizzorno, J. E. & Pizzorno, L. (2005). The Encyclopedia of Healing Foods. Atria Books, New York, U.S.A.

Nanashima, N., Horie, K., Tomisawa, T., Chiba, M., Nakano, M., Fujita, T., Maeda, H. Kitajima, M., Takamagi, S., Uchiyama, D., Watanabe, J., Nakamura, T. & Kato, Y. (2015). Phytoestrogenic activity of blackcurrant (Ribes nigrum) anthocyanins is mediated through estrogen receptor alpha. Molecular Nutrition and Food Research, 59(12), 2419–2431.

Nizamutdinova, I.T., Jin, Y.C., Chung, J.I., Shin, S.C., Lee, S.J., Seo, H.G., Lee, J.H., Chang, K.C. & Kim, H.J. (2009). The anti-diabetic effect of anthocyanins in streptozotocin-induced diabetic rats through glucose transporter 4 regulation and prevention of insulin resistance and pancreatic apoptosis. Molecular nutrition and food research, 53, 1419–1429

Norazalina, S., Norhaizan, M. E., Hairuszah, I. & Norashareena, M. S. (2010). Anticancinogenic efficacy of phytic acid extracted from rice bran on azoxymethane-induced colon carcinogenesis in rats. Experimental and Toxicologic Pathology, 62(3), 259–268.

Nwokocha, H.N. (1993). Technological packages for increased sweet potato production in Nigeria. In: F.O. Anuebunwa, C.O., Iwueke, and A. Udealor (eds). Motivating small scale farmers for effective participation in agricultural production. Proceedings of the 8th Annual Farming Systems Research and Extension Workshop in South-eastern Nigeria. Umudike: NRCRI – PCU-Southeast ADPs.

Odebode, S.O., Egeonu, N. & Akoroda, M.O. (2008). Promotion of sweet potato for the food industry in Nigeria. Bulgarian Journal of Agricultural Science, 14(3), 300–308.

Oke, M.E. & Workneh, T.S. (2013). A review on sweet potato postharvest processing and preservation technology. African Journal of Agricultural Research, 8(40), 4990–5003.

Omoruyi, F.O. (2010). Beneficial and adverse effects of phytic acid extract from Sweet Potato (Ipomoea batatas). In Biometals: Molecular Structures, Binding Properties and Applications. Nova Science Publishers, Inc., New York, 119–137.

Omoruyi, F.O., Budiaman, A., Eng, Y., Olumese, F.E., Hoesel, J.L., Ejilemele, A. & Okorodudu, A.O. (2013). The potential benefits and adverse effects of phytic acid supplement in streptozotocin-induced diabetic rats. Advances in Pharmacological Sciences, 2013, Article ID 172494, 7 pages. doi:10.1155/2013/172494

Omoruyi, F. O., Dilworth, L., Asemota, H. N., Jacobs, H. & Morrison, E. Y. (2004). An evaluation of cyanoglucoside, total phenol, protease inhibitors, phytic acid and zinc contents in some Caribbean food crops. Bioscience Research Communications, 15(3), 225–229.

Onomi, S., Okazaki, Y. & Katayama, T. (2004). Effect of dietary level of phytic acid on hepaticand serum lipid status in rats fed a high-sucrose diet. Bioscience, Biotechnology and Biochemistry, 68(6), 1379–1381.

Onwueme, I. C. (1978). The tropical root crops: Yams, cassava, sweet potato and cocoyams. John Wiley and sons Ltd., New York. 234.

Orhan, D.D., Ozcelik, B., Ozgen, S. & Ergun, F. (2010). Antibacterial, antifungal, and antiviral activities of some flavonoids. Microbiological Research, 165(6), 496–504.

Osagie, A.U. (1998). Antinutritional factors in Osagie, A.U., Eka, O.U. (Eds), Nutritional quality of plant foods, Ambik Press, Benin City, 221–244.

Owen, R.W., Weisgerber, U.M., Spiegelhalder, B. & Bartsch, H. (1996). Faecal phytic acid and its relation to other putative markers of risk for colorectal cancer, Gut, 38 (4), 591–597.

Padda, M.S. & Picha, D.H. (2008). Effect of low temperature storage on phenolic composition and antioxidant activity of sweet potatoes. Postharvest Biology and Technology, 47(2), 176–180.

Parle, M. & Monika. (2015) Sweet potato as a super-food. International Journal of Research in Ayurveda and Pharmacy, 6(4), 557–562.

Peng, L.Y., Mao, H.Y., Xiu, Y.F., Zhang, K.R. & Wang, C.X. (2012). Dyeing and anti-altraviolet properties of anthocynins extracted from purple sweet potatoes for silk. Advanced Materials Research, 441, 371–375.

Philpott, M., Gould, K.S., Lim, C. & Ferguson, L.R. (2004). In Situ and In Vitro antioxidant activity of sweet potato anthocyanins. Journal of Agricultural and Food Chemistry, 52, 1511–1513.

Philpott, M., Gould, K. S., Markham, K. R., Lewthwaite, S. L. & Ferguson, L. R. (2003). Enhanced coloration reveals high antioxidant potential in new sweet potato cultivars. Journal of the Science of Food and Agriculture, 83, 1076–1082.

Pretlow, T. P., O'Riordan, M. A., Somich, G. A., Amini, S. B. & Pretlow, T. G. (1992). Aberrant crypts correlate with tumor incidence

in F344 rats treated with azoxymethane and phytate. Carcinogenesis, 13, 1509–1512.

Raboy, V. (2002). Progress in breeding low phytate crops. Journal of Nutrition, 132, 503S–505S.

Raina, K., Rajamanickam, S., Singh, R. P. & Agarwal, R. (2008). Chemopreventive efficacy of inositol hexaphosphate against prostate

tumor growth and progression in TRAMP mice. Clinical Cancer Research, 14(10), 3177–3184.

Ramos-Escudero, F., Santos-Buelga, C., Pérez-Alonso, J.J. & Yáñez, J.A. (2010). HPLC DAD-ESI/MS identification of anthocyanins in Dioscorea trifida L. yam tubers (purple sachapapa). European Food Research and Technology, 230(5), 745–752.

Affiliated withCentro de Investigación de Bioquímica y Nutrición, Facultad de Medicina Humana, Universidad de San Martín de PorresReddivari, L., Vanamala, J., Chintharlapalli, S., Safe, S.H. & Miller, J.C. (2007). Anthocyanin fraction from potato extracts is cytotoxic to prostate cancer cells through activation of caspase-dependent and caspase-independent pathways. Carcinogenesis, 28, 2227–2235.

Redondo-Cuenca, A., Villanueva-Suarez, M. J., Rodrı´guez-Sevilla, M.D. & Mateos-Aparicio, I. (2006). Chemical composition and dietary fibre of yellow and green commercial soybeans (Glycine max). Food Chemistry, 101, 1216–1222.

Roullier, C., Duputié, A., Wennekes, P., Benoit, L., Fernández Bringas, V.M., Rossel, G., Tay, D., Mckey, D. & Lebot, V. (2013). Disentangling the origins of cultivated sweet potato (Ipomoea batatas (L.) Lam.). PLoS ONE, 8(5), e62707. http://doi.org/10.1371/journal.pone.0062707.

Saldanha, J.O. (1995). Fibre in the diet of U. S. children: Result of national surveys. Pediatrics, 96, 994–996.

Sasakawa, N., Sharif, M. & Hanley, M. R. (1995). Metabolism and biological activities of inositol *pentakisphosphate and inosito hexakisphosphate. Biochemical Pharmacology, 50(2), 137–146.*

Schmitt, E., Dekant, W. & Stopper, H. (2001). *Assaying the estrogenicity of Phytoestrogens in cells of different estrogen sensitive tissues. Toxicology in vitro, 15(4–5), 433–439.*

Scott, G.J., Otieno, J., Ferris, S.B., Muganga, A.K. & Maldonado, L. (1999) *Sweet potato in Ugandan food systems: Enhancing food security and alleviating poverty in International Potato Centre (CIP) Program Report 1997–1998, CIP, Lima, Peru: CIP.*

Scott, G.J., Rosegrant, M.W. & Ringler, C. (2000). *Global projections for root and tuber crops to the year 2020. Food Policy, 25, 561–597.*

Severini, C., Baiano, A., De Pilli, T., Romaniello, R. & Derossi, A. (2003). *Prevention of enzymatic browning in sliced potatoes by blanching in boiling saline solutions. LWT – Food Science and Technology, 36, 657–665.*

Shafie, N.H., Esa, N.M., Ithnin, H., Akim, A.M., Saad, N. & Pandurangan, A.K. (2013). *Preventive inositol hexaphosphate extracted from rice bran inhibits colorectal cancer through involvement of Wnt/β-Catenin and COX-2 pathways. BioMed Research International, 2013, Article ID 681027, 10 pages. doi:10.1155/2013/681027.*

Shamsuddin, A. M. (2002). *Anti-cancer function of phytic acid. International Journal of Food Science and Technology, 37, 769–782.*

Shamsuddin, A. M. & Ullah, A. (1989). *Inositol hexaphosphate inhibits large Intestinal cancer in F344 rats 5 months after induction by azoxymethane. Carcinogenesis, 10, 625–626.*

Shamsuddin, A. M., Ullah, A. & Chakravarthy, A. (1989). *Inositol and inositol hexaphosphate suppresses cell proliferation and tumo formation in CD-1 mice. Carcinogenesis, 10, 1461–1463.*

Shamsuddin, A. M. & Vucenik, I. (1999). *Mammary tumor inhibition by IP6: a review. Anticancer Research, 19, 3671–3674.*

Shan, Q., Lu, J., Zheng, Y., Li, J., Zhou, Z., Hu, B., Zhang, Z., Fan, S., Mao, Z., Wang, Y. & Ma, D. (2009). *Purple sweet potato color ameliorates cognition deficits and attenuates oxidative damage and inflammation in aging mouse brain induced by D-galactose. Journal of Biomedicine and Biotechnology, 2009, Article ID 564737.*

Shewry, P.R. (2003). *Tuber storage proteins. Annals of Botany, 91(7), 755–769.*

Shi, Z., Bassa, I.A., Gabriel, S.L. & Francis, F.J. (1992). *Anthocyanin pigments of sweet potatoes–Ipomoea batatas. Journal of Food Science, 57, 755–757.*

Shih, P.H., Yeh, C.T. & Yen, G.C. (2005). *Effects of anthocyanidin on the inhibition of proliferation and induction of apoptosis in human gastric adenocarcinoma cells. Food and chemical toxicology, 43, 1557–1566.*

Silva, L.S., de Miranda, A.M., de Brito Magalhães, C.L., Dos Santos, R.C., Pedrosa, M.L. & Silva, M.E. (2013). *Diet supplementation with beta-carotene improves the serum lipid profile in rats fed a cholesterol-enriched diet. Journal of Physiology and Biochemistry, 69, 811–820.*

Slavin, J. (2008). *Position of the American Dietetic Association: health implications of dietary fiber. Journal of the American Dietetic Association, 108(10), 1716–1731.*

Sobukola, O.P., Akinpelu, O.O. & Awonorin, S.O. (2010). *Functional and sensory properties of a sweet potato based extruded snack. 34th Annual conference General meeting Nigerian Institute of Food Science and Technology (NIFST), Port- harcourt. 132–133.*

Sudheer, K. M., Sridhar, R. B., Kiran, B. S., Bhilegaonkar, P.M., Shirwaikar, A. & Unnikrishnan, M. k.

(2004). *Antiinflammatory and antiulcer activities of phytic acid in rats. Indian Journal of Experimental Biology, 42(2), 179–185.*

Sun, M., Lu, X., Hao, L., Wu, T., Zhao, H. & Wang, C. (2015). *The influences of purple sweet potato anthocyanin on the growth characteristics of human retinal pigment epithelial cells. Food and Nutrition Research, 59, 27830 — http://dx.doi.org/10.3402/fnr.v59.27830.*

Sree, N.K., Sridhar, M., Suresh, K., Bannat, I.M. & Rao, L.V. (2000). *High alcohol production by repeated batch fermentation using an immobilized osmotolerant Saccharomyces cerevisiae. Journal of Industrial Microbiology and Biotechnology, 24, 222–226.*

Teow, C.C., Truong, V.D., McFeeters, R.F., Thompson, R.L., Pecota, K.V. & Yencho, G.C. (2007). *Antioxidant activities, phenolic and β-carotene contents of sweet potato genotypes with varying flesh colors. Food chemistry, 103, 829–838.*

The American Chemical Society (2013). *Purple sweet potatoes among 'new naturals' for Food and beverage colors.http://www.acs.org/content/acs/en/pressroom/newsreleases/2013/september/purple-sweet-potatoes-among-new-naturals-for-food-and-beverage-colors.html. Retrieved October 14, 2015.*

The International Potato Center, *http://cipotato.org/sweetpotato/facts- 2/#sthash.FECgKJ7p.dpuf. Date accessed September, 2015.*

Tran, T.T., Hatti-Kaul, R., Dalsgaard, S., & Yu, S. (2011). *A simple and fast kinetic assay for phytases using phytic acid–protein complex as substrate. Analytical Biochemistry, 410, 177–184.*

Udoessien, E. & Ifon, E.T. (1990). *Chemical evaluation of some malnutrition constituents in species of yam. Tropical Science, 32, 115–119.*

Ullah, A. & Shamsuddin, A. M. (1990). *Dose-dependent inhibition of large intestinal cancer by inositol hexaphosphate in F344 rats. Carcinogenesis, 11, 2219–2222.*

Underwood, B.A. & Arthur, P. (1996). *The contribution of vitamin A to public health. Federation of American Societies of Experimental Biology Journal, 10, 1040–1048.*

Vanderlinden, N. D. & Vucenik, I. (2004). *Too good to be true? Published by Bearing Marketing Communications Ltd, Ontario, Canada.*

Varadinova M.G., Docheva-Drenska, D.I. & Boyadjieva, N.I. (2009). *Effects of anthocyanins on learning and memory of ovariectomized rats. Menopause, 16(2), 345–349*

Verghesea, M., Raob, D.R., Chawana, C.B., Walkera, L.T. & Shackelford, L. (2006). *Anticarcinogenic effect of phytic acid (IP6): Apoptosis as a possible mechanism of action. LWT — Food Science and Technology, 39, 1093–1098.*

Vimala, B., Nambisan, B. & Hariprakash, B. (2011). *Retention of carotenoids in orange-fleshed sweet potato during processing. Journal of Food Science and Technology, 48(4), 520–524.*

Vinayagam, R. & Baojun, Xu. (2015). *Antidiabetic properties of dietary flavonoids: a cellular mechanism review. Nutrition and Metabolism, 12, 60–80.*

Vucenik, I., Passaniti, A., Vitolo, I. M., Tantivejkul, K., Eggleton, P. & Shamsuddin, A. M. (2004). *Anti-angiogenic activity of inositol hexaphosphate (IP6). Carcinogenesis, 25 (11), 2115–2123.*

Vucenik, I., Sakamoto, K., Bansal, M. & Shamsuddin, A. M. (1993). *Inhibition of mammary carcinogenesis by inositol hexaphosphate (phytic acid): A pilot study. Cancer Letters, 75, 95–102.*

Vucenik, I. & Shamsuddin, A. M. (2003). *Cancer inhibition by inositol hexaphosphate (IP6) and inositol: from laboratory to clinic. Journal of Nutrition, 133 (11 Suppl 1), 3778S–3784S.*

Vucenik, I. & Shamsuddin, A. M. (2006). Protection against cancer by dietary IP6 and inositol. Nutrition and Cancer, 55(2), 109–125.

Vucenik, I., Yang, G. Y. & Shamsuddin, A. M. (1995). Inositol hexaphosphate and inositol inhibit DMBA-induced rat mammary cancer. Carcinogenesis, 16, 1055–1058.

Vucenik, I., Yang, G. Y. & Shamsuddin, A. M. (1997). Comparison of pure inositol hexaphosphate (IP6) and high-bran diet in the prevention of DMBA-induced rat mammary carcinogenesis. Nutrition and Cancer, 28, 7–13.

Wallace, T.C. (2011). Anthocyanins in Cardiovascular Disease. Advances in Nutrition, (2), 1–7.

Walter, W.M. Jr., Purcell, A.E. & Nelson, A.M. (1975). Effects of amylolytic enzymes on 'moistness' and carbohydrate changes of baked sweet potato cultivars. Journal of Food Science, 40, 793–796.

Woolfe, J. (1993). Sweet potato: An untapped food resource. Cambridge University Press, Cambridge.

Wu, X., Beecher, G.R., Holden, J.M., Haytowitz, D.B., Gebhardt, S.E. & Prior, R.L. (2006). Concentrations of anthocyanins in common foods in the United States and estimation of normal consumption. Journal of Agricultural and Food Chemistry, 54, 4069–4075.

Xiuhong, Z., Yue, Z., Shuyan, Y. & Zhonghu, Z. (2015). Effect of Inonotus obliquus Polysaccharides on physical fatigue in mice. Journal of Traditional Chinese Medicine, 35 (4), 468–472.

Yang, Q., Liu, T., Kuklina, E.V., Flanders, W.D., Hong, Y., Gillespie, C., Chang, M., Gwinn, M., Dowling, N., Khoury, M.J. & Hu, F.B. (2011). Sodium and potassium intake and mortality among US adults: Prospective data from the Third National Health and Nutrition Examination Survey. Archives of Internal Medicine, 171(13), 1183–1191.

Yi, W., Fischer, J. & Akoh, C.C. (2005). Study of anticancer activities of muscadine grape phenolics in vitro. Journal of Agricultural and Food Chemistry, 53, 8804–8812.

Yoon, J., Thompson, L.U. & Jenkins, D.J.A. (1983). The effect of phytic acid on the rate of starch digestion and blood glucose response. American Journal of Clinical Nutrition, 38, 835–842.

Zaitsev, S. V., Efendic, S., Arkhammar, P., Bertorello, A. M. & Berggren, P. O. (1995). Dissociation between changes in cytoplasmic

free Ca2+ concentration and insulin secretion as evidenced from measurements in mouse single pancreatic islets. Proceedings of the National Academy of Sciences, 92 (21), 9712–9716.

Zajdel, A. Wilczok, A. Węglarz, L. & Dzierżewicz, Z. (2013). Phytic acid inhibits lipid peroxidation in vitro. BioMed Research International, 2013, Article ID 147307, 6 pages. doi:10.1155/2013/147307.

Zhang, Z., Wheatley, C.C. & Corke, H. (2002). Biochemical changes during storage of sweet potato roots differing in dry matter content. Postharvest Biology and Technology, 24(3), 317–325.

Zhang, H.Y., Yang, Q.Y., Lin, H.T., Ren, X.F., Zhao, L.N. & Hou, J.S. (2013). Phytic acid enhances biocontrol efficacy of Rhodotorula mucilaginosa against postharvest gray mold spoilage and natural spoilage of strawberries. LWT — Food Science and Technology, 52, 110–115.

Zhao, J.G., Yan, Q.Q., Lu, L.Z. & Zhang, Y.Q. (2013). In vivo antioxidant, hypoglycemic, and anti-tumor activities of anthocyanin extracts from purple sweet potato. Nutrition Research and Practice, 7, 359–365.

Zhou, J. R. & Erdman, J.W. (1995). Phytic acid in health and disease. Critical Review of Food Science and Nutrition, 35, 495–508.